HEALING OURSELVES
FROM MEDICINE

HEALING OURSELVES FROM MEDICINE

How Anthroposophy Can Save Your Life

JOAQUIN G. TAN

Foreword by Robert Sardello

GOLDENSTONE PRESS | *Benson, North Carolina*

Published by Goldenstone Press
P.O. Box 7
Benson, North Carolina 27504
www.goldenstonepress.com

ISBN: 978-0-9832261-2-3

Cover artwork: Detail, Hieronymus Bosch, *The Cure of Folly (the Extraction of the Stone of Madness)*, c. 1494 or later. Oil on board.
Cover and book design: Eva Leong Casey/Lee Nichol/Robert Sardello
Printed in USA

In *The Unknown Hieronymus Bosch*, Kurt Falk comments on *The Cure of Folly*:
"The sick human being is kept in a childlike state of consciousness through this operation and is unable to develop the faculties of his essential and complete humanity."

The information contained in this book is intended for educational use and should not replace consultation with a health professional. The content of this book is intended to be used as an adjunct to a healthcare program prescribed by a professional healthcare practitioner. The author and publisher are in no way liable for the misuse of the material.

GOLDENSTONE PRESS

GOLDENSTONE PRESS seeks to make original spiritual thought available as a force of individual, cultural, and world revitalization. The press is an integral dimension of the work of the School of Spiritual Psychology. The mission of the School includes restoring the book as a way of inner transformation and awakening to spirit. We recognize that secondary thought and the reduction of books to sources of information and entertainment as the dominant meaning of reading places in jeopardy the unique character of writing as a vessel of the human spirit. We feel that the continuing emphasis of such a narrowing of what books are intended to be needs to be balanced by writing, editing, and publishing that emphasizes the act of reading as entering into a magical, even miraculous spiritual realm that stimulates the imagination and makes possible discerning reality from illusion in the world. The editorial board of Goldenstone Press is committed to fostering authors with the capacity of creative spiritual imagination who write in forms that bring readers into deep engagement with an inner transformative process rather than being spectators to someone's speculations. A complete catalogue of all our books may be found at *www.goldenstonepress.com*. The web page for the School of Spiritual Psychology is *www.spiritualschool.org*.

10 9 8 7 6 5 4 3 2 1

To my dear family, Bella, Keegan, and Katrina,

The open-minded medical practitioners,

All those who strive to heal themselves (in spite of their doctors),

And those who have found their "participatory doctor/guide"

Table of Contents

Acknowledgements

Since 1993, there must have been several hundred individuals who took the seminar, "You Can Be Your Own Doctor," and more than a thousand who heard portions of the course through lectures delivered on various occasions in different parts of the Philippines, Asia, and Australia. The overwhelming response I received during these seminars or lectures provided me the energy and the will to write and update this book. I hope that by having something written, I will be able to reach more people and share my insights on how health can be maintained, and at the same time demystify illnesses and their treatment. To all of you, thank you for the enthusiasm you have shown.

I would like to give special mention to my friends Nicanor Perlas III and Chester Ocampo for giving encouragement and initial feedback on the contents; Mariel Francisco who made me go through the eye of the needle in the process of re-editing the manuscript—through her questions regarding a number of ideas I presented, I was inspired to rewrite some portions in order to be more precise; Sonny Yniquez for the innovative drawing in Section 1; Chestcore and Leonardo L. Co for allowing the reproduction of a number of illustrations of the plants in Section 2; the libraries of Nena Lagdameo, the British Council, University of the East Ramon Magsaysay Memorial Medical Center, the World Health Organization, and the University of the Philippines College of Medicine for making available the homeopathic literature, medical journals, books, and supporting documents used to back up the ideas presented here.

I would like to thank my dear wife, Bella, for her multidimensional and loving support in almost everything that I do. She is also my daily editor, thesaurus, and sounding board as to how I can express certain ideas to make them better understood and less threatening. I thank also my children, Keegan and Katrina, for their patience and understanding while the writing of this book was in progress.

In this updated and expanded edition, Katrina made the illustrations in Appendices 1 and 2, reworked the tables, and scanned and cleaned the illustrations in Section 2.

I would like to thank all those who sought my help for their ailments since 1989. My encounters with them helped me hone my skills in diagnosis and treatment, and later brought numerous insights mentioned in the book. Special mention must be given to those who trusted my advice against certain allopathic treatments, and rather patiently waited for the favorable results of the alternative and natural therapies they have chosen.

Lastly, congratulations to those who are developing their conscious-ness and skills in how to heal themselves, and are sharing these with others in poor communities in the Philippines. You are the living examples of how the ideas in this book have become an ideal (the guiding light) in your lives.

Joaquin G. Tan
July 1995/January 2010

Foreword

by Robert Sardello

Medicine has become one of a vast number of cultural forms that operate from the fiat assumption that all of life is a closed system. The human body is taken to be a complex relation of genetics, anatomy, neurology, and physiology, woven into a view of illness and disease as an interference in the smooth operation of an efficient civilization. This theory of the human body is now accepted as fact, carried into prominence by the support of technologies that perfectly mirror the view of body as a complex object. Centuries and centuries of understanding the body as an *open* system—that is, the view that body is soul is spirit, in manifold relations, and the medicine supporting that viewpoint—is, alas, strangely now called "alternative" medicine.

In a very short span of time, one that most readers have seen occur, a profession of great honor, respect, intelligence, and wisdom, combined with compassion and care, has lost its soul. We have seen medicine change into television and billboard advertising that promotes itself as belonging to the tradition of care, while also somehow successfully promoting treatments and drugs that carry with them the hugely multiplying phenomena of iatrogenesis—that is, illness caused by medicine. Still, the vast majority of people have been taken in by the persona which medical practice uses in order to maintain a false image of itself, since the very notion of health as it is currently conceived interweaves with a culture equally manipulated into being a closed system.

Those who belong to the "healing" professions inevitably begin the road to their career guided by the inspiration of a spiritual calling. They are filled with the idealism of helping and healing, and want to work with people, not with people-as-objects. Their education, however, is an initiation into viewing the body as a thing or process, as if the body which does the viewing of the bodies of others were not part of the circuit. This mode of consciousness is inherently oriented toward having "power-over" whatever it surveys. Such power is insatiable. When such power promotes itself as being for the "good," we are in a circuit from which it is most difficult to extricate ourselves.

A closed system is based on a mode of consciousness that looks upon a phenomenon as a mere *thing*, something "separate" and "over there"— closed in on itself, perhaps hugely complex, but not inherently in its very structure and operation anything beyond what can potentially be discovered by sensory observation and its extension through instruments. Perhaps the chief characteristic of a closed system, however, is that it views the subject of that system as a "nonrenewable resource," one that can only be fixed (when "broken") by those who have the sanctioned power and authority to do so. The moment that one walks into a medical doctor's office, the body that one lives—the body that is open to the creating currents of the cosmos—no longer belongs to that person, and one relinquishes the spiritual right to engage in any treatment that further opens body presence to the currents of wholeness. This central dimension of closed systems turns the body into an economic commodity.

Jake Tan brings a vastly larger view—a wider, broader, deeper tradition—and ways of practicing medicine in the original sense of the very meaning of the term, "the art of healing." This is the only true medicine; the rest is at best a subset of being in a healing relation with the body as inherently a structural and functional ongoing dynamic openness beyond itself, irreducible to the "only-physical." We belong, not to ourselves considered as objects, but to the mighty rhythms of the cosmos—to the movement of the sun and the moon through the sky, the rotation of the constellations, the motion of the planets, the rhythms of day and night, the seasons, the year, the interweaving of the elements of earth, air, fire, and water, the very motion of the Earth, and most of all, the continuing unfolding of body in time, as time.

To know the body as Jake Tan knows the body is a spiritual gift and a spiritual discipline, and requires inner development as well as external knowledge. If we want to know the body deeply, we must take it into our soul first with a feeling of humbleness, respect, and veneration; of wonder, with a mental silence. It requires that we are able to "touch" the bodily being and that we let it "touch" us. This "touch" is what produces the imaginations, inspirations, and intuitions through which the body reveals itself to us as a spiritual gift. Achieving such a mode of consciousness is impossible if we are not "transparent," if we do it with desire, with lust for knowledge, if we don't vibrate with the being of the others, if we don't empty ourselves first. Jake Tan is a model for this form of knowing as "being together with."

The central and essential gift of this book, coming from this kind of heart-relation with the body, is the gift of returning us to our bodies. Jake does this in ways that can be felt. That is, what we are given is something so deeply more than an "alternative" medicine. He takes us through the thick and difficult questions of what is actually going on in medicine, gained through years and years of concentrated research. The intention of this aspect of his writing concerns much more than trying to convince the reader that something is terribly wrong with medicine as currently practiced. When you carefully read what he has written, the body itself responds and begins to be able to feel more of its own inherent vital forces. Jake Tan fully understands the value of thinking—of real, vital, alive thinking—for thinking is central to medicine. It is medicine itself.

I want to emphasize this central dimension of "thinking as healing" with a story, one told hundreds of times a day, I am sure. I, like so many, have a dear, dear friend who was told by a doctor that he has cancer, and that he will ultimately die of this cancer. This alone stifles a most central dimension of the character of one who is supposed to be involved in the healing of others: *the will to heal.* When my friend went a different route altogether, this doctor went totally ballistic, pulling out every fear tactic to keep my friend from taking this path—in spite of the fact that my friend came to the quite natural strategy of continuing both forms of treatment. Having been inculcated with fear, there is an unavoidable confusion of thinking, which results in a very huge risk that one of the most important dimensions of healing for this person—thinking—is in danger. Knowing this person well, however, what seems to be happening is a change in the modes of his thinking—from thinking already completed thoughts to coming to the presence of the spiritual gift of thinking as it originates within his very being. In this instance, my friend seems to have the inner strength to avoid the tactic of fear put in his way so that the medical authority remains in power, and indeed, insulated from seeing his own narrowness. This inner strength came from the fact that the kind of treatment he elected to pursue does not view illness as an attack by an enemy, so fear was removed right at the outset of treatment.

Jake Tan's writing frees thinking from fear. It makes it possible to approach our own bodily being, and any illness that might beset us, without falling into fear. Unless fear is diminished, it is not possible to choose between one form of medicine and another with any inner clarity.

It is always better to develop the capacity of thinking before one has been given an annunciation by an "other" that one is going to die. And, one of the very best ways to be introduced into the art of thinking is by watching it happen, following one who is doing it, getting into that rhythm oneself. If one were to do no more than carefully read Part 1 of this book, a significant healing would take place. On the one hand, being held so skillfully by this writing brings about a significant "de-programming," one that helps us return to ourselves. At the same time, there is the introduction to returning to the Art of Healing, with the incredibly exciting prospect that we can become the artists!

We can, through coming into conscious connection with the spiritual center of our being, heal ourselves. Many people try to do just this and simply do not have the tools to do so, and thus, when something gets hold of them—called an illness—and they have suspicions about "standard" treatment, they end up in a cauldron of possibilities with nothing to do but try one after the other in the hope of chancing upon one that will miraculously work. Thinking, of the sort that goes on in this book, is a first and terribly necessary step in returning ourselves to ourselves! Then, of course, it is necessary to try on this kind of thinking for oneself. We could never do that if we did not see it happen and if we were not invited to engage in the dance of thinking with someone as generous as Jake Tan.

A breakthrough of consciousness concerning health and illness occurs by taking in and really digesting one of the central imaginations of medicine as an open system: that illness and disease are not enemies. We now think of health and illness as opposites, and hold to the notion that, at all costs, illness is to be eradicated so that we can live in health without opposition. Open-system medicine does not so much have an alternate theory as it does the capacity to carefully observe the way the body, and indeed, all of life reveals itself—as a dynamic polarity that is always between health and illness. There is no health without illness and no illness without health. Further, the polarity sides toward the dimension of illness, for very, very important purposes.

We are not static beings, machinery to be kept in perfect order. Rather, we are, in our very being, ever-changing, developing into new "selves." Often, when we wake in the morning and do not feel well, we say, "I do not feel myself this morning." Ah, that is the sign of a shift in the polarity, one that signals that we are changing, becoming someone new. That often does not feel good, and it is terribly important to have the right kind of support as we undergo such changes of body, soul, and spirit. It is terribly important that there is medicine available, that there is the art of healing, the art of "making wholeness" from this ever-shifting dynamic. Here is the very center of the "art" of healing that Jake Tan so closely adheres to: healing supports the evolving of the human being, rather than seeking to repair what is conceived as broken to a previous condition. If medicine is an "art," then there is, as with all art, a *making* involved. "Making" someone well concerns the skill and the genius of helping one become *more*, so that when the symptoms of the illness subside, the person sees the world differently, lives differently—more essentially, more truthfully, more wholly, more completely.

Medicine as a closed system simply does not have the conceptual tools to consider the human being in this way. Jake gives us such an open-system picture of the human being based in the anthroposophy of Rudolf Steiner. Be sure and read the short biography of our author at the end of the book. You will find that he came to this view of the human being only after searching, carefully, for many years, through many approaches to human reality. He found that anthroposophy matched what he was experiencing directly, with people with illnesses. He found that anthroposophy is not culturally bound, and that it is exactly the kind of open system that he "knew," from practice, characterized the human body. He did not first study anthroposophy and then apply that knowledge to the human being. Such abstraction was avoided, and for this reason, his approach to medicine is considerably more grounded than often found in anthroposophical medicine.

Open-system and closed-system ways of knowing remain separate as long as the value of each remains unrecognized by the other. While the first part of this book demonstrates the severe limits of a strictly closed-system of knowing, direct contact with the outside world is essential too for the "art of healing." Knowing within an open system requires that an elaboration of the impressions received be worked on inwardly, and that intuitive knowledge be developed from that elaboration. A fluid relation between the logic-field based in sensory impressions and the non-logic-field based on inner presence, and the harmonic synthesis between these two fields, can lead to the comprehension of the living human body and its illnesses. The real aid in bringing these two modes of knowing together comes from looking at the rhythmic conception of life in harmony with the harmonies of the universe. Such a comprehensive system of knowing founds the second part of this book—how to make homeopathic remedies for ourselves.

The essential principle of homeopathic medicine is "like cures like." A substance which produces the symptoms of a given illness, when sufficiently diluted through a rhythmical process, has the power of healing the given illness—in spite of the fact that not one molecule of the substance remains after the systematic, rhythmic dilution. This way of healing was discovered by Samuel Hahnemann. Anthroposophical medicine makes use of this principle in formulating its medicines. Until 1910, homeopathy was the primary way of medicine in the United States. There were homeopathic medical schools, and the system was respected and accepted and acknowledged as valid. The American Medical Association turned against this way of medicine, declaring its own methodology as the only valid medicine, for it could not understand how something that has no measurable chemical in it could possibly heal even the most serious of illnesses.

It may be helpful to state an imagination of how homeopathic remedies work, complementing the description given in this writing. When we feel ill, we have the sense that something that is felt at first as a strange and intruding part of us, is taking over. It is as if a part tries to take the place of the whole. We do not feel "ourselves." This experience is the source of the fear that comes with illness, a fear that is then literalized by medicine as a closed system that sees no value in illnesss. If something has inculcated fear and is therefore a threat to the body, then that threat has to be removed—that is the attitude of medicine as a closed system. However, when a substance is allowed to resonate its rhythmic pattern by sensitizing a medium to the vibratory action of the substance, it does so also in relation with the wholeness of myriads of other resonances, in harmony. When a part—trying to act like the whole, and thus throwing us out of harmony— is brought into relation with the resonating whole of which it is but a part, the part again finds its rhythm within wholeness, and symptoms disappear. It is not a matter of "getting rid" of an illness. We already have *all* illnesses within us. As long as these potential illnesses have not lost harmony with the whole, we do not feel ill. It is not, however, the case that being out of harmony is meaningless, and it is the task of medicine to keep us in harmonic resonance with the universe. In the polarity of health-illness, it is necessary for imbalances to occur in order that the dynamic wholeness that we potentially are can continue to develop and unfold.

In working with the various homeopathic remedies listed in Section 2 of this writing, it is important to refrain from taking a typical diagnostic medical attitude. Because medicalization of the body is now so complete, it often happens that other approaches to healing are placed within the view of the body as a closed system, and one takes herbs or homeopathic remedies as if they were simply another kind of drug. Taking remedies in this way is not very effective; indeed, if it works, it is really no different than a kinder standard medicine.

The descriptions of the mineral, plant, and animal remedies in this book begin with "symptom pictures." The symptom picture should be read through carefully. Not every symptom listed will be experienced, so the question arises how one should respond when there are only a few of the symptoms listed. The list is not a "check-list." One is not trying to determine how many of the symptoms one has. The symptom picture is simply read, carefully, slowly, taking it as if it were something more akin to a dream-picture. In fact, it is very good to be making an inner picture of a person, even of oneself, with all the symptoms, allowing that picture to live within one, much like waking with a very peculiar dream-image. The intent is to let the symptom picture, bodily felt, come into resonance with the "spirit" of the healing substance, the vibratory qualities of the substance.

When one takes a homeopathic remedy, it does not act like a drug. Symptoms are not covered over, and there may well not be the immediate cessation of the illness. Taking more of the remedy does not increase the dosage; more is not better. The symptoms may actually increase for a time. But, they begin to differ from simply experiencing the symptom without the remedy. It begins to be possible to notice and to track a sense of your own spiritual being beneath the symptom. It is as if something invisible and beautiful is developing within you, and you sense that the symptom is in some manner responsible for this emerging sense of a self that is new, vulnerable, waiting to become integral with the whole of your being. It is not as if you will ever reflectively know what this new sense of self "is," because it is not of the nature of something to be known. It is to be lived. Gradually, you have the sense that this particular illness was necessary to the unfolding of your destiny and your future, your true individuality.

Something more can be said concerning this felt-sense of the emerging and unfolding of the self. It is felt in the region of the heart; it is felt as an intimate warmth, as if the illness was a necessary purifying of the body. As the illness works its way through, one realizes how much emotional and thought illusion one has carried concerning who one thought one was. And, one realizes that there is no direct way to get at these illusions, of which there are undoubtedly more. And, one begins to deeply appreciate the gift of illness and disease as perhaps one of the few ways to clear illusory feeling and thinking concerning oneself.

There is a purity to illness. It means business, and simply sweeps through doing its work. It cares nothing of our personality, which simply gets in the way, and the stronger its resistance the stronger the illness seems to be.

There is also the other side of going through homeopathic healing, the actual bodily healing process. An astounding increase in bodily sensitivity occurs, and one experiences the actual sensation of a healing going on. It is as if the cells of the body resonate, sing, vibrate, and one recognizes the opportunity to live a different, more acute, and lively bodily existence. This new bodily life can be very hard to protect and to sustain. We now realize how harsh the present sensory world is—how much noise, absence of care, absence of a sense of nurturing goes on. To avoid being thrown right back into the sensory, emotional, cognitive chaos of stress, it becomes clear that one has to take up some kind of cultivation of the inner life. The "art of healing" is also the initiation into the inner life, or can be. The title of this book could have well been: "Medicine as a Spiritual Path."

Jake Tan has written a very multifaceted book, something like a symphony with many movements, each of incredible beauty, and if you follow the book through, step by step, more than once, you have entered medicine as a spiritual path. First, it is a book that introduces new thinking about the body, and how to think critically about current medicine. Second, it is a book with innumerable references. The references can be read on their own. You will be taken into a sense of the world of standard medicine, be able to have some sense of what lies behind it, and be introduced into the critical spirit that is always inviting us to look closely at things, and, particularly with medicine, to refrain from taking what is said without question. Then, there is the third symphonic movement of the book—the presentation, with great clarity, of a view of the human being that sees the human body as holy—not in a mystical way, but with all the precision of science, of spiritual science. The fourth movement of the book is the practical work with making remedies for healing. This part of the book can be read over and over again, slowly, as it is really something more than information; it forms the soul into coming into inner relation with the spirit, so that the true nature of medicine as the art of healing begins to dawn. A further movement of the book are the appendices to Section 1, in which the rhythmic unfolding of the development of the individual is presented. Not only does this picture help us to see that how we treat the health of our children from an early age will, in large measure, determine their future health and well-being, but the picture, as well, develops within us a living sense of the wisdom of the human being.

This is a rare and valuable book—a work of reflection, a handbook, a work of spiritual direction—and, most significantly, a book that can save your life!

Preface
2011 Updated and Expanded Edition

This book will not automatically heal your illness if you are already suffering from one. It points to everyone's potential to recognize and develop one's own healing capacities for oneself and for others later. There is no magic bullet or quick fix with regard to healing. If someone makes this claim, our first instinct is to be skeptical. It cannot be denied that part of us is also quite attracted to this idea. Why are these two general tendencies always found in one's soul: thinking, on the one hand, and feelings, on the other? The easy-going part of the self is attracted to the latter, while the more intellectual self, to the former. This is part of everyday life. We hope that someday, somehow, someone (like science) will find the panacea for all illnesses. At the same time, our mundane experiences tell us that this is a delusion. We often struggle between illusions and delusions in life. We dispel both by what we can learn from experience, either by ourselves, or from others, or by continually struggling (action/reflection) in our experience. What this book promises is the possibility to launch you into a path of healing (or improving your health further)—to have a handle to work with. We will begin from your own experience of being in an illusion about healing yourself, or in a delusion (i.e., "I cannot do without professionally trained practitioners").

Self-healing is instinctive. If in our physical body we find homeostasis—the ability of the organism to adapt to a changing environment and achieve balance—this natural instinct/ability rises up in one's feelings and consciousness as the sense of life: that is, to aspire to be better, to yearn for balance in all aspects of life, to aim for well-being, wellness, coherence, and wholeness in body, soul, and spirit. This is the essence of self-healing.

One aspect of self-healing is self-medication[1] something more people now do (especially evident since the internet began[2]). Self-medicating can take varied forms, such as taking a non-prescription drug or a multivitamin pill; not following the recommended dose of medicine prescribed by the doctor; not consulting in spite of an ill feeling; postponing an elective operation for whatever reason; sleeping off a symptom; avoiding (or eating) certain foods; surfing the internet to understand an illness or trying out other forms of medication like herbal medicine, homeopathic remedies, acupuncture; undergoing sauna baths; having a massage or a vacation—and others. Non-medicating is having the sense, consciously or unconsciously, that somehow our bodies will cope with whatever disease is being felt, that it will eventually resolve itself. Consciously reducing the pills you are taking is like having the intuition that you probably have enough (and your body can now heal itself). Understanding possible causes of an illness may actually be the beginning of self-healing (as this book will explain). Sulfur baths, regular massage, recreation, and folk herbal remedies are some of the old, pre-modern forms of self-healing.[3] Self-medication is the current expression of our instinct to self-healing. This book aims to guide us to be more aware and mindful of this instinct and direct it with conscious thought. However, a prerequisite may be a developed participative relationship with your doctor.

Informed self-medication is actually the norm today. As a matter of fact, a world body was formed to "guide" those doing self-medication (an industry-driven response to address the world trend to self-medication). This is understandable because self-medicating with chemical drugs may be disastrous, as Chapter 2 of Section 1 tries to explain. For those who want to get away from chemical drugs, however, this world body is unnecessary. Moreover, deep inside us there is the final authority that can know, deliberate, and judge/decide. This is the being I will initially be referring to as the possible point of reference within each person. This book will make this instinctive impulse towards self-medication more purposeful and conscious in relation to what you may already be doing. It will add more perspectives—more mileposts, characteristics, further indications about ourselves, and a way to process information being offered to us by insufficient but multifaceted views on health. The broader standpoints which I present in Chapters 3, 4, and 5 of Section 1 will hopefully prevent the reader from being too optimistic or pessimistic in decisions about health.

Since the first publication of this book in 1995, several young doctors have expressed to me their very positive feedback about it. One declared that after finishing the book, he "never turned back" and pursued studies of other natural forms of healing. From some community health workers, self-reliance was reinforced and the book became a constant resource for continuing study. It inspired the founding of community enterprises of safe and low-cost remedies, based on the description of remedies in Section 2.[4]

Through the grapevine, patients regularly came seeking relief from their different illnesses. I have always pointed out to them that my advice is only a first step to the true healing that can happen, mainly as I have described in this book. Those who still had a certain illusion (that I will heal them) became empowered after a month of refraining from certain foods, alcohol, or beverages; they began sleeping early, trying out creative and productive activities, and taking homeopathic remedies. Others sought more help from alternative or complementary practitioners, remaining oblivious that their healing process is generally in their hands. The rest, who stayed immersed in their illusions/delusions, continue searching for their appropriate hero. All the aforesaid are initial experiences while on a path to self-healing.

Alongside a limited practice, I prefer to give courses in order to reach more people and stimulate their instinct to self-healing. I am grateful for the enthusiastic response I get from the audience whenever I present the diverse viewpoints discussed in this book. This served as the impetus to update and expand the book.

In this new edition, I hope that the reader will be encouraged to develop more certainty in the choices they make. As we are all realizing today, every choice has a consequence for health or illness, for ourselves and our environment, sooner or later.[5] Thus, to minimize the negative effects of our choices, we have to continue striving for greater mindful living and embrace the consequences, reap the benefits, and share our two cents worth of insights with others so they too may begin to become aware of their choices in life.

Please take the ideas presented here as hypotheses. This is the open-minded way of grappling with new thoughts. Like any modern-day person, we all need to digest new ideas so that we can test them, make them our own, and eventually (hopefully) become our ideal in life.

Notes

1 Fifty-nine percent of Americans polled say they are more likely to treat their own health condition now than they were a year ago. Seventy-three percent would rather treat themselves at home than see a doctor, and 6 in 10 say they would like to do more of this in the future. See World Self-Medication Industry website at *http://www.wsmi.org*.

2 One research firm estimated that 65% of people who visited the internet in a 12-month period went to health-related sites. See World Self-Medication Industry website at *http://www.wsmi.org*.

3 Other old forms of self-healing are meditation, prayer, and developing harmonious

relationships with one's neighbors and with the environment.

4 Another skill participants learn in the seminars I give, other than making and using homeopathic remedies, is ear acupressure. This is a very simple and safe way to balance initial weaknesses of the life body. The points can be used for diagnosis and treatment. The principle behind ear acupressure is holographic science—where the part mirrors the whole; thus in the ear one will find the whole of the human being. For more information about auricular therapy, just type *ear acupressure* in your internet search engine and download an ear diagram.

5 For example, every time we buy something, we are buying not just the product, but the whole ideology behind the company making the product. If the product is produced at the expense of the environment, then buying the merchandise supports the degradation of the environment. If the bank where you deposit your money lends to companies who make guns and war machinery, then you are also supporting war (or being an accessory to it). In the same light, buying goods that are produced with mindful care for the environment support such causes. See *greenfund.com* or type *ethical investments* or *socially responsible investments* in your internet search engine for more ideas about mindful living—how your daily purchases can support the development of healthy living and environment.

Introduction

Today, orthodox[1] medical science appears to be at its peak. There are more and more diagnostic technologies introduced, with digital and automated sophistication and compact, futuristic looks, promising ever-greater accuracy. Very detailed studies of bacteria, viruses, and human genes give doctors no doubt as to what they are up against. Additional—and bigger—hospitals are being constructed to serve more patients. Drugs are being sold in unprecedented quantities in almost every country in the world. The knife, though feared by many, is the magic wand of medical practice. To undergo surgery connotes a new lease on life, a reprieve from the darkness of disease. These are just some of the hallmarks of progress which medical science boasts of.[2]

However, all these seeming wonders can be viewed in another way. The increasing number of surgical operations implies that doctors are failing to stop or reverse the progress of diseases, thus resorting to excising the organ or tissue (and in an increasing number of cases, replacing them with mechanical ones, or organs from donors). Surgery is, in a sense, an act of desperation, more like a crude slash and burn strategy—often prolonging the dying process rather than extending life.[3] Proliferating hospitals indicate not only that wellness has become a commodity, but also that physicians now find it difficult to treat diseases at home, since they rely more on sophisticated equipment and instruments rather than on their own capacities or simple common sense. Such medical equipment does not necessarily mean more accurate diagnoses;[4] it can also mean that medical training is not adequately preparing doctors to be confident of their diagnostic skills. Therefore, they need various machines that will tell them whether they are right or wrong. Ultimately, the physician is transformed from a healer to a mere technician. "Surgeon" becomes the glamorous name for a bio-mechanic. Moreover, chemical drugs are automatically considered an absolute necessity to effect a "cure," conditioning one to be oblivious to the risks involved (such as new illnesses which may be caused by the drug).[5]

Thus, if one views the health situation from other perspectives— the sophistication, greater organization, grandiose structures, increased expenditures for health care, the long queue of patients in the doctor's office, and hospitals that are almost always filled to capacity—these may indicate that true healing is eluding the public, including the doctors themselves. In 1976, Ivan Illich[6] started the introduction to his book, *Limits to Medicine*, by saying, "The medical establishment has become a major threat to health." In 1980, Robert S. Mendelsohn, MD, stated, "I do not believe in modern medicine. I am a medical heretic.[7]" Around the turn of the 21st century, Dr. Joseph Mercola, DO, writes in *www.mercola.com*, "The existing medical establishment is responsible for killing and permanently injuring millions of Americans…[8]" What would make these sane people say these things? Modern medicine is idolized and idealized by people all over the world as part and parcel of modern life.[9]

What are the facts behind these assertions? For us ordinary folks, these are indicative of an urgent need to rethink the matter and start seeing through the veils of glamour and "scientific" pronouncements. Where do we find true healing? In medical science? In religion? In drugs? In political authorities? In traditional medicine or healers? In alternative medicine? It is time to take a look at how we can be in charge of our own health. How do we avoid developing an illness which may require hospitalization? How do we approach the treatment of an illness without automatically running to a physician? How can we remain healthy in spite of our polluted environment, alongside the threat of the medical establishment and the unnecessary fear it has created about lurking bacteria and viruses in one's environment (particularly from fellow human beings) and our hereditary predispositions?

This book is about rediscovering the healing powers within us as well as in nature, and how we can harness them again. Various healing arts through the centuries have alluded to and attempted to work with these twin powers. A significant part of this inner power has been called *homeostasis* by other schools of medicine. Walter B. Cannon first coined the word in 1930 and described its effects in *The Wisdom of the Body*.[10] It is the higher principle/intelligence working in each organism. Homeostasis is the ability of the organism to adapt to a changing environment and achieve balance. The immune system is only a part of this. Scientists describe how wise our bodies are and how creative the processes evoked. For example, enzymes or peptides are created at will, simultaneous to one's inner activity, or to address a particular deed as a response to certain environmental signals like danger or bliss.

Sadly, orthodox medical science has lost the understanding of this wisdom. Instead, it has developed an arsenal of therapies and technologies that suppress this creative inner power. Ironically, these therapies are all in the guise of saving lives and eliminating or preventing disease. They may be important at certain times, but unnecessary most of the time, as this book will attempt to elucidate.

The power of minerals, plants, and animal products to heal has been ridiculed and discarded in modern therapy, while their synthesized chemical counterparts are believed to be more potent and beneficial. Chapters 2 and 3 of Section 1 will attempt to dispel this delusion and place these chemical drugs in an appropriate perspective.

This book may seem to be anti-doctor as well as anti-scientific research. It is so to the extent that doctors have become no longer healers, but mere prescription dispensers—so much so that researchers are practically wasting money in researching diseases whose causes may be imaginary, or at most reveal only a small part of the total reality.[11] As for the zeal and determination shown by doctors and scientists in the search for true healing, very little can be said against it. Despite the fact that vested interests (whether for financial gain or for power) play a large role in molding the direction of today's research, current practices, and standard procedures, the will to heal among doctors is seldom lost. However, good intentions are not enough. There are some crucial elements missing in the whole quest of medical science to eradicate diseases. Because of these missing elements, medical science has developed a distorted concept of health and illness, and has applied a therapy that produces new diseases rather than true healing. Worse, human dignity is constantly being sacrificed.

Every now and then, some scientists propose to rethink the scientific paradigm and point to some of the missing elements.[12] But orthodox science has failed miserably to rectify itself. It insists on its conservative position and outdated worldview, and flaunts statistics showing that the world's health is at its best. Its proponents present an arsenal of technology; voluminous, specialized, but often reified scientific findings; and an army of committed and dedicated personnel as further proofs. These authoritarian declarations have not done much to make people healthy, but rather have mesmerized the public and cultivated a monocropped mindset. Worse, the fear generated by these declarations has made the consuming public subject to manipulation by the vested interest groups (and have invoked in many people their Pavlovian instinct[13]). How can we break free from this captivity and appreciate other viewpoints and discover our own center again?

Others who have already been awakened may be expecting that this book will proclaim a dawning new age in medicine, a paradigm shift.[14] Many books have already done that. This one is about developing a viewpoint, a thinking mood and perspective. It is about nurturing a willful mind and heart that can go in and out of any paradigm and see its limitations, strengths, and meanings in relation to healing and development. Only a willful mind and heart engaged in living thinking can bring about a healing process. If orthodox science sticks to its present assumptions, which fail to appreciate the wisdom of the body, it will fail to understand this healing mind and heart.

This book is about working out what each one of us already possesses, but has failed to recognize. It is acknowledging and nurturing the existing capacities we have within us. Using this force for health and willful deeds are just two of the possibilities.

We are fortunate that within the human spirit, we can still find the yearning and the aspiration to do the good and be better persons. We are not only learning from our own experiences, but also from the experiences of other fellow human beings—especially those who are victims of today's modern lifestyle. In medicine, we can avoid the high cost of health care, minimize cancerous and degenerative diseases, prevent the unnecessary mutilation and poisoning of our physical bodies, and stop the consequent degradation of human dignity. We should then start somewhere. We can start with ourselves.

There are two sections in this volume. The first serves as the background to the second, and gives the foundation for a holistic view of medicine and healing. The second compiles the medicinal actions of minerals, plants, and animals which may be found in your garden, your immediate environment, in the supermarket or health food shops, and that are proven on the basis of a principle of medicine called the Law of Similars.

For those unfamiliar with other schools of medical thought, there are two new concepts that must be understood. They are the Law of Similars, or *similia similibus curentur* ("like cures like"), and the Process of Provings. These two concepts were formulated by Samuel Hahnemann, MD, in the 1790s. His discoveries led to the founding of a school of medical thought called *homeopathy*.

Section 1, Chapter 1 expounds on these two concepts and their implications for humanity's search for true healing. I will also discuss a third concept called *potentization* or *dynamization* of remedies, another offshoot of Hahnemann's work. I will compare these principles with the prevailing dominant medicine, known as *allopathy*, which involves the use of remedies that produce effects opposite to the disease.

My position with regard to allopathy is that it has a place in the whole spectrum of healing, but just like anything else, it has its limitations. Knowledge of these limitations is important for putting allopathy in perspective. From here, one can judge where it can be of value. (Appendix

2 of this book is an attempt to put the healing arts and schools of medicine in a spectrum.) Research shows that the extensive use of the allopathic principle is a main factor in the rise of the degenerative, sclerotic, and cancerous illnesses among today's young generation.[15] A few decades ago, these diseases afflicted only the older generation of 60 years and above. In fact, we are conditioned to believe that degenerative illnesses are part of aging. This need not be so. One can be old without necessarily becoming sclerotic or suffering from one of the dreaded diseases. This is another reason why orthodox medicine is in a crisis. Chapter 2 of Section 1 elaborates on this crisis. Without full understanding of this situation, humanity's health is endangered.

In leading toward a holistic understanding of medicine, I have included in the discussion an expanded image of the human being taken from the fundamentals of anthroposophic medicine. This expanded image—which includes bodily "sheaths"—is necessary to fully comprehend the different aspects of our being. The way these bodily sheaths interact with each other is inhibited or promoted through mindful nutrition and lifestyle, equanimity of emotional life, and harmony with the diverse conditions of the environment. This interaction is eventually taken hold of, integrated, and given coherence and meaning by an inner striving self. This determines one's disposition and susceptibility to illness or well-being. Chapter 3 of Section 1 gives as comprehensive a picture as possible to illumine the reader on the role of constitution and disposition in the genesis of a disease. This discussion is not exhaustive, but it will be broad enough to challenge the reader to fill in the details on his own.

At the end of Section 1, I suggest some steps for anyone who would like to develop his skills in healing himself and eventually help others heal themselves.[16] The discussion is centered on how to creatively work with our inner doctor and not resort to remedies which would suppress that faculty. Let me emphasize that the remedies from the animal, plant, and mineral kingdoms described in Section 2 are only necessary while we are still mastering this proficiency. Proficiency in working with and/or calling forth the healing forces within is the ultimate goal.

I also offer some suggestions on what one can do to effect policy changes in our health care system. This should pave the way for the pluralistic and eclectic practice of medicine we need in our societies. These steps must be taken to ensure that patients have real choices in the kind of therapy to pursue for their ailments. As a prerequisite, doctors should be free to practice without prejudice for one particular school of medical thought. To reeducate the medical community towards a holistic understanding of medicine and healing is a most urgent need. Since reform will probably not come immediately from within the medical establishment itself, ordinary people should take the initiative.

Section 2 gives instructions for preparing your own homeopathic remedies. Chapter 1 of Section 2 shows how to prepare "mother tinctures" and how they can be potentized for home or community use. The whole procedure is actually very simple. I thought hard about why homeopaths of the past did not teach people how to do it. I came to a very simple conclusion: the profit motive prevented the "secret" from being shared. Another possible reason is that healing the sick has always been relegated to the "priests" or "doctors." Ordinary people are almost always dependent on them. Because of this relationship, ordinary folks do not feel competent to handle healing themselves. This need may no longer be the case today. One aim of this book is to break this mental block. Through our willful thinking capacity, learning from our own experience and that of others, and the knowledge generated by various researchers through the centuries about the processes in the body, soul, and spirit (now conveniently accessible through the internet), we are able to think through and have a sense in our heart of what may be inharmonious, inconsistent, and incoherent in our being—the true origin of illnesses. From this understanding and profound comprehension, we can arrive at how we can treat ourselves by using the various suggested means discussed in Section 1 and/or through the use of remedies described in Section 2.

The extensive endnotes deal with parenthetical, supplementary, and other points of view which would distract the reader if kept in the main text. They also provide bibliographical guidance for those who would like to go deeper into the subject. In this updated and expanded edition, I decided to put the notes after every chapter to encourage the reader to read them along with the main text. Many of the updates I made are found in the notes, while the expanded portions of the book are in the appendices.

The use of the word "he" in this book is used in the sense of both male and female and therefore gender neutral, unless from the context the meaning is clearly masculine.

My hope is that this book, like other manuals which aim to stimulate self-help in medicine, will further encourage ordinary people to consciously take their healing into their own hands.

Notes

1   I have opted to use the word "orthodox" to describe the kind of science that today's medicine is following. There are new findings in science that are already departing from some of the basic premises of orthodox science. Consequently, new therapies and technologies are being developed from the results of these new findings. Chapter 2 of Section 1, entitled "The Crisis of Orthodox Medicine," will provide a more detailed description of what this orthodox science is really about.

2   We often hear medical science's claim that the overall improvement in life expectancy is brought about by medical intervention. However, sociologists John and Sonja McKinley calculate that less than four percent of the decline in mortality between 1900 and 1975 in the US is due to medical measures. Scholars now agree that the additional breakthroughs in reduced mortality were due to better housing, hygiene, and nutrition. Vaccination, an over-emphasized medical success, was introduced only when the diseases were already well under control. See McKinley S, McKinley J. The questionable contribution of medical measures to the decline of mortality in the United States in the twentieth century. *Milbank Memorial Fund Quarterly.* 1977;(summer):405-430. See also Cowley G. What high tech can't accomplish. *Newsweek.* October 4, 1993:42-45.

3   See Siegel BS. *Love, Medicine and Miracles: Lessons Learned about Self-Healing from a Surgeon's Experience with Exceptional Patients.* New York: Harper & Row; 1990:17. Siegel asks, "How can we say we're prolonging life when a person has become no more than a valve between the intravenous fluids going in and the urine coming out? All we're prolonging is dying."

4   It has not been proven that many costly medical diagnostic technologies are more advantageous than the least expensive ones, for example, a fetal electronic monitor over a stethoscope. The former reinforces the doctors' dependency on machines, making them lose their innate ability. The process of doctoring also becomes more impersonal. See ibid, p. 44; Bucker HC, Schmidt JG. Does routine ultrasound screening improve outcome in pregnancy? Meta-analysis of various outcome measures. *British Medical Journal* 1993;307:13-17. The procedure does not improve the outcome of pregnancy in terms of an increased number of live births and of reduced prenatal morbidity. Worse, the new devices may even have after-effects. See Newnham JP et al. Effects of frequent ultrasound during pregnancy: a randomized controlled trial. *Lancet* 1993;342:887-890; Mark J, Keise DC. Frequent prenatal ultrasound: time to think again. *Lancet* 1993;342:878-879. Ultrasound does not always ensure an additional benefit. In fact, frequent ultrasound may even negatively influence fetal growth. In the book *What Doctors Don't Tell You: The Truth About the Dangers of Modern Medicine,* Lynne

McTaggart exposes the possible inaccuracy of CAT (computer axial tomography) scan and MRI (magnetic resonance imaging), the proverbial diagnostic equipment of today's orthodox medicine. "The initial reports that MRI gave more detailed images than CAT were 'overly optimistic.' All the initial fanfare, which came from individual cases of patients, could not be confirmed by subsequent larger studies using full scientific methods. The earlier studies turned out to be not well controlled." Is this finding of "studies not well controlled" to introduce new equipment, medical procedures, or drugs symptomatic of today's medical science? Why were drugs withdrawn from the market previously, and continue to be to this very day? Is financial and political interest taking over human safety and rigorous scientific pursuit? This is one of the main delusions this book wants to dispel. See also *New Scientist,* September 17, 1994:23. It was announced on the cover of this prestigious British magazine that *80 percent of existing medical procedures have never been properly tested.*

5   Balancing risk and benefit is a part of the process one goes through when taking any course of action. Taking risk is part of progress and development. However, orthodox medicine has taken this principle quite out of hand. From their perspective, the risks of chemical drugs and other interventions are necessary because there are no other options. But from other perspectives, there are a number of options available. This is a recurring theme of this book. The risks have been too great (premature deaths, mutilated bodies, and the emergence of new diseases) while the benefits are practically nil. (A number of emergency therapies, the mending of bones, trauma care, and plastic surgery are a few of the areas where orthodox treatment seems to be at its real best.)

6   Illich I. *Limits to Medicine, Medical Nemesis: the Expropriation of Health.* New York: Penguin Books; 1976:11.

7   Mendelsohn RS. *Confession of a Medical Heretic.* Warner Books: 1980:11.

8   Moreover, Dr. Mercola's passion is to transform the traditional medical paradigm in the United States. His website is now among the top 10 health sites on the internet: *www.mercola.com.* He not only has an extensive and updated critique about today's orthodox medicine, but also offers simple, practical health solutions and natural organic products to replace whatever orthodox medical procedure or drug one is currently using. Subscribing to the website's newsletter is free of charge.

9   For example, as early as 1995, the Ministry of Public Health of the People's Republic of China reported that 2.5 million Chinese were hospitalized annually after taking the wrong medicine, and 100,000 died from violent reaction to drugs. "More and more people are suffering bad reactions because of their blind faith in new and imported medicine." (See 100,000 Chinese dying from wrong medicine. *The Philippine Star.* May 23, 1995:25. Reported by UPI.) This is how much western orthodox medicine is idolized

by (or has deluded) the people of the world. Quarter-truth advertising, propaganda, films, and television shows on heroic medicine have contributed immensely in the creation of the myth. This book attempts to put orthodox medicine in its proper perspective.

10 Cannon WB. *The Wisdom of the Body*. New York: WW Norton; 1932. Quoted in Strohman R. Ancient genomes, wise bodies, unhealthy people: limits of a genetic paradigm in biology and medicine. Presented at: International Conference on Redefining the Life Sciences; July 7-10, 1994; Penang, Malaysia. The Third World Network.

11 A continuing theme of this book is that diseases are multifactorial. Germs and mutated genes may be present but are not sufficient factors to cause diseases. The billions of dollars being spent in researching these alleged causes of disease (as orthodox medicine continues to assert) may be considered wasted resource which could have been allotted to raise the quality of life of poor people to a more humane level.

12 For example, see Engel GL. The need for a new medical model: a challenge for biomedicine. *Science* 1977;196:129-136. "Engel proposed that health and disease should be seen as arbitrarily defined states determined by biological, psychological, and social factors. The relative importance of each set of factors should be taken into account for the specific disease and the particular patient, but the specific contribution of each factor should be taken into account in considering aetiology, diagnosis, prognosis, and prevention of any given medicine." Quoted in Boyle C. Diseases with passion. *Lancet* 1993;342:1126-1127. See also Davisson CT. Is clinical medicine a science? Application of some of the ideas of Owen Barfield to clinical medicine [doctoral thesis]. New Haven, Conn: Yale University School of Medicine; 1978. "It is not now a science." Davisson suggested steps on how it can truly be what it claims to be.

13 The recent "threat of epidemics" like SARS, bird flu, and swine flu is an indication of how fear induced by medical declarations can easily make people resort to mass immunization or wear "protective masks" for any sign of colds or cough. People are oblivious that the fear itself can cause an illness, that wearing a mask does not help much (after 10 minutes the mask becomes a culture medium for germs), that vaccination does not always protect but may even induce new illnesses. See note 31, Ch. 3 on this, and *mercola.com* newsletter. Here are just some of the titles particularly devoted to the H1N1 "pandemic": *Many Health Workers Won't Take Swine Flu Vaccine; Shocking Swine Flu Vaccine Miscarriage Stories; Swine Flu is NOT the Problem—It is the Vaccine that May Harm or Kill You; Nanoparticles Used in Untested H1N1 Swine Flu Vaccines; Thimerosal Law Changed for H1N1 Vaccine; Swine Flu—One of the Most Massive Cover-ups; CDC Documents Reveals Shocking Information; Shocking Swine Flu Vaccine Miscarriage Stories; Do NOT Let Your Child Get Flu Vaccine; Flu Vaccine Exposed; Obama Declares Swine Flu Emergency.*

14 In the more affluent countries, patronage in alternative medicine (particularly acupuncture, homeopathy, herbal medicine, and manipulation therapy) has increased sharply in the last two decades. The percentages of public patronage are as follows: Belgium, 31%; Denmark, 23%; Germany, 46%; Holland, 20%; UK, 26%; US, 34%; France, 49%; Sweden, 25%. See Fischer P, Ward A. Complementary medicine in Europe. *British Medical Journal.* 1994;309 107-110. There is definitely a paradigm shift in these countries. This data may also be indicative of the failure of orthodox medicine to deliver what it has promised.

15 This poorly understood epidemic of the 20th century, labeled as "degenerative diseases," indicates that the functions of bodily organs deteriorate progressively as if aging is accelerated. There is still no unified theory of causation, and heated debates on the matter continue to take place around the world. Some scientists have hypothesized that synthetic (artificial) chemicals may cause these illnesses. See Kilburn KH. Epidemic then and now: chemicals replace microbes and degeneration oust infection. *Archives of Environmental Medicine.* 1994;49(1):3-5. This paper supports that hypothesis but does limit itself to a single class of causes (for reasons which will be mentioned). Other factors would also be discussed in order to arrive at a thorough, coherent understanding. From this understanding, one can then resort to preventive measures more wisely and intervene in healing degenerative diseases more fruitfully than the way orthodox medicine does it now.

16 At this point, I would like to caution the reader that the path to self-healing will be full of obstacles and trials. The first obstacle to heal oneself is one's tendency to egotism. One facet of egotism is commonly experienced by everyone as over-estimating (thus we subject ourselves to illusions and optimism) or underestimating (thus we are in a certain state of delusion or pessimism) oneself. An example of the former state of consciousness is to say, "I know myself and what my body needs, thus I do not need those self-help books!" An example of the latter attitude is, "I am not ready to do something about my situation because I do not know much about it." These two tendencies can be found in varying degrees in most of what we do, especially in trying out new things. Some kind of egotism is normal to most adult situations today. This is not necessarily all negative, because egotism develops in each and every one of us a sense of "self." In self-healing, we all need a point of reference (as the book will elucidate later) and this point is the "self." What we need alongside our current notion of self is to cultivate objectivity with respect to our personal experiences, as well as humility and eventually selflessness; these all help in avoiding the pitfall of egoism.

One of our tasks in the process of healing ourselves is to bring the "little egotistic self" to a continuing search, discovery, and realization of a *higher* notion of self, which the book will explain, especially in Section 1, Chapter 4.

Section One

Towards a Holistic View of Medicine and Healing

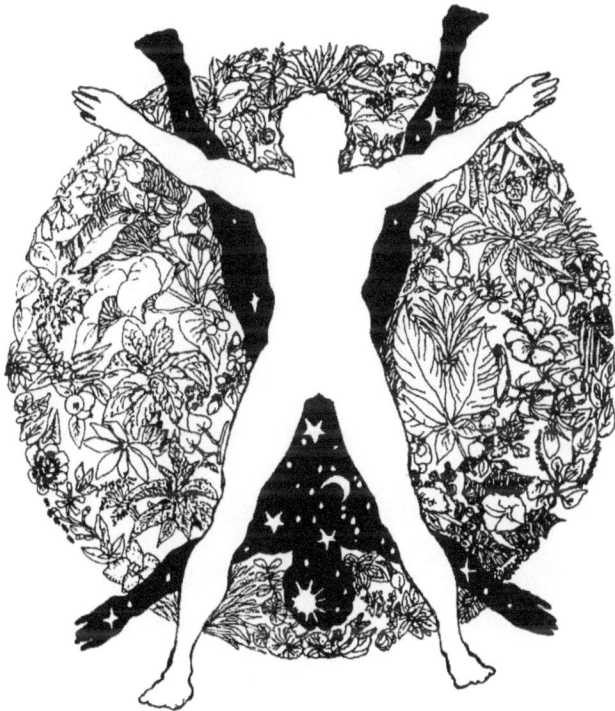

Chapter One

❧

The Contribution of Homeopathy

The Law of Similars, The Process of Provings,
and the Potentization of Remedies:
Samuel Hahnemann (1755-1843)

The Law of Similars is closely related to the meaning of the word *homeopathy*. The latter is derived from two Greek words, "omeos" (similar) and "pathos" (suffering), or "similar suffering." Homeopathy is a system of medicine which treats an illness with a substance that produces an effect similar to that of the illness being suffered. To understand how Samuel Hahnemann, MD, arrived at this principle, let us relive the context of Hahnemann's search for an efficacious art of healing.

Hahnemann lived in an age when broad discoveries in physics and chemistry were sweeping Europe, and natural science was still relatively new.[1] Medicine as a science was also in its infancy. The works of medical giants, such as Hippocrates of the Greek period and Paracelsus during the Renaissance, had lost their meaning in this new age. Medical science had to reconceptualize the origin of illnesses and postulate how these could be cured.

The folk medicine which was extensively used at that time began to be questioned. Without clear knowledge of the active ingredients of medicinal plants (which chemistry was only starting to examine), medical practitioners began to refuse to make use of them. To medical science, folk medicine was superstitious, despite the actual cures it brought about. Moreover, many of the folk practitioners had either lost the wisdom behind their remedies or failed to adapt their explanation to scientific terminology.[2] Worse, a number had fallen into degenerate practices which reinforced the misgivings of scientists. Traditional wisdom and the new form of analytical thinking inevitably clashed.

This was the situation when Hahnemann qualified as a physician at the University of Leipzig in 1779. After several years of medical practice, Hahnemann became unhappy with the situation. This was the era when blood-letting, using lancets and leeches, was predominant. Cupping, blistering, sweating, and other strenuous and often fatal measures were also used.[3] Discoveries in the chemistry of compounds paved the way for various concoctions called polypharmacy, administered in large doses to induce vomiting, to evacuate the bowels, or to produce sweating. These were ineffective at the least, but more often hazardous, based on Hahnemann's experience. The following quotation from *The Life and Letters of Dr. Samuel Hahnemann* shows his frustrations:

> It was agony for me to walk always in darkness, when I had to heal the sick, and to prescribe, according to such or such an hypothesis concerning diseases, substances which owe their place in the Materia Medica to an arbitrary decision... Soon after my marriage, I renounced the practice of medicine, that I might no longer incur the risk of doing Injury, and I engaged exclusively in chemistry, and in literary occupation. But I became a father, and serious diseases threatened my beloved children... My scruples redoubled when I saw that I could afford them no certain relief.[4]

Voltaire (1694-1778), the French writer and philosopher who also lived during this era, opined the following about the practice of medicine: "Physicians have been pouring drugs about which they know little for diseases about which they know less, into human beings about whom they know nothing."[5]

Due to this grim situation, Hahnemann resorted to translation work as his sole means of livelihood. This was when he discovered the Law of Similars.

A. THE DISCOVERY OF THE LAW OF SIMILARS AND THE PROCESS OF PROVINGS

While doing translation work, Hahnemann never ceased to examine and inquire. He wanted to understand the basic principle of healing which eluded medical science at that time. In the process of translating Cullen's *Materia Medica*, he reacted to Cullen's assertion that success in the treatment of intermittent fevers using the Peruvian bark *Cinchona*, was due to its bitterness. This was not exact thinking. In his dissatisfaction, he took the medicine himself. He described the results as follows:

> I took by way of experiment, twice a day, four drachms of good China, my feet, finger ends etc., at first became cold; I grew languid and drowsy; then my heart began to palpitate, my pulse grew hard

and small; intolerable anxiety, trembling, prostration throughout my limbs; then pulsation in the head, redness of my cheeks, thirst, and in short, all these symptoms, which are ordinary characteristic of intermittent fever, made their appearance, one after the other, yet without the peculiar chilly, shivering rigor... This paroxysm lasted two or three hours each time, and recurred if I repeated this dose, not otherwise; I discontinued it, and was in good health.[6]

Through this experiment, Hahnemann gained valuable insight into the foundation of folk medical practice in various cultures of the world. That is, *a remedy for a disease produces similar symptoms in a healthy organism.* (For example, the indigenous people of the Philippines, called Hanonoo Mangyans, practice the same principle.[7]) Hippocrates was known to have said: "Through the like, disease is produced, and through the application of the like it is cured." Likewise Paracelsus wrote in his *Doctrine of Signatures*: "You bring together the same anatomy of the herbs and the same anatomy of the illness into one order. This simile gives you an understanding on the way in which you shall heal."[8] A Chinese proverb states too: "To counteract a poison, a similar poison must be used."[9] In this sense, Hahnemann rediscovered for modem humanity a lost principle of healing which orthodox medicine was then unable to understand. He also pioneered the *process of proving*, that is, testing a remedy on a healthy human being rather than on diseased humans—the general practice at that time and carried on till today.[10]

Hahnemann's Law of Similars can be considered a discovery as significant as Archimedes' law of buoyancy and Newton's law of gravity. However, it was not immediately acceptable to the prevailing allopathic school of thought and the materialistic science at that time.[11]

B. THE FOUNDING OF HOMEOPATHY

Hahnemann shared his findings with other disgruntled physicians whom he came in contact with. For six years they experimented on themselves, taking different plant, mineral, and animal extracts, including poisonous ones. They kept scrupulously detailed accounts of the symptoms produced by each drug taken, and published the detailed results in small bulletins. In doing so, this ragtag group of physicians recognized the symptoms of many illnesses for which they had in vain been seeking cures. They discovered specific remedies (from minerals, plants, and small animals) capable of effecting cures.

In 1796, Hahnemann and his group publicly proclaimed homeopathy as their system of medicine. In 1812, Hahnemann compiled the results of the numerous drug tests and published them as the first *Materia Medical Pura* in six volumes. Some of the remedies I describe in this book were part of this first materia medica. These medicines have cured millions in more than 200 years of the practice of homeopathy.

C. THE DISCOVERY OF POTENTIZED OR DYNAMIZED REMEDIES

Proceeding to Hahnemann's discovery of the third principle, i.e., the principle of dynamized or potentized remedies, first we must picture the enthusiasm of these physicians/scientists with regard to their newly found (rediscovered) laws. Reinspired with the "will to heal," Hahnemann and his colleagues administered the preparations to their patients. They observed an initial aggravation of the symptoms, then eventually a cure. However, some tinctures often caused intense aggravation of the symptoms, and another dose was considered hazardous. The aggravation was understandable because of the toxins of the remedies which were producing the symptoms.

This made Hahnemann quite depressed. For many years this problem was a living question for him. Then one day, he started diluting the tinctures to one tenth of the original amount, and submitted each dilution to a series of vigorous shakes which he later called "succussion." When Hahnemann gave these diluted remedies to his patients, the aggravation of symptoms was lessened, and he still got the desired cure. He continued diluting the remedies following the same ratio and procedure. He reached a point where he made a cure without any aggravation of the symptoms. He even went further in his dilution, so that theoretically the substance is no longer present, and yet the mixture became more potent! This was a critical juncture for Hahnemann and his group. How could he explain the principle behind this phenomenon in a society where the dominant thinking is "more is might"?

To answer this question, we must go back to the debate among scientists at that time regarding what constituted life. This was the debate between materialism and vitalism. The materialists asserted that chemical processes produced the phenomenon of life; to the vitalists a non-sensible vital body was responsible for it. Hahnemann and his colleagues may have taken their argument from the vitalists. Thus homeopaths explained that "there lies hidden in every substance in nature some inner life, and that we can mobilize and use this force if we know how to process the substance."[12] The rigorous shaking or succussion of the diluted solution releases "the spirit-like" qualities of these substances, Hahnemann wrote later on. This explained why the higher dilutions are actually more potent than the original tincture. In other words, ingesting the spirit, vital force, or energy rather than just the substance that is found in the minerals, plants, and animals is what stimulates healing.[13]

For the die-hard materialists of yesterday or today (who considered only physical and chemical processes as real), homeopathic remedies were utter nonsense and "quackery." For the more open-minded, the spirit or vital force found in these remedies is an imponderable, i.e., it cannot be weighed or measured or conclusively explained by a materialistic paradigm of thought. For those of us who are able to transcend the orthodox scientific way of thinking, it is quite easy to follow Hahnemann's logic.

For others who have been exposed to an indigenous culture where the spirit in nature is still recognized, Hahnemann's explanation is palpable. There are indigenous people in every society or country who still practice and preserve their traditional culture and beliefs based on this notion. Their worldview and knowledge about nature and the human being is now more commonly called by social scientists, Indigenous Knowledge System. However, most of the established medical institutions have lost their appreciation of living nature and have unwittingly adopted the materialist scientific view of orthodox science.

How has orthodox science affected our way of thinking? What are the consequences of orthodox science for our way of life, particularly with regard to health and illness? This is the subject of the next chapter.[14]

Notes

1 The use of the laws of physics and chemistry (derived from the inorganic, dead, mineral world) to explain living processes is the primary cause of the crisis in orthodox medical science. Natural science is still unable to satisfactorily explain life. This brought about the mindset of those living in more affluent countries to view nature as a mere resource, e.g., the forest is seen simply as board feet of lumber instead of a habitat of biological diversity. In medicine, this way of thinking is exemplified by doctors who justify the use of chemical drugs to inhibit or replace biochemical secretions of the body, or often use unnecessary surgery to remove or replace "defective parts," as if bodies were machines.

2 Those who were able to explain the wisdom behind their therapies banded together

and called their medicine the science of *naturopathy*. The word naturopathy was first introduced by a 19th century homeopath, John H. Scheel, to connote promoting the health of the whole person through natural means. Later on, herbal medicine became a discipline distinct from naturopathy. Naturopathy is briefly discussed on page 27. See Olsen KG. *The Encyclopedia of Alternative Health Care*. New York: Pocket Books; 1990:208-226. Type *naturopathy* in your internet search engine or go to *naturopathyonline. com.*

3   Weiner M, Goss K. *The Complete Book of Homeopathy*. Bantam Books; 1982:237-243. Here it is mentioned that George Washington was not spared from the fatal measures of the allopaths. "Despite the continually shifting theoretical ground of medicine in Hahnemann's time, regular medical practitioners generally resorted to the methods of 'heroic' medicine: blood-letting, cupping, blistering, purging, sweating, and other strenuous and often fatal measures. In an effort to draw off what they considered excess blood, physicians would open a patient's veins and remove anywhere from several ounces to several quarts of blood. Leeches were sold in great quantities for the same purpose... Harsh substances were placed or burned on the skin, and when the resulting second-degree burn became infected, the pus that exuded was taken as evidence that the infection was being drawn out of the body... Not even the wealthiest and most powerful figures with the best medical care available to them were exempted from the dangers of such treatment. George Washington died following a sore throat and breathing difficulties, probably due as much to the heroic treatment he received as to his actual illness: during the afternoon and evening of the last day of his life, he was bled three times, having had at least four pints of blood removed, treated with blistering, and dosed with calomel." See also Coulter HL. *Homeopathic Influences in 19th Century Allopathic Therapeutics: A Historical and Philosophical Study*. St Louis: Formur, Inc., Publishers; 1973. Coulter went through documents written by both allopathic and homeopathic practitioners in the early 19th century and gave an idea of how these physicians were thinking.

4   Bradford TL. *Life and Letters of Dr. Samuel Hahnemann*. Philadelphia: Boericke and Tafel; 1895. Quoted in Vithoulkas G. *Homeopathy Medicine of the New Man*. New York: Avon Books; 1971:20-21.

5   Quoted in Mendelsohn R. *Mal(e) Practice: How Doctors Manipulate Women*. Chicago: Contemporary Books, Inc.; 1982:59. Mendelsohn quoted Voltaire to point out that what the latter had said 200 years ago "is even more appropriate today because there are so many more drugs to abuse."

6   Vilhoulkas, p. 23.

7   From a lecture delivered by Robert Kasberg, Jr., PhD (Anthropology), during the

symposium on Indigenous Knowledge System in conjunction with the Sustainable Agriculture Fair held at University of the Philippines, Los Banos, Laguna, October 21, 1991. Dr. Kasberg, who is married to a Hanunuo woman, stayed with the Hanunuos for more than 12 years. His doctoral dissertation is on the medicinal system of this same tribal group.

8 Quoted in Panos M, Heimlich J. *Homeopathic Medicine for the Home.* Los Angeles: J.P. Tarcher; 1980:ll.

9 Based on a conversation with Leonardo Co, taxonomist and expert on Chinese medicine. When I told him about the Law of Similars, he remembered the Chinese proverb approximately as quoted.

10 When a drug is withdrawn from the market because of its adverse side-effects and eventual death from its continuous use, this is, in a sense, the final test conducted on diseased human beings. Tests done on animals to show drug efficacy and/or toxicity are actually not conclusive (but it is one of the main bases to show that the drug is ready to be used on human beings), because we all know human beings would react differently from animals. Human beings have "I"s as their highest principle and the main determinant of the immune system, which animals do not have. This will be explained further on in Chapters 3, 4, and 5 of Section 1.

11 Throughout the 19th century, allopaths ridiculed homeopaths and homeopathy, denoting their disapproval (more out of prejudice and ignorance) of the Law of Similars. For example, in 1838 a professor at the University of Pennsylvania joked about the "little fist" which homeopathy shakes at the "giant" disease. Another example: "[Allopaths] deal with realities and not with subtleties, and use remedies that are capable of visibly affecting the bodies of their patients... No one can persuade himself for a moment that bloodletting, tartar emetic, calomel, opium, quinine, etc. are not powerful agents, capable of exerting a decided control over the course and events of diseases." Quoted in Coulter HL. *Homeopathic Influences in Nineteenth Century Allopathic Therapuetics.* St. Louis: Formur Inc., Publishers; 1973:5. See also Nicholls PA. *Homeopathy and the Medical Profession.* London: Croom Helm; 1988. This book is the tortuous history of homeopathy from the 19th century to the present, where it is now part of complementary medicine in most developed countries.

12 Vithoulkas, p. 31.

13 This is a bibliography of studies on the efficacy of potentized remedies. Some are published in reputable medical journals like *Lancet*. Most are double-blind studies to allay the fears of skeptics that the cures are merely due to the placebo effect. They should be read by those who want to face the truth squarely. Reiley D et al. Is evidence for homeopathy reproducible? *Lancet* 1994;344:1601-1606; Jacobs J et al. Treatment

of acute childhood diarrhea with homeopathic medicine: a randomized clinical trial in Nicaragua. *Pediatrics* 1994;93:719-725; Kleijnen J, Knipschild P, ter Riet G. Clinical trials of homeopathy. *British Medical Journal* 1991;302:316-323; Davenas Elizabeth D, Poitevin B, Buenaviste J. Effect on mouse peritoneal macrophages of orally administered very high dilutions of silica. *European Journal of Pharmacology* 1987;135:313-319; Dorfman P, Lasserre MN, Tetau M. Preparation for birth by homeopathy: experimentation by double blind versus placebo. *Cahiers de Biotherapie* 1987;94:77-81; Ferley JP et al. A controlled evaluation of a homeopathic preparation in the treatment of influenza-like symptom. *British Journal of Clinical Pharmacology* 1989, 27:329-335; Gibson RG, Gibson SLM, MacNeil AD et al. Homeopathy therapy in rheumatoid arthritis: evaluation by double blind controlled trial. *British Journal of Clinical Pharmacology* 1980;9:453-459; Gibson RG et al. Salicylates and homeopathy in rheumatoid arthritis: preliminary observation. *British Journal of Clinical Pharmacology* 1978;6:391-395; Guttentag OE. Homeopathy in the light of modern pharmacology. *Clinical Pharmacology and Therapeutics* 1966;7:426; Lewith G, Brown PK, Tyrell DAJ. Controlled study of the effects of homeopathic dilution of influenza vaccine on antibody titres in man. *Complementary Medicine Research* 1989;3:22-24; Mayaux MJ, Guihard-Moscato ML, Schwarz D et al. Controlled clinical trial of homeopathy in post operative ileus. *Lancet* 1988;xxx:528-529; Reiley DT, Morag A, Taylor MA, McSharry C, Aitchison T. Is homeopathy a placebo response: controlled trial of homeopathy potency, with pollen in hayfever as model. *Lancet* 1986;(October):881-886; Reiley DT et al. Is homeopathy a placebo response? A controlled trial of homeopathic immunotherapy (HIT) in atrophic asthma. *Complementary Therapies in Medicine* 1993;l(suppl.):24-25; Reiley DT. Young doctors' views on alternative medicine. *British Medical Journal* 1983;287:337-339; Riebel L. A homeopathic model of psychotherapy. *Journal of Humanistic Psychology* 1984(Winter);24:9-48; Sacks A. Nuclear magnetic resonance spectroscopy of homeopathic remedies. *Journal of Holistic Medicine* 1983(Fall-Winter);5:172-175; Slonim D, White K. Homeopathy and psychiatry. *Journal of Mind and Behavior* 1983(Summer);4:401-410; Wiesenauer M, Gaus W. Double-blind trial comparing the effectiveness of the homeopathic preparation Galphimia Potentization D6, Galphimia Dilution 10 and placebo on pollinosis. *Ar Vleimittelforschung* 1985;35:1745-1747; Buckman R, Lewith G. What does homeopathy do—and how? *British Medical Journal* 1994;309:303-306; Cazin JC et al. A study of the effects of decimal and centimal dilution of arsenic on retention and mobilization of arsenic in the rat. *Human Toxicology* 1987(July).

The succeeding list consists of studies on the effects of potentized substances. A brief commentary is likewise given to give the reader some idea of the report. Amato. Molecular divorce gives strange vibes. *Science News* 1986(November 1):277-278. This study by chemists working for the US Government's National Bureau of Standards, and who knew nothing about potentization, noted that when they shook the coupled molecules of nitric oxide, the units did not weaken and break into parts, but rather developed stronger molecular bonds. Buenaviste J et al. Human basophil degranulation triggered by very diluted anti-serum against IgE. *Nature* 1988(June);333:816-818. This experiment duplicated seventy times around the world discovered that human blood serum full of white blood cells and Immunoglobulin E Type (IgE) antibody continue to react to a solution of anti-IgE antibody even though the solution has been diluted 1: 10^{120} parts water—or one to ten followed by 120 zeros. Smith RB, Boericke GW. Changes caused by succussion on nuclear magnetic resonance patterns and bioassay of bradykinin triacetate (BKTA) succussions and dilution. *Journal of the American Institute of Homeopathy* 1968(Nov-Dec);61:197-212. This study using nuclear magnetic resonance (NMR) showed that twenty-three different homeopathic medicines and potencies had distinctive readings of subatomic activity, while a placebo did not. Sainte Laud J, Haynes D, Gerswin G. Inhibition of whole blood dilutions on basophil degranulation. *International Journal of Immunotherapy* 1986;2:247-250. These scientists provided evidence that potentized doses of blood (5x, 7x) demonstrated an inhibiting effect on basophil degranulation. This effect was evidenced after exposure to fourteen of eighteen allergens, including tree pollens, mold, mites, house dust, Penicillin, Candida albicans, and aspirin. Stebbing ARD. Hormesis: the stimulation of growth by low levels of inhibitors. *The Science of the Total Environment* 1982;22:213-234. Stebbing, a British scientist (not a homeopath), has referenced over 100 studies from various scientific fields which show that microdoses of certain substances can have even greater effects upon a system than larger doses. Type *emoto water* in your internet search engine for the effect of an intangible, like thoughts on water.

In this age of freedom to speak one's mind out, the abovementioned studies can be "refuted" by other well-funded studies whose motive could be to protect the current dominance of orthodox science (and the financial and power reward it has hitherto gained). At some point, it is best to rely more on our inner sense for truth rather than just on voluminous studies and statistics. Resorting only to endless studies and statistics (quantity) to discover the truth is a convenient trap set by the materialistic mindset of today.

14 Many philosophers and scientists have criticized the unfounded assumptions and inadequacies of materialistic science. See Berman M. *The Reenchantment of the World.* Ithaca, NY: Cornell University Press; 1981; Roszak T. *Where the Wasteland Ends.* Garden City, New York: Doubleday and Co.; 1972; McLaughlin A. Images and ethics of nature. *Environmental Ethics* 1985;7(4):293-319, in Perlas N. *The Second Scientific Revolution and the Center For Alternative Development Initiatives,* Unit 718 Cityland Mega Plaza, Ortigas, Pasig City, Philippines, or see *www.cadi.ph.* Continue reading Chapter 2 and the notes to get a clearer idea of the inadequacies of orthodox materialistic science as the basis of understanding life.

Chapter Two

❧

The Crisis of Orthodox Medicine

Unknown to many, orthodox medicine actually is in a crisis. Generally, this crisis has two facets: (1) a crisis in the practice of medicine, and (2) a crisis in the science itself. Without an understanding of both, we endanger the health of humanity.[1]

A. CRISIS IN THE PRACTICE

What are the inadequacies and excesses of today's medical practice? In 1995, when I made reference to Robert S. Mendelsohn, *MD's Confessions of a Medical Heretic* (1979), it was thus far the most comprehensive critique of today's medical practice.[2] Since then others have followed suit, like Stuart M. Berger, MD, *What Your Doctor Didn't Learn in Medical School* (1988); Dr. Joe Collier, *The Health Conspiracy: How Doctors, The Drug Industry and the Government Undermine Our Health* (1989); and Joseph Mercola, DO, in *www.mercola.com* (2000). From the side of investigative journalism and victims of medical practice, we have Hans Ruesch, *Naked Empress or the Great Medical Fraud* (1982) and Lynne McTaggart, *What Doctors Don't Tell You: The Truth About the Dangers of Modern Medicine* (1996). These are just a few of the more courageous individuals who declared in their written works that "the Emperor has no clothes."

Most of the aforementioned authors reiterated and elaborated on what Dr. Mendelsohn had already said. Naturally, they gave their own updates, nuances, and examples to the different issues discussed. A quotable quote comes from Dr. David Greer, Dean of Medicine of Brown University, addressing a graduating class: "Fifty percent of what we taught you is wrong. Our problem is that we don't know which fifty percent."[3] These words depict in a nutshell the mood of this chapter. I hope that after reading this book, you will have a fairly good appreciation of Dr. Greer's dilemma.

The subtopics discussed below come from the pioneer medical heretic, Dr. Mendelsohn, who summed it all up quite comprehensively. Although the data to support his arguments are mostly from the United States, I think the situation in other countries is not much different. If intensive studies are conducted in less affluent countries (which usually do not have budgets for research), it may be a worse picture. I will briefly discuss the more important conclusions of the studies cited, adding findings from other sources to support his point.

1. Many Drugs May Cause More Problems Than They Cure

A common experience among those who take drugs is that these may trigger various side-effects. One who is taking a drug for a particular ailment needs to take another to remedy the side-effects of the first, and then a third one to alleviate the side-effects of the second. In the end this person could be taking six to eight different drugs.[4] There have also been cases of drugs being withdrawn from the market because of observed adverse side-effects.[5] Worse, most drugs can lead to sclerosis, degeneration, or cancer of particular organs—yet the public is informed only much later (or not at all) of these after-effects.[6]

For example, aspirin, when given to suppress children's fever, has been found to lead to Reye's syndrome, a potentially fatal neurological condition. It is not uncommon for chloromycetin to interfere with the bone marrow's production of blood. Tetracycline is deposited in the bones and teeth. Intake of an antibiotic may encourage a worse infection due to the development of a strain of bacteria resistant to the drug.[7] Individuals who resort to antibiotics have 2.9 times the risk of reinfection. Taking steroids for a long period of time causes the adrenal cortex to shrink and shrivel. Reserpine, a drug to lower high blood pressure, subjects the user to tripled risk of breast cancer.[8] Insulin can cause diabetic blindness. The synthetic hormone DES (diethylstilbestrol), found in contraceptive pills and menopausal estrogen, causes cardiovascular diseases, liver tumors, headaches, depression, and cancer in the users as well as in their children.[9]

The side- and after-effects of drugs are further compounded by our pill-popping reflex that is largely propagated through advertisements and by our own doctors. There is a term for doctor- or drug- induced diseases: *iatrogenic illnesses*. A study published in the *New England Journal of Medicine* in 1981 showed that 36% of all cases admitted in a respected university's hospital were iatrogenic in nature.[10] On July 26, 2000, the *Journal of the American Medical Association (JAMA)* reported that medication errors are the third leading cause of death in the US. In 2000, a presidential report described iatrogenic error and illness as "a national problem of epidemic proportions," causing up to 98,000 annual deaths. The report estimated the cost of lost income, disability, and health care costs to be $29 billion a year.[11]

Studies are accumulating, linking the use of modern chemotherapeutics (including synthetic vitamins) to genetic damage.[12] Once damage is done, the development of tumors and cancer cannot be far behind. Worse, the danger to human heredity, i.e., the transmission of recessive mutation through whole generations, cannot be ignored.[13]

2. Hospitals Are Dangerous Places for the Sick

The word "hospital" comes from Latin meaning "guest," but seldom is this place truly hospitable. The meaning has been totally turned around. Little attention is given to the caring or healing of patients as opposed to medicating them.[14]

The sick person who is already weak is exposed to a lot of other possible sources of illness in the hospital.[15] Air-conditioning ducts distribute the contaminants. Nurses and doctors who regularly go in and out of the room carry with them the contagions. After ten minutes of use, a surgical mask becomes vulnerable to bacterial colonies, instead of serving as a shield. The nursery can be the most dangerous place in the hospital for the newborn.[16] Infants (particularly those who are denied breastfeeding) have not yet developed their immune system, so they are more susceptible to infection. Sadly, hospital procedures have absolutely no respect for human dignity.[17] You have to take off your clothes and wear a hospital gown, leaving you vulnerable to inspection by innumerable doctors, nurses, and technicians. You have to lie down most of the time and eat what they serve you. If you do not have enough money, you sleep in a room with sick strangers.[18]

A lengthy stay in the hospital is often unnecessary. You are probably better off spending the time and money in a resort! Accidents involving children seem to occur more often in hospitals than in any other place. The survival rate of patients in the intensive care unit is the same as for those who are cared for at home.[19]

More than 95% of births to healthy women should have been outside the hospital. Babies born in the hospital are six times more likely to suffer distress during labor and delivery, eight times more likely to get caught in the birth canal, four times more likely to need resuscitation, four times more likely to become infected, and thirty times more likely to be permanently injured. Mothers are three times more likely to experience hemorrhage in hospitals than in home births.

There is now a term for hospital-acquired infection: *nosocomial diseases*. A cross-sectional survey of 18,163 patients in 43 hospitals in the United Kingdom in 1980 showed that 9.3% of the infections were hospital acquired.[20] The actual figure is probably higher. Hospital officials will be the last to admit that their hospitals are sources of infection.

At the turn of the century, the Centers for Disease Control and Prevention (CDC) in the US estimated that each year nearly 2 million people acquire infections while hospitalized, and about 90,000 die from those infections. This was followed up in 2004 by HealthGrades' *Patient Safety in American Hospitals* study entitled "In-Hospital Deaths from Medical Errors at 195,000 per Year."[21]

Worst of all indicators, the death rates in hospitals declined as much as 50% during doctors' strikes (for example, in Israel the death rate dropped 50% in 1973; in Bogota, Colombia, 35% in 1976; and in Los Angeles County, 18% in 1976).[22] When the doctors went back to work, the death rates rose again to their normal level.

In 2008, California hospital workers were on strike. The death rate in the state of California suddenly plummeted. The strike was so effective at reducing deaths that certain sectors are proposing hospital workers stay on strike permanently as a new system of "health care."[23]

3. Most Operations Do Little Good and Many Do Harm

An estimated 7.5 million unnecessary medical and surgical procedures are performed each year, writes Gary Null, PhD, in *Death by Medicine*. Rather than reverse the problems they purport to fix, these unwarranted procedures can often lead to greater health problems and even death. A 1995 report by Milliman & Robertson, Inc., concluded that nearly 60 percent of all surgeries performed are medically unnecessary, according to *Under The Influence of Modern Medicine* by Terry A. Rondberg.[24]

Mendelsohn asserts that surgery can be cut down by as much as 90% if doctors' decisions are subjected to peer reviews, and if doctors know and recommend alternative treatments. Women and children are the unwitting victims of many unnecessary operations. The usefulness of tonsillectomies, for example, has never been proven. Most hysterectomies have been found to be unnecessary.[25] Coronary heart surgery provides little benefit.[26] A radical change of diet proved more effective and long lasting.[27]

Part of the problem is the fact that there are too many surgeons. If one consults a surgeon, it is but logical to expect he will recommend an operation. Moreover, teaching and research hospitals increase the danger

of the patient being used for the doctor's own purposes.[28] The best way
to deal with surgery is to ask questions, scrutinize test results, and solicit
second and third opinions from various schools of thought in medicine. It
is likely that other therapies can provide a genuine cure, whereas allopathic
doctors presume surgery is the only answer.

4. Medical Testing Laboratories Are Scandalously Inaccurate

Medical testing laboratories are another area of concern. Consider the
following findings.[29] Surveys of laboratories across the US demonstrated
that 10% to 40% of their work in bacteriologic testing was unsatisfactory;
30% to 50% failed various simple clinical chemistry tests; 12% to 18%
flubbed blood grouping tests and typing; and 20% to 30% botched
hemoglobin and serum electrolyte tests. Fifty percent of the "high standard"
laboratories licensed for Medicare work failed to pass careful scrutiny.
Retesting of results revealed that only 20% of them produced acceptable
results more than 90% of the time. Only half passed the test 75% of the
time. Simple tests such as blood cell count, urine analysis, tuberculin test,
and chest X-rays are so controversial and difficult to interpret that their
usefulness is extremely limited. Part of the problem is that doctors rely too
much on quantitative information provided by these tools.[30] In the end,
these doctors lose their ability to diagnose without the use of such tests.
This is an offshoot of a materialistic science way of thinking.

If the above is happening in a so-called highly affluent country like
the US, can less affluent countries be better off—considering that they
may be using secondhand equipment, making do with inadequately trained
personnel, and are unable to conduct thorough retests to verify the results?

5. Annual Physical Examinations Are a Health Risk

The entire diagnostic procedure—from the moment the patient enters
the doctor's office to the moment he leaves clutching a prescription or a
referral slip—is seldom a useful ritual. We are conditioned to think that
the more tests one undergoes, the more thorough the examination, the
better off one is. This is nonsense, and in certain cases dangerous. One
should approach the diagnostic procedure with careful scrutiny rather than
full trust and confidence. The doctor sets the limits of what is normal
and abnormal, what is good or bad. However, doctors are not trained to
recognize wellness, but rather to detect disease. Therefore they are more
apt to pronounce one sick than well. If one's condition is diagnosed as

"abnormal," one is asked to undergo a battery of tests that could be inaccurate and may lead to false conclusions. Worse, one may end up with a prescription, with its accompanying adverse side- and after-effects.[31]

6. The X-Ray Machine Is the Most Dangerous Tool in a Doctor's Office

How about the X-ray machines that doctors depend on so often? Doctors tend to prescribe an X-ray as a routine procedure, oblivious to the side-effects. Exposure to X-rays can cause thyroid lesion, cancer, high blood pressure, cataracts, diabetes, and cardiovascular diseases. A fetus exposed to X-rays will have six times the probability of acquiring childhood leukemia.[32] Mammography will cause more breast cancer than it can detect.[33] Early this century the US Department of Health and Human Services listed X-ray and gamma rays as one of the major carcinogens.[34]

Many of the X-ray machines in less affluent countries may be secondhand. They may have leaks or may not be properly calibrated. One exposure is about 10 millirad. Depending on the operator and the quality of the machine, it may emit as much as 100 millirad in one picture. This means that one may get an overdose of radiation with just one session. As for the interpretation of X-ray pictures, a study revealed that the experts contradict each other 24% of the time. Given the same pictures at another time, each expert contradicted himself 31% of the time. Worse, 32% of chest X-rays showing definite abnormalities in the lungs were misdiagnosed as negative.

7. Authoritarianism in Organized Medicine

Mendelsohn further provides the context of today's medicine. He likens today's medical institutions to a church where the doctors are priests, or rather *Medical Deities* (as Bernie Siegel, MD,[35] would like to put it). What they say should be swallowed hook, line, and sinker. "Doctor's orders!"—we frequently hear. The term used to describe the impact of doctors' negative statements is "nocebo effect." In the "placebo effect," anything which a doctor says or prescribes has a healing effect; in the "nocebo effect," a doctor's statement such as, "You have only 6 months to live!" creates such a psychological impact that even before the end of the sixth months, the person dies. This absolute image of the man or woman in white and their tendency to authoritarianism, is a large part of the problem.[36] It evokes in us a corresponding attitude of diffidence and blind faith in the doctor, so we, as patients, also become part of the problem.

Corollary to this is the issue of who controls the whole medical enterprise. Doctors are only the lowly priests. Behind them are the pharmaceutical companies, medical research institutions, state agencies and medical schools that provide the latest research on various drugs and illnesses, and a regular supply of indoctrinated doctors, pharmacists, nurses, and other allied medical professionals. Furthermore, there are the colleges of medical scientists who ultimately endorse what is "scientific." They play "god" and control the direction to be taken by research institutions, or determine which disease should be given priority of investigation.[37] The findings are presented as scientific declarations or "revelations." These declarations eventually become dogmas, whose main effect is the increased power of the physicians and the whole orthodox medical establishment.[38] Naturally, the funds for research are provided by the state or philanthropic institutions and individuals that are either conscious or unconscious of the implications of the "help" that they extend.

In 2001, Thomas Szasz referred to the modern affluent societies' inclination for transforming human problems into "diseases" and judicial sanctions into "treatments," replacing the rule of law with the rule of medical discretion. This situation leads to a type of government Szasz called "Pharmacracy." In this "therapeutic state," healthcare providers have far more power than consumers. The lopsided power may make consumers vulnerable to iatrogenic illness, which becomes an important cause of illness and death.[39]

This leads us to the other crisis in medical science, that is, the science itself. Many civil society organizations in various countries around the world involved in social change have fallen into the trap of thinking that by wresting control of the science and technology (e.g., the nationalization of the drug industry, or bringing down the cost of medicine by legislating the use of generic drugs), they are able to remedy the inequity in the health care delivery system, or make people healthy.[40] The discussion that follows indicates that this is still an inadequate strategy (if not worse), and would continue to erode humanity's health.

B. THE CRISIS OF ORTHODOX MEDICAL SCIENCE

Some medical historians believe that today's orthodox medicine has no professed therapeutic principle from which it prescribes.[41] Ironically, this is the medical system which claims for itself the monopoly of the word "scientific." Medical scientists argue that medicine benefits from discoveries made in all branches of science. However, the fact remains that it may not have any professed, coherent, or comprehensive principles according to which they apply these discoveries. What really is the basis of what we call science today?

There are four essential assumptions or worldviews underlying what we are all conditioned to consider as science.

1. Materialism—Matter as the Only Reality

The first assumption is: what is real is only that which can be seen by the physical senses. To a scientist, reality is what can be counted, weighed, and measured.[42] Thus, orthodox medical science always boasts of the increase in human life expectancy or quantity of life, rather than its quality. We commend someone who lives till his seventies or eighties despite his regular intake of various maintenance medications, dependency on insulin injections, or use of a dialysis machine. We think of someone who has great material wealth as successful, disregarding how he feels inside. All other qualities such as taste, smell, beauty, or ugliness, which cannot be quantified, are considered unworthy of scientific investigation.[43] Purpose or meaning in life, including human consciousness and spirit, are banished as "subjective." Prayer is considered an "arbitrary optional frill that simply is not in the same league as drugs and surgery."[44] This habit of thinking is extended not only to medicine, but to all other disciplines including biology, history, economics, and politics. By assuming that matter alone explains the natural world, most of us are continually being led to view materialism as part of the scientific method itself. A more recent example can be found in the science of genetics: diseases are now being explained by cellular genetics, which in turn is understood in terms of molecular or atomic laws of physics.[45] The idea of the human being is lost in the process.

2. The Human Body and Nature as Machines and as Mere Chemicals

The second assumption of orthodox science is: reality is mechanical. The human body is thus viewed as a great machine. Energy, measured by one's calorie intake, is used up to produce movement. People are able to think because of chemical reactions in the brain. Carl Sagan's book, *The Dragons of Eden*, displays this dismal viewpoint. To Sagan, the working of the brain (considered as synonymous with the mind) is a consequence of its anatomy and physiology, nothing more. This viewpoint is the basis of orthodox medicine for administering chemicals as remedies to human beings.

Likewise, we have been conditioned to see nature as a mere assembly of chemicals. We complacently allow the use of chemicals in agriculture, thinking that the soil and the plants are basically only of chemical nature. It is interesting to note that the same manufacturers that poison the environment are also responsible for the drugs that poison human beings.[46]

This mechanistic viewpoint also justifies the practice of either removing or replacing bodily organs when they are no longer functional— just like replacing a part of an automobile. The science of genetics has carried the assumptions of materialistic science too far into the field of human life. Genetic engineers are eyeing human clones as a reliable source of spare organs (oblivious to the fact that human souls are in them). We should be militantly critical of such indiscriminate applications.[47]

3. The Method of Reductionism

The third assumption is reductionism: every phenomenon has a single cause. The germ theory of disease is an example of this way of thinking. Let us put this in historical context.

a. The Germ Theory of Disease

In 1876, when Louis Pasteur discovered bacteria and Robert Koch made his fundamental studies on the biology of anthrax, the *contagium* (postulated by Fracastorius 100 years before the invention of the microscope) was finally verified. As I mentioned earlier, natural science, at its infancy, tended to oversimplify. Therefore, it hypothesized that disease could only have one cause, not several. Moreover, the inner logic of materialistic science then dictated that one must concentrate on discrete, observable phenomena such as microorganisms.[48]

In earlier times, it was believed that disease was caused by the wrath of God, or the work of the devil. (As late as 1632, the townspeople of Oberammergau, Germany, made a solemn pledge to elaborately reenact the life, passion, and death of Christ every ten years, due to their belief that the plague which affected their village and eventually spread to most of Europe was a punishment from God.)

The scientific-minded naturally wanted a more rational explanation. Thus, various theories were forwarded to account for the genesis of infectious diseases. Before 1876, the dominant theory of the origin of

epidemics came from Thomas Sydenham (1624-1689). He attributed them
to a combination of temporal, climatic, and telluric influences, which he
termed "epidemic constitution." In 1840, the work of Jacob Henle first
indicated that epidemics are not due to atmospheric or chemical causes,
but are brought about by a parasitic "contagium vivum." He stated that
"investigation of the cause of miasmatic-contagious disease must begin
with the contagium." Thus in 1876, the contagium was finally verified, and
bacteria became the object of research.[49]

Orthodox science still did not adequately explain why in an epidemic
not everyone succumbed to the disease. It is important to recall here the
debate in 1876 between Robert Koch and Max von Pettenkofer. Pettenkofer
and other clinicians disputed the claim that bacteria were the sole factor
behind a disease. They argued that the environment and each person's
disposition and constitution were as important in the genesis of infectious
diseases as bacteria. This explained why not everyone succumbed during
an epidemic.

Pettenkofer was able to eliminate cholera infection in Munich,
Germany by providing clean water and ensuring proper waste disposal.[50]
Incidentally, in the midst of the debate between Pettenkofer and Koch
about bacteria, the 74-year old Pettenkofer drank a suspension of *vibrio
cholerae* to prove his point. As he predicted, he remained well. A similar case
was reported by Letterer, whose colleague injected himself with a virulent
culture of *tubercle bacilli* as an act of suicide. To his surprise, he did not even
become ill.[51]

Before his death, Louis Pasteur admitted that germs may not be the
cause of disease after all, but may simply be another symptom of the
disease. He realized that germs led to illness when the person's immune
or defense system is not strong enough to overcome them. Factors that
comprised the quality of host resistance to germs included hereditary
endowment, nutrition, stresses in life, and psychological state.[52]

Numerous current and past experiments have consistently shown
that germs do not spontaneously grow inside the human body. As a matter
of fact,

> One milliliter of blood from a healthy human being kills more
> than ten million influenza agents in vitro. Human albumin destroys
> certain staphylococci at body temperature in one-and-a-half hours,
> and is thus a stronger bacteriostatic than penicillin.[53]

Scientists had transplanted the cold virus in the lining of sinuses of
various individuals and only 12% of them caught a cold![54]

Other schools of medical thought (homeopathy, naturopathy, homotoxicology, and anthroposophic medicine) have argued that there is an inherent law in living tissues that governs invading microorganisms. All foreign elements are subordinate to the host organism's higher principles or structural plan. (See the discussion on an expanded image of the human being in Section 1, Chapter 3 to get a clear picture of what these higher principles are.) The predisposition and constitution of a human being, therefore, are as important, if not more important, than pathogenic factors. If pathogens have found a medium in which to grow inside our bodies, it is because we have created the conditions ("food") for them to grow. We have made part of our body the medium for their growth.

Homotoxicologists and naturopaths further argue that the real material cause of disease is a chemical which they call homotoxin (in Latin: *homo*, human; *toxin*, poison). Fever, inflammation, and allergic reactions are normal body reactions to remove homotoxins.[55] If these reactions are suppressed, the toxins will be pushed deeper into the tissues to arise later as chronic diseases, tumors, degenerated organs, or cancer. Moreover, homotoxicologists have discovered that bacteria actually perform a beneficial function in an illness:

> They secrete the enzyme hyaluronidase which dissolves connective tissue. Homotoxins stored in the connective tissue are set free as well. The homotoxins, not the bacteria, are the decisive factor in inflammation.[56]

If homotoxins make our body react with a fever or an inflammation, then orthodox medicine is barking up the wrong tree. This also means that many of their therapeutics such as antipyretics, antihistamines, and antibiotics are actually harmful. They suppress the body's normal process of removing toxins. That is exactly why they are immuno-suppressants![57] Need we wonder, then, why autoimmune diseases are increasing in number, and are striking a younger and younger section of the population?

b. The Gene Theory of Disease

A more recent explanation by orthodox science of the origin of cancer and other degenerative diseases is that they are caused by the mutation of genes, and that they are hereditary. This explanation is a step deeper into reductionism, a modern-day expression of jumping from the frying pan into the fire. What are the dangers in believing that genes cause diseases, old age, and other undesirable human experiences? Why is medical science so desperate in selling this new view of disease and worldview of life to us?

We have already mentioned the worldwide trend of increased patronage of alternative medicine. Another main reason for this (and the loss of faith in conventional medicine) is the failure of modern drugs to cure cancer and degenerative diseases. This failure is, however, rarely admitted in public. We are led to believe that the battle against these diseases is being won.[58] But what is the real score, for example, in the case of cancer?[59] Cancer has been studied for more than a hundred years now. In 1990, about 8,000 oncologists from all over the world gathered at an International Cancer Congress in Hamburg, Germany. Ironically, all that their press statement essentially said was that in spite of the tremendous amount of research done in the technologically developed countries, little is known about the real causes of cancer, and the only reliable finding is that smoking contributes to the development of cancer.[60] Moreover, "the contribution that chemotherapy makes in the treatment of organs affected by cancer is practically nil," commented the news magazine *Der Spiegel* in the press statements.[61]

After 20 years, the list of carcinogens has finally been expanded, but the main therapies are still chemotherapy (a neurotoxin—carcinogenic[62]) and radiation (toxic, carcinogen, mutagen—causing mutation in the DNA, and teratogen—causing defects in offspring). Research on AIDS (as discussed in note 76 of this chapter) is coming to a dead end, although most scientists and doctors do not know (or admit) this. Orthodox science is putting all stakes on genetic science to provide the knowledge, and genetic engineering the therapy. For example, the Institute of Cancer Research in the UK has redirected its research into gene functions and regulation and molecular biology.[63]

We are being conditioned to think that science has not yet uncovered enough facts, and therefore needs more time and resources to unravel how genes create diseases.

The Human Genome Project, which started in 1990, has finished mapping the 100,000 genes of the human being. This genetic research project hopes to eliminate disease and extend life significantly beyond current expectancy. It assumes that non-infectious diseases are caused by defective genes; that diagnosis and therapy are possible only through genetic analysis; that aging and other complex human behaviors are traced back to genetics; and that all genes may be mapped into Mendelian factors (i.e., unique gene = unique effect or characteristic).

However, an emerging body of evidence showing functional

informational redundancy in cell regulation is undermining the
"uniqueness assumption" of genetic determinism.[64] The genes and their
products (i.e., enzymes, hormones) are interactive with each other and
with the environment. This network of interactions is called the *epigenetic
system*. Human behavior or complex diseases like cancer cannot be traced
or encoded in a gene, but rather in the environmentally interactive cellular
epigenetic network. This is a chaotic system, and to predict the role of a
particular gene in the whole system is a difficult task.

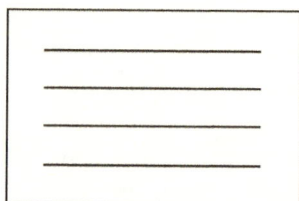

a. One to One (Haldane)

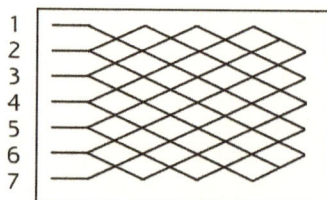

b. Network: Polygenic,
Peliotropic, Interactive
(Wright)

In the above figure, a linear connection between genes and disease
may only be correct for less than 2% of our current diseases. Biomedical
geneticists would have us think that with the intensive mapping of the
human genes, they will be able to figure out a one-to-one correspondence
between gene and disease. From the viewpoint of the epigenetic
informational systems, 98% or more of our current diseases are multifactorial, influenced by a network of genes interacting with one another
and with environmental signals. In other words, the disposition to a disease
is at the level of the epigenetic system, not the single gene. For example,
if gene 5 has mutated or is missing, its effect may be neutralized or coped
with by the combined actions of the other genes. Conversely, whatever
process is affected by gene 5 is also affected by the other genes. Thus
even though this gene is mutated (upon biochemical analysis), one can
never be sure if it contributes directly to a cancer, arteriosclerosis, or a
mental disease (as orthodox science claims).[65] In other words, a mutated
gene—just like a germ—may be a necessary but not a sufficient factor.
The promise by biomedical determinism of a more exact, linear diagnosis
(where one can confidently point an accusing finger to a responsible gene)

is problematic, and may lead to an erroneous therapy (and its side- and after-effects) and a false sense of security.[66]

It is obvious that oversimplifying the cause of a disease can never explain the real nature of an illness. Even though orthodox medicine acknowledges the constitution and susceptibility of an individual as important factors in the onset of a disease, their genetic explanation is acceptable only to the gullible and uncritical mind. Others, however, are asking: why is it that with a mere change of diet or attitude to life, heart disease, cancer, or even AIDS is reversed?[67] If a degenerative ailment is reversed, then the mutated cell (which allegedly caused it) has been repaired! Orthodox science seldom asks this question, and is trapped in its own reductionism.

Chapter 3 will discuss an alternative view of the role of constitution and disposition in the genesis of a disease. But first, let us look at how reductionism is applied in pharmacology.

c. Active Ingredient Syndrome in Pharmacology

Orthodox pharmacologists can be certain about the effectiveness of a drug only if they are able to identify its active ingredient or chemical. Once this is identified, they can isolate the chemical and perform tests on animals and animal tissues. The idea behind this is to be able to use a single chemical substance to produce a chemical reaction. Thus, bacteria or proliferating cells are destroyed by an active substance that blocks a reaction or replaces a missing substance. This approach is considered to be the most effective and only way worthy of development. However, there are problems related to this approach.

Firstly, because of the direct intervention of a concentrated single active ingredient and its apparent effectiveness, the patient and his reactions are bypassed. These reactions are ignored since only the anticipated effects are taken into consideration. Doctors and patients are blinded by momentary successes without regard for the consequences that follow a suppressed illness. Moreover, iatrogenic (drug-induced) damage is disregarded, usually resulting in the taking of more drugs, or in new illnesses.

Secondly, in the biological realm an isolated maximum principle is not the norm. Seemingly antagonistic substances occur together in nature and preclude the damages of one-sidedness. For example, vitamin D is produced in nature with vitamin A—its antagonist—thereby preventing the dangers of hypervitaminosis D. In other words, introducing an isolated active ingredient in an organism can result only in a highly specialized effect that neglects or ignores the wholeness of the organism.[68] This is exactly what happens when we use allopathic drugs.

As I pointed out earlier, the method of testing is itself part of the problem. Furthermore, this isolated active principle testing procedure presumes that less active substances must be less effective. On the contrary, such substances can work synergistically and bring about effects that are much more comprehensive. It is already known that along with the "primary active substance" of a plant, there are constituents working synergistically. This explains why whole extracts can have stronger physiological effects than isolated substances.[69]

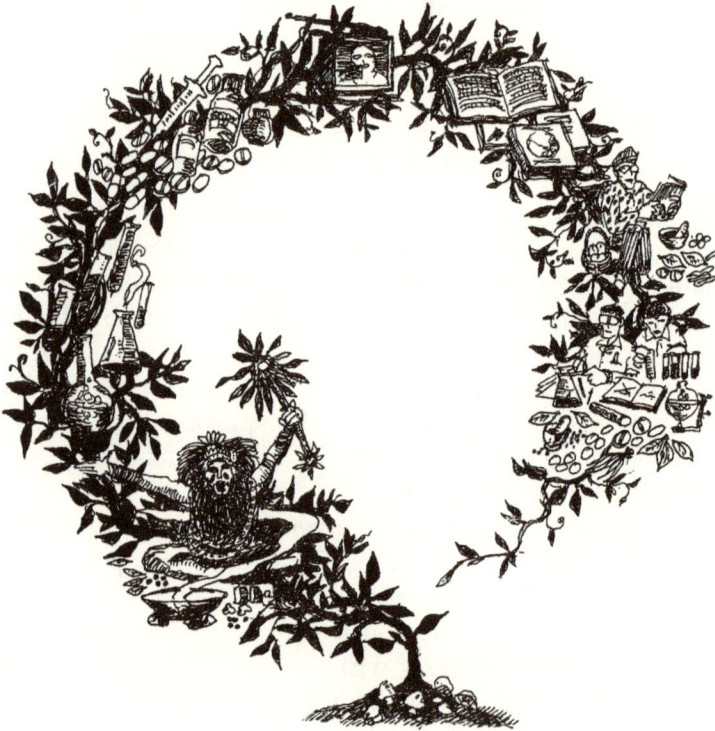

The therapeutic principle advocated in this book is that the remedy should work on the broadest possible supra-order basis. The remedy should work protectively and intervene the least. It should stimulate and work with the person's immune system rather than suppress it. Thus the basic gesture in therapy should be to strengthen what is *within*, in order that the organism will be capable of warding off any influence from the outside. The issue behind therapeutics is therefore not a question of dosage but rather of method. The method that takes into account the whole organism and how its parts are affected can better guide the organism to fully overcome the illness, and thus achieve true healing.[70]

The parameters used by the US Food and Drug Administration in determining the validity of active ingredients and the efficacy of drugs are based on this isolated approach. Current herbal medicine research tends to be trapped in this one-sidedness.[71] Without a rethinking of the reductionist method in science, there will always be the danger of unwanted results arising from non-recognition of the effects on the rest of the organism.

4. Darwin's Struggle for Existence and Orthodox Medicine's War-like Stance

The last assumption in science involves its whole attitude towards illness, namely, a war-like stance reminiscent of Darwin's "struggle for existence." Such a struggle exists to a certain degree. But orthodox medicine has blown this principle out of proportion. The problem arose when orthodox medicine confused the symptoms—fever, inflammation, and allergic reaction—for the disease. The symptoms were suppressed with antipyretics, antibiotics, or antihistamines. This approach can be designated as symptomatic therapy, and can be traced back to Galen (130-201 A.D.), who expounded the principle *contraria contrariis curari*, that is, the giving of remedies that produce an effect opposite the symptom. This principle was earlier espoused by Hippocrates (5 B.C.), who saw it working with other principles such as *similia similibus curentur* ("like cures like," rediscovered by Samuel Hahnemann in 1797). Galen, however, first re-presented it with an almost dogmatic one-sidedness which has affected the subsequent practice of medicine (and the loss of understanding and appreciation for the other principles of medicine). His writings became the basis of medieval medicine, from which allopaths have inherited their view of therapy.[72]

The Galenic principle is emphasized in our whole society, for example, in the use of pesticides to eliminate pests. Advocates of sustainable agriculture argue that the problem is by no means solved with their use. The problem is postponed and made worse because beneficial insects are also killed, resulting in an imbalance in the ratio of pests and beneficial insects. This leads to the further use of pesticides and the evolution of more virulent strains of pesticide-resistant pests. The brown plant hopper, which infests rice crops, is a case in point.[73] After a few crop cycles, large-scale infestation occurs, with heavy damage to crops.

In the long run, this *symptomatic* approach to nature is not only extremely costly, but dangerous to both the environment and human nutrition. A new way of healing in this area must originate from the idea of community ecology—taking into account the whole community of plants and animals, their interaction with each other, and their relationship to their habitat.[74] In other words, farmers must develop the proper respect for the laws of the living, granting them preference over short-term economic gains.

Another example is taken from what is presented as preventive medicine, or disease control, to promote "public health." In the villages of Borneo, insecticides were used to control malaria mosquitoes. The residues then accumulated in the cockroaches, which are resistant to the insecticide. Geckoes fed on these cockroaches and became lethargic. They eventually were eaten by cats, and the cats died. Rats then freely multiplied and brought the threat of an epidemic of bubonic plague, unheard of in the tropical jungle. Ultimately, the only solution the government thought of was to drop cats into the villages by parachute![75] This is indeed a heroic, Hollywood-film-quality image—but pathetic if one sees the picture from a broader perspective.

Could there be other undocumented cases where an epidemic was induced because of orthodox science's war-like stance against disease? Could AIDS and other autoimmune diseases be the beginning of this iatrogenic epidemic?[76]

The Galenic principle in our way of thinking must be de-emphasized with regard to living systems, especially human beings. Orthodox science presumes that the consequence and goal of this war-like comprehension of illness is the extinction and prevention of all illnesses.[77] This is not merely an illusion, but also a negation and circumvention of the meaning and purpose of illness. (See the subsection "Meaning of Illness.")

At this point, it is also important to comment on another therapy which orthodox medical science often prescribes. This is *substitution* therapy—the replacement of a substance we may be missing in nutrition, like vitamin supplementation or glandular product supplementation, such as insulin in diabetes.[78] Symptomatic and substitution therapies have their proper place in the broad spectrum of possible therapies. Both practices can save and prolong life. However, substitution therapy promotes the eventual atrophy of the organ and a lifelong dependency on the substituted product, to say the least.

It ought to be understood, therefore, that these measures have nothing to do with true healing. If healing occurs from their use, it is only because a crisis has been handled with a substitution, or the reaction of an individual has been temporarily relieved until self-healing can take place. However, orthodox medicine would have us think that when an organ's product has been substituted or surgically removed, or a reaction has disappeared (i.e., suppressed), healing has taken place. This is a major delusion.

Orthodox medical science does have a coherent and comprehensive principle in therapeutics, although it may not have been clearly articulated. Orthodox medicine has unwittingly taken on the hidden assumption of the materialistic science of the 19th century. It is the science of the dead and inorganic world brought into the living realm. This science is unable to understand living systems. It has brought with it a mode of thinking that brings death and more illnesses. What we need is a new medical science that can harmonize with the living.

C. OTHER SCHOOLS OF MEDICAL THOUGHT

It is not generally known that there are other schools of medical thought that have survived the dominance of orthodox medical science. We have so far only tackled the principles of homeopathy. There are other schools of thought, which, if taken together, can give us a holistic picture of the living human being and a coherent, comprehensive principle of therapeutics (Appendix 2 elaborates on this). Once we survey and understand the principles behind these other schools of medical thought, we will be able to discover how the various therapeutics have a place in giving human beings the opportunity to heal themselves, along with the creative use of symptomatic and substitution therapies.

1. Naturopathy

Naturopathy was the first to expound the idea that toxins are the main cause of illnesses, and that fever and inflammation are the body's attempts to eliminate them. Natural forms of therapy are generally resorted to. These include: proper nutrition, or eating fermented products like yogurt and sour vegetables and abstaining from meat; cleansing through fasting, sitz baths, and warm linen wrappings; using hot and cold compresses; hydro-therapy; massage; herbal medicine, and others. Naturopaths believe that the human body possesses tremendous power to heal itself by means of its homeostasis. This mechanism restores the body's balance in structure and function, and its capacity to adapt to environmental changes. The healing power of nature—the vital force—is the foundation of naturopathic philosophy and practice. Naturopathic doctors use only those therapeutic substances and techniques which act in harmony with the body's self-healing processes. Recently, they have incorporated other complementary natural methods such as chiropractic, homeopathy, and acupuncture in their range of therapies.

2. Chiropractic

Chiropractic takes the view that illnesses arise from misplacement of the nerves in the spine and joints. Thus chiropractors align the relationship of the bones along the joints and the spine. Any interference with the nervous system will lessen its ability to function internally and to adapt to the environment and social stresses. The chiropractic philosophy is based on the deductive principle that the universe is perfectly organized, and that each individual is an extension of this principle designed to express life (health) and the universal law.[79] It is important to note here that a great clinician named Alexei D. Speransky, MD, was successful in producing a typical syndrome of infectious diseases in the complete absence of bacteria by directly stimulating the nervous system. This led him to conclude that infectious diseases are based on the disturbance of the nervous system.[80] Thus, Speransky unwittingly gave chiropractic clinical and experimental evidence to support its diagnostic and therapeutic principle. Chiropractic is currently prescribed by holistic doctors to relieve backaches, or for conditions that require alignment of the spine and joints.

3. Acupuncture

Acupuncture makes use of the Chinese concept of the vital force which they call "chi." There are essentially twelve regular meridians and two extra ones where "chi" is circulated by the body. Each meridian has a set of points; here, very thin needles are inserted to stimulate the point and the meridian. Disease arises when there is a block or an insufficiency in the flow of "chi" affecting a particular organ or tissue. To restore the normal flow of chi, the acupuncturist stimulates particular points along different meridians diagnosed to be connected to the block. Acupuncture is the most popular therapy in traditional Chinese medicine. Chinese herbal medicine, massage, and culinary art are also used by traditional Chinese doctors in conjunction with acupuncture, or prescribed separately, depending on the severity or character of an illness. Traditional Chinese medicine should not be divorced from its essential philosophy of Taoism. In this worldview, the human being is a microcosm of nature. Human beings represent the juncture between heaven and earth, the offspring of their union, a fusion of cosmic and terrestrial forces.[81]

4. More on Homeopathy

Earlier we discussed how Samuel Hahnemann came to discover the therapeutic principle of like cures like. One could ask the question: what, therefore, is homeopathy's understanding of disease? Hahnemann classified diseases into two types: the acute and the chronic. "Acute diseases usually run their course within a period of variable duration, [while chronic illnesses] often seem trifling and imperceptible in the beginning but... act deleteriously upon the living organism... insidiously undermining its health... resulting in the final destruction of the organism."[82] All illnesses result from the derangement of the vital body, or life force, in man. This dynamic force makes the difference between a corpse and a human being.

Hahnemann wrote extensively on these two types of diseases. However, it is beyond the scope of this section to go into his insights as to how the vital body becomes deranged. The reader is encouraged to read more on this topic, as well as on the other schools of thought in medicine described above. My own version of how and why our interweaving bodies get deranged or out of balance is discussed in Section 1, Chapter 5, and in Appendix 1.

Notes

1 This crisis forced the US federal government to enact a law establishing an Office of Alternative Medicine (OAM) in 1992. It is now called the National Center for Complementary and Alternative Medicine, or NCCAM. NCCAM brings together other medical schools of thought, and all kinds of therapies not utilized by orthodox medicine but widely patronized by the American public. This includes chelation and bio-oxydative medicine (whose principles can still be explained by orthodox science), and all mind/body therapies, as well as traditional and new systems of medicine such as acupuncture, homeopathy, naturopathy, anthroposophic medicine, biologically-based therapies, various manipulation therapies, and energy medicine. The NCCAM staff meets regularly to discuss how their work can be incorporated into mainstream medicine. These practitioners are no longer called "quacks," as they had been referred to since allopathy became the dominant medical thought in the US. In Europe, these

therapies have always been tolerated as complementary to orthodox treatment.

2   In discussing the adverse effects of orthodox medicine, I do not mean to imply that doctors have bad intentions. In fact, most doctors only mean well and take their career seriously as one of service to humanity. However, the practice of medicine has developed in such a way that doctors exercise nearly absolute power over their patients. The famous Chinese proverb, "Absolute power corrupts absolutely," has a lot of truth in it. This, alongside the other reasons discussed in this section, contributes to the overall ill effects of the practice of orthodox medicine.

3   Quoted in Berger S. *What Your Doctor Didn't Learn in Medical School.* New York: Avon Books; 1989:9.

4   See Martin E. *Hazards of Medications.* Philadelphia, PA: JB Lippincott; 1910:5; Garb S. *Undesirable Drug Interaction.* New York: Springer, 1975; or Graedon J. *People's Pharmacy.* New York: Avon Books; 1976.

5   "The adverse effects of drugs are only one reason for withdrawing drugs from the market. A more serious but less talked about reason is the unethical practices of doctors and scientists who test the drugs. A commission of distinguished scientists, including 4 Nobel laureates, studied the drug problem and found the culprits are the doctors and scientists who test the drugs. They found clinical trials of new drugs were 'a shambles.' The [US Food and Drug Administration] spot-checked the work of some doctors doing such clinical trials, and found 20% guilty of a wide range of unethical practices, including giving incorrect dosage and falsifying records. In a third of the reports checked by the FDA, the trial had not been carried out at all. In another third, the experimental protocol was not followed. In only a third of the tests could results be considered scientifically worthwhile!" Mendelsohn RS. *Confessions of a Medical Heretic.* 1979:74.

   In England, pharmaceutical companies do not behave any better. See Collier J. In the pocket of the industry. In: *The Health Conspiracy: How Doctors, The Drug Industry and the Government Undermine Our Health.* London: Century Hutchinson Ltd.; 1989:29-87. See also Hampton JR, Julian DG. Role of the pharmaceutical industry in major clinical trials. *Lancet* 1987;2:1258-1259; Lauritsen K et al. Withholding unfavorable results in drug company sponsored clinical trials, *Lancet* 1987;1:1091. In drug advertisements, these companies are more notorious. See Collier JG, Pilkington TRE. Human insulin: a misleading advertisement. *British Medical Journal* 1984:289-291; Collier JG, New Illegibility of drug advertisements. *Lancet* 1984;1:341-342; Collier JG, Herxheimer A. Roussel convicted of misleading promotion. *Lancet* 1987;1:113-114.

6   Reputable medical journals continue to warn doctors of the damage drugs can cause the organs of the body. Going through some issues of the *British Medical Journal*, I

found these alarming studies: Olsson R. et al. Centrolubar liver cell necrosis, myocardial infarction, and hyperamylasaemia after high dose of corticosteriods; and Smith GW et al. Hyperkalaemia and non-oliguris renal failure associated with Trimethoprom. *British Medical Journal* 1994(February);308:454. Both studies cited not just the development of degenerate organs and tissues, but also the death of particular cells and the organ itself.

Why are these warnings seldom heeded? One main reason is that doctors tend to think that these drugs are the only ones available. They are modern, the result of scientific progress, and only the uneducated do not believe in them. An added fact is that most doctors hardly upgrade their knowledge by reading relatively independent journals. They rely mostly on what representatives of various drug companies give them. The real issue is that doctors are not aware of any alternative treatments. Had their eyes been opened to other schools of therapy, many would probably abandon these drugs. However, vested interests (under the guise of science) have their way of not letting this happen. See Collier J. *The Health Conspiracy: How Doctors, The Drug Industry and the Government Undermine Our Health.* London: Century Hutchinson Ltd.; 1989; Carter JP. *Racketeering in Medicine: The Suppression of Alternatives.* Norfolk, VA: Hampton Roads Publishing Co. Inc.; 1992. See also Note 40.

7   The effectiveness of antibiotics is still under question. One study concluded that there is no evidence that antibiotics reduced the incidence of mastoiditis. Other researchers found out that antibiotics provide relief of symptoms, but subsequently there is no difference from those given a placebo. In treating sore throats, research has determined that today's strain of streptococcus very rarely causes rheumatic fever, and that antibiotics do not even eradicate the strep in 25% to 40% of the cases. Furthermore, 33% to 50% of the cases of rheumatic fever occur without sore throat symptoms. Ulman D. *Homeopathy: Medicine for the 21st Century.* North Atlantic Books; 1988:121-124.

Worse, the use of antibiotics and other chemical drugs leads to the emergence of fungal infections such as candida or aspergillus (a hospital spread fungus) considered more lethal. See Haney DQ. Fungal infections emerge as major health threat. *The Philippine Star.* October 28, 1993.

8   Another example involves diuretic drugs given to patients with hypertension. A drug to control hypertension may end up causing it. This is what happens: these drugs take water from the cells and pass it out through urination. "A diuretic, however, has only one idea in mind, and obsessed with that one idea, it careens through the body, demanding, 'water, water!' from every cell it meets. The result is that the fluid tension in the blood vessels is reduced, which is what the doctors want to happen, but the water level everywhere else is affected at the same time. The brain will be forced to give up some of its water, which under normal conditions it does only in direst emergency,

causing the patient to feel dizzy and drowsy." This is a normal "undesirable" side effect of diuretics. But if analyzed further, "a diuretic basically works by latching onto sodium atoms, causing the body to discard excess salt, and this in turn indirectly brings down the water level in the tissues, since water is bound up with salt in our bodies... The diuretic cannot help it if too much sodium is taken where water is still needed. Since potassium is close to sodium in its atomic structure, the diuretic causes it to be depleted, leading to weakness, fatigue, and leg cramps... ironically, a potassium deficiency is now suspected to be a causal link in high blood pressure, which means that the diuretic may be promoting the very condition it was meant to cure." From Chopra D. *Quantum Healing: Exploring the Frontiers of Mind/Body Medicine*. Bantam Books; 1989:44-45.

9 "Menopausal estrogens have been implicated so strongly in the causation of gall bladder disease and cancer of the uterus... that the USFDA has been forced to issue warnings to doctors and patients... which remain unheeded... instead... most doctors use them routinely, supposedly to prevent the mildest of menopausal discomforts. Estrogen is used to preserve youth, for cosmetic purposes, to relieve depression, and for the prevention of cardiovascular disease—all for which its effectiveness has been disproved. Estrogens are also used to prevent bone demineralization in older women. Exercise and diet also can prevent demineralization, and they do not cause cancer." Mendelsohn RS. *Confessions of a Medical Heretic*. 1979:64-65.

10 Steel K et al. Iatrogenic illness in general medical services at a university hospital. *New England Journal of Medicine* 1981(March);304:638-642.

11 See American Iatrogenic Association, 2513 S. Gessner, No. 232, Houston, TX 77063-2096; *www.iatrogenic.org.ic*

12 In 2001 the researchers at the University of Pennsylvania found out that "the nutrient (ascorbic acid) can act as a catalyst to help make a toxin that can injure DNA, the body's genetic code. More recently, the Hayden Institute website reports, "Ascorbic Acid (Synthetic Vitamin C) May Damage DNA." See *www.haydeninstitute.com/index. php?option*. For other articles, search the Web for *vitamins and genetic damage*.

13 See Reckeweg. *Homotoxicology: Illness and Healing through Antihomotoxic Therapy*, pp 124-125, for further discussion on the adverse effects of chemicals and chemical drugs.

14 See Siegel B. *Love, Medicine and Miracles*, p 17.

15 The Harvard Medical Practice Study I recently revealed that "there is a substantial amount of injury to patients from medical management, and many injuries are the result of substandard care." Brennan TA et al. Incidence of adverse events and negligence in hospitalized patients. *New England Journal of Medicine* 1991(February);324:370-376. See note 29 for the results of Harvard Medical Practice Study II.

16 See Haney DQ. Fungal infections emerge as major health threat. *The Philippine Star.* October 28, 1993. These new classes of disease are mostly spread in hospitals and as a result of the widespread use of antibiotics and other chemical drugs; Pillay D et al. Parvovirus B19 outbreak in a children's ward. *Lancet* 1992(January);339:107-109.

17 For a discussion of why doctors fail as human beings, see Weatherball DJ. Inhumanity of medicine. *British Medical Journal* 1994(December);309:1671-1672.

18 Mendelsohn RS. *Confessions of a Medical Heretic.* 1979:131.

19 Hospital treatment of patients with pneumonia increases the risk of re-infection 5.45 times! See Hedlund JU et al. Risk of pneumonia in patients previously treated in hospital for pneumonia. *Lancet* 1992(August);340:396-397.

20 Ayliffe GAJ et al. *Hospital Acquired Infection: Principles and Prevention.* 2nd ed. Wright: London; 1990. See also Nosocomial infection with respiratory syncytial virus. *Lancet* 1992(October);340:1071-1073; Polish LB et al. Nosocomial transmission of Hepatitis B virus associated with the use of a spring-loaded finger-stick device. *New England Journal of Medicine* 1992(December);3263:721-725; Pillay D et al. Parvovirus B19 outbreak in a children's ward. *Lancet* 1992(January);339:107-109; Pittet D et al. Nosocomial bloalstream infection in critically ill patients: excess length of stay—extra cost and attributable mortality. *Journal of the American Medical Association* 1994(May);271:1598-1601.

21 See American Iatrogenic Association, 2513 S. Gessner, No. 232, Houston, TX 77063-2096; *www.iatrogenic.org.ic*

22 *Newsweek* magazine, October 4, 1993, featured the Los Angeles County doctor's strike and the corresponding phenomenon of lower death rate as an inadvertent result of the strike.

23 See NaturalNews.com, "California Health Workers Are on Strike Today"; *bmj.com*, "Doctors' strike in Israel may be good for health."

24 See Natural News at *www.NaturalNews.com/unnecessary_surgery.html*

25 See also *www.lprww.com* and download the article "Up to 90% of certain surgeries performed in the US are unnecessary," by Alan Inglis, MO.

26 Even if it did, the bypass itself can become clogged and leave the patient right back where he or she started before the operation.

27 Many recent studies prove that change of diet has a more lasting effect than drug treatment. See Watts GE et al. Effects on coronary artery disease of lipid-lowering diet plus cholestyramine, in the St. Thomas Artherosclerosis Regression Study (STARS). *Lancet* 1992(March);339:563-569 ("Dietary change alone retarded over-all progression

and increased over-all regression of coronary artery disease."); Rivellese AR et al. Long-term metabolic efficacy of two dietary method of treating hyperlipidaemia. *British Medical Journal* 1994(January);308:227-231 (The two diets are: low in fat but rich in carbohydrates and fiber and low in carbohydrates and rich in polyunsaturated and monosaturated fatty acids.); Kjeldsen-Kragh J et al. Controlled trial of fasting and one-year vegetarian diet in rheumatoid arthritis. *Lancet* 1991(October);338:899-902 ("Benefits were still present after one year, and evaluation of the whole course showed significant advantages for the diet group on all measured indices."); Singh RB et al. Randomized controlled trial of cardioprotective diet in patients with recent acute myocardial infarction: results of one year follow-up. *British Medical Journal* 1992(April);304:1015-1019 (Comprehensive dietary change significantly reduced complications and mortality after one year.); East Anglian Multicenter Controlled Trial: Treatment of active Crohn's disease by exclusion diet. *Lancet* 1993(November);342:1131-1134 (Diet provides a further therapeutic strategy in active Crohn's disease.).

28 See Scully D. *Men Who Control Women's Health: The Miseducation of Obstetrician-Gynecologists.* Boston: Houghton Mifflin Company; 1980. Ms. Scully, a sociologist, intimately looked at the apprenticeship of ob/gyns for two years in several teaching hospitals. "I saw women talked into surgery they didn't need. I saw procedures forced on women who didn't understand them." Ms. Scully's observations reveal how institutional patients are used as teaching materials by inexperienced physicians and surgeons, and how, for the poor, the cure can be worse than the disease.

29 The Harvard Medical Practice Study II revealed that the proportion of adverse events due to negligence was highest for diagnostic mishaps (75%), non-invasive therapeutic mishaps (errors of omission, 77%), and events occurring in emergency room (70%); errors in management were identified for 58% of the adverse events. Leape LL et al. The nature of adverse events in hospitalized patients. *New England Journal of Medicine* 1991(Febrary);324:377-384. Search the web for *epidemiology of medical errors* or *errors in laboratory medicine* for more updates on this issue.

30 "Labs tests and diagnostic machines wouldn't be so dangerous if doctors were not addicted to the quantitative information these tools provide. Since numbers and statistics are modern medicine's language of prayer, quantitative information is considered sacred, the word of God indeed, the last word in a diagnosis. Whether these tools are simple, like thermometers, scales, or calibrated infant bottles, or complicated, like x-ray machines, EKGs, EEGs, and lab tests, people and doctors are dazzled into crowding out of the process their own common sense and the qualitative judgment of doctors who are real diagnostic artists." Mendelsohn RS. *Confessions of a Medical Heretic.* 1979:31.

31 The benefit of annual physical examination continues to be challenged, but largely remains standard procedure by a "scientific" establishment that is addicted to and dependent on quantitative data and statistics. A recent example is from Schmidt JG. Epidemiology of mass breast cancer screening: a plea for valid measure of benefit. *The Journal of Clinical Epidemiology* 1990;43(3):215-225. The author argues that "Many thousands of mammograms are needed to prevent one cancer death, and for each woman who can derive a direct benefit in terms of a prevented cancer death, hundreds of women have to suffer the anxiety of a positive screening mammography. Moreover, it is possible that adverse effects of breast cancer screening may contribute to mortality from other causes." The author concluded that "It may be an error to recommend mass breast screening." This is one good reason why ordinary folks must take health care into their own hands. For more recent discussion on this see the McDougall Newsletter at *drmcdougall.com.*

32 Women's reproductive organs are most vulnerable to radiation-induced damage because the ovaries contain all the eggs the female will ever have. See Caufield C. *Multiple Exposures.* London: Secker and Warburg; 1989:224-235.

33 It was estimated that a mammography screening program will produce five cases of cancer for every one detected (ibid, p 232). Women of less affluent countries are fortunate that routine mammography is still not possible because of lack of funds. Physical examination of the breast is still the best screening process and avoids the risk of inducing cancer from the X-ray radiation in mammography. See Mittra I. Breast screening: the case for physical examination without mammography. *Lancet* 1994(February);343:342-344. The question to ask is not how to refine mammography screening but whether it is needed at all ("Physical examination is as effective as screening mammography."); Fentiman IS. Pensive women, painful vigil: consequences of delay in assessment of mammographic abnormalities. *Lancet* 1988;ii953. The anxious waiting period can be a traumatic experience.

34 Exposure to X-rays has been finally listed as one of the major carcinogens by the US Department of Health and Human Services; see *www.cancer.org/.../PED_1_3x_ Known_and_Probable_Carcinogens.asp*

35 See Siegel B. *Love, Medicine and Miracles,* p 19. One of the rude awakenings of Dr. Siegel when he first attended a workshop on Psychological Factors, Stress, and Cancer was, "Here I was, an M.D., a 'Medical Deity,' and I didn't know what went on in the head at all! The literature on mind-body interaction was separate, and therefore unknown to specialists in other areas. I realized for the first time how far ahead theology, psychology, and holistic medicine are in this respect."

36 One possible consequence of the almost absolute power of doctors is abuse of

discretion. The Chinese proverb "Absolute power corrupts absolutely" is appropriate here. The people in the Philippine provinces are particularly vulnerable. In almost all the seminars I conducted in various provinces, a number of participants narrated incidents of doctors resorting to surgery for abdominal pains. A common theme of the story is that the patient's family is unable to produce the money for the cost of surgery, thus the operation is postponed. Due to the postponement, the patient just rested and the following day he got well. In some cases, the accompanying friend stated that the patient is an indigent and requested the doctor to put the patient under observation rather than immediately operate. The doctor agreed and the patient got well just the same. This seems to be outright malpractice! Poor rural folks are the unwitting victims.

Every week, four to five cases of malpractice are reported to the Philippine Department of Health (personal communication). The complaints are passed on to the Professional Regulatory Commission but we hardly hear of doctors being punished for their misdeeds. Only those who have the money to pursue the case in court are given some chance to seek redress. The poor, as always, are unable to protect their rights. If the doctor you consult says you need surgery, always seek a second or even a third opinion, preferably from doctors who are not colleagues of the first one you consulted. By not informing the other doctor of the diagnosis of the first doctor you can prevent the second doctor from a biased diagnosis. You will find out that their diagnosis can be very different. See also Socrates JAU. Surgical malpractice in Puerto Princesa: the sinister side of a noble profession [photocopy]. Palawan: Provincial Health Office; 1995.

37 Whoever is in control allots funds to the research of diseases which affect his immediate constituency. Why is this so? Joe Collier's answer is quite blunt. "Why study the diseases of the third world... if the victims are mostly too poor to pay for the treatment?" Collier J. The *Health Conspiracy: How Doctors, The Drug Industry and the Government Undermine Our Health*. London: Century Hutchinson Ltd.; 1989:51. There may also be racial underpinnings in the practice of medicine. See Littlewood R, Lipsedge M. Psychiatric illness and British Afro-Carribeans. *British Medical Journal* 1988;296:950-951; Lakhani SR et al. Differences amongst Asian patients. *British Medical Journal*, 1986: 293: 1169; Bhate, S. "Prejudice Against Doctors and Students from Ethnic Minorities", *British Medical Journal* 1987;294:838; Smith R. Deception in research and racial discrimination in medicine. *British Medical Journal* 1993(March);306:668-669; Esmail A, Everington S. Racial discrimination against doctors from ethnic minorities. *British Medical Journal* 1993(March):306:691-692.

38 Ironically this power is set against those who do not toe the line. A basic dissatisfaction with the practice of orthodox medicine brought about the evolution of a number of alternatives. Orthodox doctors quickly label them as quackery, without bothering to

know the principles of medicine they operate on. See Carter JP. *Racketeering In Medicine: The Suppression of Alternatives.* Norfolk, VA: Hampton Roads Publishing Co. Inc.; 1992. He wrote a 360-page exposé on how organized medicine orchestrated financially motivated cover-ups to control medical care and ease out emerging alternative forms of treatment. By "organized medicine" he is referring to the American Medical Association, State Board Examiners, medical schools and teaching hospitals, the American Hospital Association, the National Health Insurance Association (representing 1,500 companies), and the entire drug, pharmaceutical, and medical equipment industry. The mudslinging continues, in spite of the organization of the Office for Alternative Medicine. Like all reforms, it takes a lot of time for the people in power (especially orthodox doctors) to change—even until they have grown old or have been removed from office.

39 Szasz T. *Pharmacracy: Medicine and Politics in America.* Syracuse University Press: Syracuse, NY; 2003.

40 In Bangladesh, the nationalization of the drug industry encouraged doctors to prescribe drugs left and right, oblivious of their adverse effects. This excessive drug use may have weakened the constitution of the Bangladeshi and at the same time promoted the development of the new strain of *cholera vibro.* It is normal for the Bangladeshi to have diarrhea twice a year. See New cholera strain is difficult to kill: Bangladesh researchers. *The Phillipine Star,* September 29, 1993:5.

41 Vithoulkas, p 20. He investigated the work of Sir Stanley Davidson, *The Principles and Practice of Medicine,* a standard textbook, and discovered that in its 1262 pages not a single line expounded any principle of medicine. He went through the other textbooks and obtained the same result.

42 Augros RM, Stanciu GN. *The New Story of Science.* New York: Bantam Books; 1986:3.

43 The denial of these qualities can be traced to Descartes in 1630: "Neither beautiful nor the pleasant signifies anything other than the attitude of our judgment to the object in question." Spinosa agrees: "Beauty... is less a quality of the object studied than the effect arising in the man studying that object." Two centuries later Charles Darwin writes: "The sense of beauty obviously depends on the nature of mind, irrespective of any real quality in the admired object." Freud followed through by saying: "Psychoanalysis, unfortunately, has scarcely anything to say about beauty... All that seems certain is its derivation from the field of sexual feeling." Ibid, pp 37-38.

44 Quoted in Dossey L. *Healing Words: The Power of Prayer and the Practice of Medicine.* New York: Harper Collins Publishers; 1993. Dr. Dossey probes the scientific literature for proof of prayer's efficacy. "I found an enormous body of evidence: over one hundred experiments exhibiting the criteria of 'good science,' many conducted under stringent

laboratory conditions, over half of which showed that prayer brings about significant changes in a variety of living beings." Why is this not common knowledge among scientifically trained physicians? "I came to realize the truth of what many historians of science have described: A body of knowledge that does not fit with the prevailing ideas can be ignored as if it does not exist, no matter how scientifically valid it may be. Scientists, including physicians, can have blind spots in their vision. The power of prayer, it seemed, was an example." Ordinary folks know that prayer heals. But the current notion of what science is (ingrained in our education and maintained by continuous scientific pronouncements), is slowly eroding this—if it is not already lost—in all of us.

45 Perlas N. The Second Scientific Revolution and the Center for Alternative Development Initiatives, Unit 718 CityLand Megaplaza, Ortigas Avenue, Pasig City, Philippines, or *www.cadi.ph*. This belief is articulated to the fullest extent in the writings of Harvard sociobiologist E. O. Wilson. However, even Karl Marx, a believer of dialectical materialism, attacked this crude form of atomic materialism. Unfortunately, Marx fell into the opposite trap of sociological reductionism and materialism. Marx taught that all content of human consciousness arose out of the material conditions obtaining in the modes of economic production. Marx was correct to the extent that human beings are "behavioralist" in the sense of B. F. Skinner, that is, are passive receptors of contents of consciousness. However, the Marxist-Skinnerian doctrine no longer applies to cognitively active human beings who are reflective and creative. See Sorokin PA. *Social and Cultural Dynamics*. New York: Bedminster Press; 1963 [4 vols].

46 I purposely omitted the discussion on the hazards of chemical pollution on health for obvious reasons. This is currently a hot environmental issue and a number of books have already been written about this threat to human health (please see the bibliography). Thus implicit in this book is the need to work for a healthy environment free from chemical pollutants. For studies on the relationship of pollution and health see Purdey M. Degenerative nervous disorders and chemical pollution. *The Ecologist* 1994(May/June);24(3). Exposure to chemicals including solvents, organophospates, and pyridine compounds has a role in the increasing incidence of Parkinson's disease, multiple sclerosis, motor neuron disease, and myalgic encephalomyelitis. His extensive bibliography is also worth looking into; Saracci R et al. Cancer mortality in workers exposed to chlorophenoxy: herbicides and chlorophenols. *Lancet* 1991(October);338:1027-1032. Risk appears to be increased for cancer of testicle, thyroid, other endocrine glands, and nose and nasal cavity; Carpenter L. Cancer in laboratory workers. *Lancet* 1991(October);338:1080-1081. Those aged 15 to 64 had increased risk of cancer of the brain, nervous system, stomach, pancreas, bone, skin and haematopoietic system; Breast Cancer Prevention Collaborative Group. Breast cancer: environmental factors. *Lancet* 1992(October);340:904. See also Needle HL.

Raising Children Toxic Free: How to Keep Your Child Safe from Lead, Asbestos, Pesticides, and other Environmental Hazards. New York: Avon Books; 1995. For an updated list of possible chemical carcinogens please see *msdschem.ox.ac.uk.carcinogens.html.*

47 See Fischer JA. *Our Medical Future: Breakthroughs in Health and Longevity by the Year 2000 and Beyond.* New York: Pocket Books; 1992:50-53. Cloning human beings seem to be a far-fetched idea. *Newsweek* magazine, however, reported that scientists have actually cloned the human embryo despite protests from various sectors on ethical grounds. See Adler J et al. Clone hype. *Newsweek.* November 8, 1993:42-44; and Gelman D et al. How will the clone feel!? *Newsweek.* November 8, 1993:46-47.

An equally horrifying trend is towards the commodification of the human body. The commercial trade of body parts is affecting mostly the poor people who are particularly encouraged to sell a kidney or lend a womb to those who can afford it. See Kimbrell A. *The Human Body Shop: Engineering and Market of Life.* Penang, Malaysia: Third World Network; 1993; India probes kidney transplant scam. *The Philippine Inquirer.* February 5, 1995:14; Hong Kong to ban Chinese human organ trade. *The Philippine Star.* October 31, 1994:2.

48 Husemann F, Wolff O. *The Anthroposophic Approach to Medicine* (3 vols). Anthroposophical Press Inc.; vol 3:12.

49 Ibid, p 12.

50 See Von Pettenkofer M. The Value of Health to a City: Two Lectures Delivered in 1873. Quoted in Illich I. *Limits to Medicine.* Penguin Books; 1977:25.

51 Op cit, p 14.

52 Ullman, p 119.

53 Quoted in Husemann F, Wolff O. *The Anthroposophic Approach to Medicine* (3 vols). Anthroposophical Press Inc.; vol 1:7.

54 Chopra D. *Quantum Healing: Exploring the Frontiers of Mind/Body Medicine.* Bantam Books; 1989:142.

55 During a fever, the organism's white blood cells become more mobile and active, and secrete the enzyme interferon. Interferon inhibits virus multiplication (Ullman, p 93). In animal tests, temperature is an important factor in their survival. The mortality rate goes up to 100% if animals infected with virus are left at low temperature. If the animals are kept in room temperature up to 38 degrees centigrade, all or many survive. A decrease of body temperature of only one-tenth degree causes an increase of virus by a factor of 2. Thus, the lower the temperature, the more virulent the viruses are (Husemann F, Wolff O. *The Anthroposophical Approach to Medicine* [3 vols]. Anthroposophical Press Inc.; vol 1:171-172). For the role of fever in bacterial

infections see two studies by Matthew Kluger: Kluger M. Fever and survival. *Science* 1975(April);188:166-168; and Kluger M. Fever: effect of drug-induced anti-pyresis on survival. *Science* 1976(July);193:237-239. In both studies, Dr. Kluger affirmed that fever increases host survival and stressed in the second study that "the prevention of fever by the use of an anti-pyretic drug... increases the mortality rate from bacterial infection." *Lancet* came out with an article renewing the warning on the use of antipyretics. See Shann F. Antipyretics in severe sepsis. *Lancet* 1995(February);345:338. See also Graham NMH et al. Adverse effects of aspirin, acetaminophen, and ibuprofen on immune function, viral shedding, and clinical status in rhinovirus-infected volunteers. *Journal of Infectious Diseases* 1990;162:1277-1282; and WHO Programme for the Control of Acute Respiratory Infections. The management of fever in young children with acute respiratory infections in developing countries. Geneva: World Health Organization; *WHO/ARI* 1993;93:30.

The standard text on pathology describes the process of inflammation as the manner in which the body seeks to wall off, heat up, and burn out infective agents or foreign matter (Ullman, p 5). But the way orthodox doctors treat infection is contrary to this understanding. Antibiotics block the enzymes that break down toxic protein in the process of catabolism. This results in the accumulation of more toxic protein or homotoxins and may lead to new infections (Reckeweg, *Homotoxicology: Illness and Healing through Antihomotoxic Therapy,* p 37). In other words, antibiotics replace the action of white blood cells. Consequently, they suppress our own bodily processes.

Histamine is produced by mast cells which are secreted when exposed to allergens. Histamine dilates capillaries, which then increase the blood supply to peripheral parts of the body in defense against allergens. It constricts the respiratory bronchules, tubes that help the body cough and expel the allergens. Lastly, it causes increased gastric secretion in the effort of the body to digest the allergens (Ullman, p 140). If one takes antihistamine, all of these are negated and more toxins remain in the body.

56 Quoted in Reckeweg, *Homotoxicology: Illness and Healing through Antihomotoxic Therapy,* pp 62-63. Worse still, the killed bacteria turn into endotoxins. Who do you think does the cleaning up in a massacre of bacteria? Our immune system must eliminate them through normal channels, or call for another inflammation or fever. This is one reason for the phenomenon of relapse (retoxification) and/or the emergence of new illnesses. See also Brandtzaeg P et al. Plasma endotoxin as a predictor of multiple organ failure and death in systemic meninggococcal disease. *Journal of Infectious Diseases* 1989;159:195-204; Anonymous. A nasty shock from antibiotics. *Lancet* 1985; ii:594; van Deventer SJH et al. Endotoxaemia: an early predictor of septicaemia in febrile patients. *Lancet* 1988;i: 605-609.

57 See Husemann F, Wolff O. *The Anthroposophic Approach to Medicine* (3 vols). Anthroposophical Press Inc.; vol 3:32. He concluded his discussion on chemical drugs

by saying that "[a]ntibiotics negatively influence the organism's healing reactions and are thus opposite of a true remedy... To the extent that bacteria are only a symptom of the underlying disease, antibiotics act only symptomatically. They also reduce some of the effects of the organism's reaction to infection by suppressing immunity." Symptomatic therapy is discussed on p 24. See also Kilburn KH. Epidemics then and now: chemicals replace microbes and degeneration oust infections. *Archives of Environmental Medicine* 1994(January/February);49(1). He mentions that many antibacterial and antifungal agents like penicillin and streptomycin are neurotoxic chemicals. Thus, using these chemicals may lead to degenerative diseases. He also reported that "surgical operating room personnel exposed to anesthetic gases have increased incidences of spontaneous abortions, leukemia, and lymphoma; and they score poorer on psychometric tests. Exposure to sterilants, especially ethylene oxide, propylene oxide, and formaldehyde, has been associated with cancer, especially leukemia. Chemicals appear to have replaced bacteria and fungi as hazards to hospital personnel," and others as well.

58 See Nash JM. Stopping cancer in its tracks. *Time.* April 25, 1994:38-44. "New discoveries about wayward genes and misbehaving proteins show how cells become malignant, and perhaps how to bring them under control." This new understanding, as always, promises new solutions to cancer. If only they ask why genes become wayward and proteins misbehave, they will realize that X-rays, excess protein consumption, chemical drugs, and chemical food additives (among others) are the culprits. Cancer would have been checked years ago. To study genes and how they mutate may only be a waste of time and money which can be used for other more worthy pursuits like eradicating poverty.

59 See Bailar JC, Smith EL. Progress against cancer? *New England Journal of Medicine* 1986(April);314:1226-1232. These awakened scientists had pushed the warning button nine years ago. "We are losing the war against cancer... a shift in research emphasis from research on treatment to research on prevention, seems necessary if substantial progress against cancer is forthcoming." See also Astrow A. Rethinking cancer. *Lancet* 1994(February);343:494-495.

60 In 2009, or nearly 20 years after this International Cancer Congress, the National Institutes of Health in the US finally expanded the list of risk factors to the development of cancer. See *www.nih.gov.news/carcinogens.* But more are suspected. See *msds.chem.ox.ac.uk/carcinogens.html* for a more extensive list of carcinogens.

61 Annual Report of Institut Hiscia, the Society for Cancer Research. Arlesheim, Switzerland; 1991:3. An internationally renowned professor of oncology also confessed that he could no longer ask his patients to undergo chemotherapy, which he would have firmly advocated just a few years ago. To most, this is thought-provoking. For others, it is about time!

62 See *cancerlaw.net/chemo.htm* for more information about the toxic and carcinogenic effect of chemotherapy and radiation.

63 See Institute of Cancer Research in the UK at *www.icr.ac.uk* to see the list of their research priorities. The International Agency for Research in Cancer is a little more innovative and is looking at cancer prevention as its priority for research. The agency is hosting conferences and workshops on environmental exposures to carcinogens and making people know more about these carcinogens.

64 See Strohman R. The epigenesis: the missing beat in biotechnology? *Biotechnology* 1994(February);12:157. For example, gene 4 may itself be redundant in the epigenetic system. A single mutation of this gene may not have an effect in the overall system, since the system contains alternating gene elements and gene products which may perform identical functions. Moreover, even if the gene is mutated but not redundant, the epigenetic network may reset itself when given appropriate environmental signals. This is how intelligent our formative force body is in managing our physical body. However, orthodox science doubts this intelligence and has developed a whole arsenal of immune-suppressing drugs to fight the system it is supposed to assist. The next thing they will announce is the development of a synthetic gene product to substitute for the supposedly mutated gene. See Nash JM. Stopping cancer in its tracks. *Time.* April 25, 1994:44. This is the promise of orthodox science in cancer control. They do not aim for true healing, but only to control. Anyway, we are all doomed to die with cancer or other diseases, as orthodox science wants us to believe.

65 On the other hand, genetic damage may be reversed by mere diet in a cardiovascular disease. For example, see Watts GE et al. Effects on coronary artery disease of lipid-lowering diet plus cholestyramine: the St. Thomas Arteriosclerosis Regression Study (STARS). *Lancet* 1992(March);339:563-569. "Dietary change alone retarded over-all progression and increased over-all regression of coronary artery disease." See also note 27 for more studies on the long-term effect of diet in other diseases. If there is remission then there must have been repair done to the genes. If this is so, how come very few scientists are asking how diet could possibly regress cardiovascular disease if there are mutated genes involved? Everybody wants to understand how disease occurs, but not how people get well. This attitude reveals that even scientists are trained for disease and not wellness. Or is it also because there is more money in the research of disease than wellness? The answer to the first question may actually be very simple: the life force or vitality of the food heals. But without a concept of the life force/life body, orthodox science will *never* find the answer.

66 Biomedical geneticists are actually in conflict with the recent findings in molecular and developmental biology; in conflict with cell and molecular studies of disease and adaptation; in conflict with population genetics; and in conflict with studies in

disease distribution. See Strohman R. Ancient genome, wise bodies, unhealthy people: limits of a genetic paradigm in biology and medicine. Presented at the International Conference on Redefining the Life Sciences, July 7-10, 1994, Penang, Malaysia: Third World Network, for a more detailed discussion on these conflicts. The Human Genome Project then is an attempt to ram through a hypothesis despite very clear fundamental disagreements with orthodox science's own findings. We can only expect more reified facts and expensive therapy, which will again be unnecessary.

A much worse effect of therapy coming from this flawed science is the intake of genetically engineered products. Sometime in the 1980s, pharmaceutical companies sold genetically engineered amino acids such as L-tryptophan (classified as food additive) and insulin (for insulin dependent diabetics), using bacteria to produce the said products. They assume that bacteria can produce the same biochemical gene product as a human system would do. The adverse effects, however, can be horrifying. As of June 1992, genetically engineered L-tryptophan resulted in an epidemic of an apparently new illness to thousands, crippling of hundreds, and death to 38 innocent users. Its symptoms were eosinophilia, a blood disorder marked by abnormally high counts of white blood cells, and myalgia, severe muscle pain. See Talman S, Puckey H. Bio-engineered drug kills 38, harms thousands. *Third World Resurgence* 1993;38:17.

"Human" insulin mass-produced by genetically engineered bacteria has resulted in British patients suddenly dropping unconscious due to inadequate physiological feedback from the artificial insulin. See Perlas N. When what could go wrong, did go wrong... *Third World Resurgence* 1993;38:38; Overcoming illusions about biotechnology. Penang, Malaysia: Third World Network; 1994.

See also, The need for greater regulation and control of genetic engineering: a statement by scientists concerned about the current trends in the new biotechnology. Penang, Malaysia: Third World Network; November 1994 (The Third World Network, 228 Macalister Road, 10400 Penang, Malaysia). "Many of the claims about the benefits of genetic engineering... have been exaggerated, or have not been based on adequate scientific foundations. Many scientists are increasingly questioning the scientific validity of the basic premises of the paradigm underpinning genetic engineering." See Hubbard R, Wald E. The eugenics of normalcy: the politics of gene research. *The Ecologist* 1993(September/October);23. "The myth of the 'all powerful gene' threatens to impose a new eugenics—with 'normality' defined by arbitrary models of a standard human." Black W et al. Advance in diagnostic imaging and overestimation of disease prevalence and the benefits of therapy. *New England Journal of Medicine* 1993(April);328:1237-1243. "...these technological advances... create confusion that may ultimately be harmful to patients." Duesberg PH, Schwartz JR. Latent virus and mutated oncogenes: no evidence for pathogenicity. *Progress in Nucleic Acid Research and Molecular Biology* 1992;43:135 204.

67 Recent studies point to the presence of polysaccharides and phytochemicals in whole herbal extracts and in edible plants as the "active ingredients" in a range of bioactivities such as anti-virus, anti-bacteria, anti-inflammation, anti-hypoglycemia, anti-coagulation, anti-phagocytotic, and anti-tumor activities. See Waldron KW, Selvendran RR. Bioactive wall and related components from herbal products and edible plant organs as protective factors. In Waldron KW, Johnson LT, Fenwick GR, eds. *Food and Cancer Prevention: Biological Aspects.* Cambridge: Royal Society of Chemistry, 1993; Begley S. Beyond vitamins. *Newsweek,* April 25, 1994:42-47; Schardt D. Phytochemicals: plants against cancer. *The Philippine Star* August 20, 1994:27-29. See also Chapter 3, Notes 63-65. See also Callen M. *Surviving Aids.* New York: Harper Collins; 1996. The survivors interviewed "had what is commonly referred to as 'the right attitude,' which basically meant that they had hope. All the survivors had dabbled with what are generally referred to as holistic approaches to healing... Openness to holistics was indicative of a more general open-mindedness... a sudden interest in spirituality and religion was another pattern that emerged... Finally, nearly all of the survivors were involved to some extent in the politics of AIDS" (or social transformation).

68 Husemann F, Wolff O. *The Anthroposophical Approach to Medicine* (3 vols). Anthroposophical Press Inc.; vol 2:51.

69 Ibid, p 51.

70 Ibid, p 52.

71 Most herbal books have to refer to the discovered active ingredients found in the plant as the justification for its healing effect. This indicates how medicinal plant research is caught in the active ingredient syndrome. Why can scientists not acknowledge the experiences of countless generations in the use of these plants? Experience is still the best way to know that something is real or effective.

72 Rhodes P. *An Outline History of Medicine.* London: Buttersworth;1985:29.

73 Kenmore PE. Indonesia's integrated pest management: a model for Asia. FAO Rice IPC Programme, Manila, 1991. In this study, Kenmore showed that the extensive use of pesticides resulted in the brown plant hopper infestation of 1976-77 in Indonesia and of 1990-91 in Thailand.

74 Based on Nicanor Perlas's seminar on biodynamic agriculture, the basic ingredient in community ecology is good soil fertility. With good soil, 100% of diseases and about 80% of pests can be avoided. If pests come and proliferate, the predators are induced to multiply too. Thus, a balance in the ratio of insect populations is achieved. Crop rotation, diversity of species and variety of planting material, and meticulous selection of quality seeds are also part of this new approach to pest management.

75 See Illich I. *Limits to Medicine.* Penguin Books; 1977:29.

76 Take note that the HIV virus as the cause of AIDS is only a hypothesis. To view the HIV virus as the sole cause of AIDS is a clear indication that today's science is still stuck in one-sided thinking. There are other hypotheses with regards to the cause of AIDS. See Dresberg P. *Is Aids Virus a Science Fiction?* Berkeley: University of California; 1990. His position is that HIV has no role in AIDS. Or write to The Group for the Scientific Reappraisal of the HIV/AIDS Hypothesis, 2040 Polk Street, Suite 321, San Francisco, CA 94109, US. There are personal accounts of AIDS victims recovering from the illness (Mark Griffin is one of them) through regeneration therapy, i.e., prolonged period of eating living foods, deprogramming of negative thought patterns, and experiencing a gentle, non-sectarian spiritual awakening which enables one to be in harmony with oneself, humanity, and the environment. See also Mark Griffin, *AIDS: The Apprenticeship,* for testimonies of people who have recovered from life-threatening disease (20, route du Vallon, CH-1224 Chene-Bougeries, Switzerland).

See also Dickson D. Critic still lays blame for AIDS on lifestyle, not HIV, *Nature* 1994(June);369:434. He reported the talk of Kary Willis, recipient of the 1993 Nobel Prize for Chemistry, who reiterated the points discussed above and suggested that "the deaths of HIV positive children were caused by their treatment with the drug AZT." The AIDS epidemic in Africa was "probably the result of misleading AIDS test due to cross-reaction with malaria anti-bodies which look like AIDS antibodies." For a critique of the current AIDS testing system see Mortimer PP. Fallibility of the HIV western blot. *Lancet* 1991(February);337:286-287. "This test has been used as the 'gold standard' for other assays and the possibility that it might itself be inaccurate has been largely ignored."

In 1992, moreover, a series of cases were reported of AIDS without HIV. This brought in the possibility of other viruses and factors in AIDS. See Lauren J et al. Acquired immunodeficiency syndrome without evidence of infection with HIV type 1 and 2. *Lancet* 1992(August);340:273-274; AIDS minus HIV. *Lancet* 1992(August);340:280; and Hishida O et al. Clinically diagnosed AIDS cases without evident association with HIV type 1 and 2 infections in Ghana. *Lancet* 1992(October);340:971-972. The Japanese scientists reported that 135 of 227 Ghana AIDS patients diagnosed by using the WHO clinical criteria were negative of HIV. For other possible pathogens involved in AIDS, see Kyle W. Simian retroviruses, polio vaccine and the origin of AIDS. *Lancet* 1992(March);339:600-601. His hypothesis is that virus particles found in polio vaccine produced before 1985 were HIV (or some variant, e.g. retrovirus) when tested with reverse transcriptase analysis. "A critical look should now be taken at all such vaccines," Dr. Kyle warned.

See also Murphy B. The politics of AIDS. *Third World Resurgence* 1994;47:33-40. He argues that "the factors that give rise to the development of AIDS are largely social and political, rather than biological... [he supports the view] that HIV by itself is neither necessary nor sufficient to cause AIDS... A host of other 'opportunistic' infections can also result and give rise to such immunodeficiency and even where HIV is present, it is invariably found in combination with these other infections. Since most of these other infections are quite often the by-product of the material conditions of the poor... what is required is not medicine, but social justice."

With the above discussion, AIDS should be seen as resulting from a host of factors. Other factors include malnutrition (i.e., devitalized food) and the periodic suppression of the immune system with chemical drugs. They are all synergistic contributors to AIDS. Thus to blame only one cause (a virus) is again an orthodox medical syndrome of barking up the wrong tree, as we have mentioned earlier. For a more elaborate discussion on how modern chemical drugs can induce AIDS, see Root-Bernstein R. Do we know the cause(s) of AIDS? *Perspectives in Biology and Medicine* 1990(April);33:481-494. See also Callen M. *Surviving Aids.* New York: Harper Collins; 1996. Callen tells both his own story and, through in-depth interviews, the stories of other long-term survivors: women, gay, straight, bisexual, black, white, and brown. "AIDS has taught me the preciousness of life and the healing power of love... (it) forced me to take responsibility for my own life—for the choices I had made and the choices I will still make."

The website *www.virusmyth.com/aids/controversy.htm* will give you an update on this ongoing issue. Also search the web for *iatrogenic epidemic* to get an idea of suspected epidemics caused by today's medical procedures.

77 Orthodox doctors often resort to prophylaxis using chemical drugs, while claiming this to be prevention of disease. Studies reveal that chemical drugs or chemical supplements as prophylaxis may be dangerous to one's health. For example, see Fugh-Beman A, Epstein S. Tamoxit: disease prevention or disease substitution. *Lancet* 1992(January);340:1143-1145; CLASP (Collaborative Low Dose Aspirin Study in Pregnancy) Collaborative Group. A randomized trial of low-dose aspirin for the prevention and treatment of pre-eclampsia among 9364 pregnant women. *Lancet* 1994(March);343:619-629. Their findings do not support routine prophylactic or therapeutic administration of aspirin; Van der Meer JTM et al. Efficacy of antibiotic prophylaxis for prevention of native-valve endocarditis. *Lancet* 1992(January);339:136-137. Antibiotics might do little to decrease the total number of patients with endocarditis in the community; Simmons NA et al. Case against antibiotic prophylaxis for dental treatment of patients with joint prothesis. *Lancet* 1992(February):339:301; Stansfield SK et al. Vitamin A supplementation and increased prevalence of childhood diarrhea and acute respiratory infection. *Lancet* 1993(September);342:578-582; de Francisco A et al. Acute toxicity of vitamin A given with vaccines in infancy. *Lancet* 1993(August);342:526-527; Jacobus CH et al.

Hypervitaminosis D associated with drinking milk. *New England Journal of Medicine* 1992(April);326:1173-1177. See also Note 78 on iron supplements given to children.

78 Mineral supplements like iron sulfate should always be critically viewed. See Idjradinita P et al. Adverse effects of iron supplementation in weight gain of iron-replete young children. *Lancet* 1994(May);343:1252-1254, a study which proved that iron can in fact retard the growth of healthy children; for pregnant women, iron supplement is also not necessary if the diet is adequate. An increase in the absorption of iron from food is a physiological consequence of normal pregnancy. Barrett JER et al. Absorption of non-haem iron from food during normal pregnancy. *British Medical Journal* 1994(July);309:79-82. Moreover, iron supplementation results in the inhibition of the absorption of zinc from the intestine.

79 Bauman E et al. *The Holistic Health Book*, p 80.

80 Husemann F, Wolff O. *The Anthroposophical Approach to Medicine* (3 vols). Anthroposophical Press Inc.; vol 3:26-27. See also *www.gohlchiropractic.com/index_files/ site2/gohlmind.html* for more discussion of Speranksy's *A Basis of the Theory of Medicine* and its relation to the principles of chiropractic. You can still ask the question: who is (the being) using the nervous system that causes the misalignment or misplacement of the nerves? Understanding this being and how one can regulate his nerve impulses is the subject of later discussion.

81 Beinfield H et al. *Between Heaven and Earth: A Guide to Chinese Medicine*. New York: Ballantine Books; 1991.

82 Hahnemann S. *Organon of Medicine*. Quoted in Vithoulkas, pp 46-47.

Chapter Three

❦

Understanding Constitution and Disposition in Relation to Health and Illness

A. AN EXPANDED IMAGE OF THE HUMAN BEING

As we go through the aforementioned schools of medical thought, we can discern that they all point to an image of a human being that is made up of more than chemical or physical processes. They lead to something more than just the physical body. The concept of the vital-life body is common to all these schools. They all acknowledge the contribution of emotions, mind, and nutrition in the processes of maintaining health, and in the genesis of illnesses. Germs or mutated genes may be present, but are not sufficient factors to cause any disease.

Their therapeutics are also consistent with this view. These schools have been ridiculed by orthodox medicine as quackery—having no "scientific" basis whatsoever, thus unworthy of being called medicine. Being put down by orthodox medicine, contemporary practitioners of these schools are now trying to rearticulate their principles of medicine using conventional terminology and adapting to some of the current findings of science. However, in the process they get caught in materialistic thinking. For example, some acupuncture books postulate a neural theory of action.[1] This is perhaps a way to make the scientific community understand how acupuncture works. However, this is also a half truth. Most of those who are articulating this position have lost (or are unable to comprehend) the idea of the vital-life body. Conventional terminology cannot approximate the idea of the vital-life body. Thus in the course of time, some of the literature has been rewritten to conform to an orthodox scientific way of presentation. A number of original ideas have been lost this way. It is therefore important to be discerning with the materials we read, and develop other capacities to renew the meaning of the old texts.

At this point, let me introduce a relatively new school of thought in medicine—*anthroposophic* medicine—which to my mind renews and invigorates the understanding of the worldviews of the above schools of medicine. Also, this new medicine can serve as the broad framework in which the other schools of thought in medicine and their therapies can be meaningfully situated. But more importantly, I believe, this new school of thought in medicine broadens the comprehension of the human being, society, and nature, and introduces new therapies as well.

1. The Emergence of Anthroposophic Medicine

Anthroposophic medicine was founded in 1920 by Rudolf Steiner, an Austrian philosopher, educator, spiritual scientist, and researcher. It is based on a body of knowledge which Steiner developed and called *anthroposophy*,[2] literally translated as "wisdom of human being." Steiner's works not only renewed medicine, but also served as the foundation of various initiatives for social transformation which include the Waldorf or Steiner system of education,[3] the biodynamic agriculture movement,[4] the Camphill movement (a way of working with the mentally handicapped and other children with special needs),[5] architecture,[6] and various arts such as speech, painting, music, and sculpture.[7] The renewed artistic impulses are also prescribed as therapy to patients by anthroposophic doctors. Steiner also introduced a new form of movement called *eurythmy*, or "visible speech." Eurythmy is used today as a performing art, as part of Steiner pedagogy for both youth and adults, and in curative and social therapy.[8]

Let us look into the life of Rudolf Steiner, and the context in which he made his contribution to practically every aspect of human life.

Rudolf Steiner lived between 1861 and 1925. This was the period when orthodox materialistic science was at its peak. Steiner had two important faculties—a clairvoyant capacity, also described as picture consciousness (to put it simply), and a capacity for logical and analytical thinking suitable for scientific investigation.[9]

Most people today, except perhaps some of the traditional healers of indigenous peoples and cultures, have lost the clairvoyant capacity common among our forefathers. This is the main reason why folk remedies are no longer understood. The people of ancient times knew the healing power of herbs because their clairvoyant capacity beheld the inner power of the plants.[10] (In an interview with one local healer in the Philippines, I asked how he knew which plant to prescribe. He replied that an inner voice [clairaudience] tells him which one.) The ancient Greeks saw and conversed with their gods Athena or Apollo to know their wishes, and to learn from them music, warfare, handicraft, and reason. The way

Hippocrates and Paracelsus articulated their systems of medicine (or even traditional medicines like acupuncture or ayurveda) was still reminiscent of this form of consciousness. For example, the points and the lines of the meridians in acupuncture were discovered not by trial and error, as taught in schools, but by ancient practitioners who actually beheld (saw) the "light" that radiates out of the points. (The light—biophotons—emitted by the acupuncture points can be verified by a new technology.)[11] Thus, reading original literature on traditional Chinese medicine is not easy, because what the ancient Chinese writer wanted to describe is how the "chi" flows, circulates, and metamorphoses into yin and yang (modified by human consciousness), in and out of the organs and the whole body through the meridians, creating illness or health.

Orthodox science, which uses purely logical-analytical thinking, cannot understand the pictures being described by the ancient Indians, Persians, Egyptians, Greeks, Chinese, or indigenous communities. This is how the ancient peoples approached the world so differently from the way modern humanity views reality today.[12]

Through various consciousness exercises which he developed, Rudolf Steiner was able to fully realize his clairvoyant faculties. He described these faculties as having three levels: imagination, inspiration, and intuition.[13] He then used these faculties to understand the spiritual forces interweaving the material world and to conceptualize the deeper meaning of human existence, nature, and the evolution of the cosmos.[14] Out of this understanding, he was able to illuminate and renew many branches of art and science. In addition to the initiatives already mentioned, we have today anthroposophic medicine, nutrition,[15] epistemology,[16] psychology and psychiatry,[17] natural science,[18] the three-fold social order (insights into how society can be restructured in order that human beings may live creatively and harmoniously),[19] and many other initiatives addressing various aspects of human life.[20]

Steiner also had a well-developed faculty for logical-analytical thinking. As a student, he was most attracted to geometry and the natural sciences, in which he excelled. He was awarded the title Doctor of Philosophy in 1891 at the age of 30, and was frequently in the company of distinguished scientists and philosophers of his time. He reached the peak of his scientific involvement when Karl Julius Schroer, an authority of Goethe's literary works, asked him to edit Goethe's scientific works. He worked on this for seven years. From his understanding of the scientific works of Goethe, he formulated what is now termed Goethe's scientific approach to natural science, or Goethean science. Goethe, who was known more as a poet, was misunderstood as a scientist because his work did not fit into the prevailing theory of his time. Even scientists after Goethe had difficulty reading his scientific work because they could not grasp his way of thinking. Steiner restored the prominence of Goethe's scientific work when he published the book, *Goethe the Scientist: A Theory of Knowledge Implicit in Goethe's World Conception.*[21] This work paved the way for further understanding and recognition of Goethe's thought and scientific accomplishment.

For more than 25 years until his death in 1925, Steiner wrote over 40 books and gave more than 6,000 lectures on almost any subject matter he was asked to expound on. This collection became the body of knowledge called anthroposophy. In 1920, he gave his first lecture to medical doctors who sought his help on how to renew the art of healing based on the findings of his spiritual research.[22]

With his clairvoyant capacity he was able to see, experience, and behold the supersensible processes intrinsically weaving in matter. Alongside this vision, he used his analytical-logical thinking to formulate a coherent concept about what he saw, experienced, and beheld. Thus, unlike many clairvoyants, he was able to express the concepts and ideas of his visions and experiences in a language understandable to modern humanity.[23] One who reads his work with an unprejudiced mind will sense the truth in what he communicates. Our current faculty of thinking at this point in human evolution—grappling with ideas and concepts—is the commonly shared way to arrive at knowledge and eventually discover and realize truths, an approach supported by Steiner.

Here I would like to emphasize that anthroposophic medicine is not just another system of medicine. It may well be the most holistic approach to healing in the full sense of the word. In the words of Francis X. King, Steiner's anthroposophic medicine "is perhaps the most holistic of all philosophies of healing, for it is not just concerned with the whole body as a unity, or even with the mind and body as a unified and self-contained biosystem, but with body, mind, and spirit—the soma (body), psyche (soul), and pneuma (spirit) of the New Testament's Greek original."[24]

This is the main reason why I regard anthroposophic medicine as an integrating framework for the other schools of thought in medicine for this modern time. It can include, understand, and use allopathy; traditional medicine like Chinese medicine, ayurveda, and medicines of indigenous peoples; the various streams of modern psychology; and other new and emerging therapies found today in the world.

As we go over the fundamental ideas of anthroposophic medicine, we will see that all the other therapies and schools of thought in medicine

can be situated in one whole spectrum of the principles of healing and
therapeutics.[25] Appendix 2 puts in a schematic picture the various medicines
and therapies hitherto in the world, and what aspect of the interweaving
bodies of the human being, described below, they intend to address.

2. The Four-fold Human Being

Here it is necessary to put forward an expanded image of the human
being.[26] As I said earlier, orthodox medicine is still trapped in recognizing
only the physical body as the sole reality. The expanded image we use here
does not deny the physical body, but acknowledges that it is only the visible
part of the human being. It consists of substances which also make up
the external world, but its form and functions cannot be fully explained
in the mechanistic and chemical terms used to describe inanimate mineral
substances. We can better understand the functions of this physical
body if we keep in mind that every form and every process should be
comprehended as an expression of the soul and spirit. Thus, everything
that a human being is—the way he speaks, thinks, feels or moves, his
uprightness, and the way he looks at the world—is an expression of his
soul and spirit. None of this arises from the physical body. But the physical
body is a necessary vehicle for such expression. In the anthroposophic
view of the evolution of humanity and the cosmos, the physical body was
created out of the deepest wisdom in order to serve as tool for the soul
and spirit. Moreover, the physical body is directly related to carbon, and
the lungs are the cardinal organ that manages this substance.

Interwoven within this physical body is the *formative force body*. This
force gives form to the physical-chemical substances. The physical body is
perpetually in the process of becoming and passing away. As a matter of
fact, orthodox science has discovered that we renew parts of our body every
day, and thus have a totally new body every seven years. This is the basis
for the daily requirement of substances such as protein, carbohydrates,
and fats. The formative force body is what gives permanence to our form
in the course of changing every molecule of the body. Consequently, the
formative force also governs this process itself. It is the bearer of growth,
regeneration, and procreation, and therefore life. It stimulates and guides
metabolism. For example, if we picture in our mind's eye the processes of
becoming and passing away, we see a fluidic process. The formative force
body is synonymous with the fluid or water organization. Every fluidic
process that dissolves substances and then renews them is part of the
formative force body, and makes one alive and maintains life.[27]

The liver is the cardinal organ directly related to the formative force body. It is the main anabolic organ and directly manages water in the physical body.

Plants as well as human beings possess a formative force body. In the Eastern tradition, this is equivalent to the concept of the etheric body (*oikos* from the Greek). But we will not use that term here because it has connotations which may confuse our current description. Incidentally, without the formative force body, the physical body will decompose into a corpse, in accordance with the law of the mineral world. The formative force body is similar to what the other schools of medical thought refer to as the vital force, homeostasis, the wisdom of the body, or the healing power of nature (*vis medicatrix naturae*). To the Chinese, it is the totality of the "chi" that is found in all cells and organ systems, including its continuous circulation and its radiation in and out of the body.

The anthroposophical approach to medicine further differentiates the third and fourth bodies, or members, of the human being. They are the *sensitivity body*, and the *ego* or "*I*," the immortal spirit of the human being.

The sensitivity body is the bearer of pain and pleasure, drives and emotions, joy and sorrow. This is connected to the air element, and therefore is also called the "air organization." Air passages in our physical bodies are easily affected by whatever this body experiences. If we are anxious or are in fear, our breathing becomes heavy. Our sinuses can even become clogged. We sigh when relieved of certain tensions.

Air is actually 80% nitrogen. Thus this body has a direct affinity with protein metabolism, the substance that has incorporated nitrogen in its structure. It is directly related to the cardinal organ of the kidneys, which eliminate nitrogen in the form of urea and uric acid. This sensitivity body is what humans have in common with the animal kingdom. The capacity to experience pain and pleasure produces consciousness, a consciousness that is experienced from within an enclosed body. This consciousness is known as the soul in contemporary religion. In the Eastern tradition, this is called the astral body, referring to light, like the stars. A clairvoyant would see this body like a luminous star, inherently interweaving with the physical body.[28]

The ego or the "I" is the spiritual core of a human being. Only humans are able to say "I" to refer to themselves. Moreover, each ego is unique, as each one is able to say "I" only to oneself. The "I" uses the faculties of thinking, feeling, and willing to gain experiences of the world processes; it develops capacities and abilities, and thus enriches and ennobles itself. The "I" can think—and know why he knows. He can even think about his own thinking process. Animals know (consciousness). But they do not know that they know (self-consciousness), and they do not know why they know (reflective consciousness). The "I," being the highly self-individualized aspect of a human being, stamps its uniqueness on the physical body. We each have our own fingerprints and unique features. Lately scientists have detected that each individual has his own individualized protein. Even though we eat the same food, each person will digest it differently and synthesize its own life substance from it. This is the basic force behind our immune system. That is, we reject or react to a substance that is foreign to our body.

The "I" lives in warmth. This is the reason why we need a body temperature of 37 degrees centigrade. Too low or too high a temperature would mean death, meaning that the ego is unable to inhabit the body. There is an ego organization which the "I" uses to affect the physical body. It is also called the *warmth body*. The cardinal organ related to the "I" is the heart, and the element it manages is hydrogen.

Disease occurs when the interaction of the different members is unduly disturbed and one member becomes more active than the others. For example, in a stomach ache, the sensitivity body is more active than it should be. We thus feel pain. In a tumor, the formative force body continues to stimulate the physical body to produce growth which is supposed to be held in check by the sensitivity body. The therapy then is to strengthen that which is weak, or divert the excess strength of the other. This is done by the various therapies discussed in "An Overview of the Anthroposophic Approach to Therapy" later in this chapter.

In diagnosis, a further application of the four-fold principle of the human being can be seen in an inflammation. An inflamed part is warmer than the rest of the body (indicating the presence of the ego organization). It is more sensitive and/or more painful (due to the presence of the sensitivity body). It has more water (because of the formative force body), and the color changes into reddish brown (a sign of a change in material). Here we can see that all the four aspects of the human being are active in the process of healing. Inflammation is only an outward manifestation or label. Thus if we suppress this natural healing process, we are literally suppressing our own individuality. The therapy in any inflammation is always to apply more warmth to augment the body's own warming process. With more warmth, healing can be enhanced. However, the application of warmth should not be too much or too long, to the point that it will offset the process.

3. The Constitutional Temperaments and the Four-fold Human Being

In equating the elements of mineral-earth, earth, water, air, and warmth with the specific bodies, anthroposophic medicine indicates that these elements have reflective qualities similar to processes operating in the various bodies. Moreover, these qualities can be found in the constitutional temperaments. These are: *melancholic, phlegmatic, sanguine,* and *choleric* temperaments. Constitutional temperaments are the product of the interaction among the various bodies, such that one "fold" or bodily sheath of the human being tends to dominate the others. The qualities or characteristics related to a particular bodily sheath (which I describe below) are more readily expressed by the organism than the others.

For example, the phlegmatic has a strong formative force body and is like water. He can flow in and out of any situation but is placid like a stagnant body of water. This placidity can be disturbed by wind, but will eventually calm down. Water is universal solvent: it has a balanced ph (alkalinity and acidity). Mediating various viewpoints is the strength of a phlegmatic. The liver is the organ in the body that makes water alive, and balances for the organism what food it needs. Any imbalance in nourishment of the organism can be traced to the dysfunction of the liver. A phlegmatic will have a strong liver but may unduly overburden the other organs. If he indulges too much in rich food, he may have liver problems later in life.

The melancholic is more influenced by the material body. He is more inward, introverted, as if enclosed in a cube. His attention is not easily aroused but is most persevering. He likes to stay at home more than to go out. He is rigid and fixed in his ideas, interested in natural science, history, or anything involving the study of matter and various materials. He is prone to infection (the lungs being the main organ that manages the material body), congestion, and depression. Depression is being enclosed in the darkness of matter. He cannot see (inner) light. Worse, he can bring himself to a state of delusion and extreme melancholia.

The sanguine temperament is like air. The sanguine person wants to be everywhere and to experience everything. He is the great generator of ideas, plans, and programs. His attention is easily aroused but has little strength or perseverance. He wants to please everyone, and is jolly and happy to be with. He accommodates all ideas and points of view but may not choose one for fear that it might alienate some of his friends. This may lead him to character instability, or worse, to lunacy and insanity. In such situations, he may have hyperactive kidneys that need to be toned down. Potentized calcium carbonate may be necessary to bring him down to earth.

Finally, the choleric temperament is very warm, protective, and dependable. He is a doer, the commander, the boss, the pusher of initiatives. In pushing, he usually wants to have his way of doing things; he has a tendency towards egoism. His attention is easily aroused and he is most strongly persevering. The unformed choleric will have an uncontrolled temper. He can be the fanatic, and in the extreme, a maniac. His heart will suffer in the process and/or his gall bladder can be exhausted from over-activity.

The table below summarizes the organization of the four-fold human being and its various correspondences.

Member	Organization	Element	Cardinal Organ	Temperament
Physical Body	Mineral	Carbon	Lung	Melancholic
Formative Force Body	Water	Oxygen	Liver	Phlegmatic
Sensitivity Body	Air	Nitrogen	Kidney	Sanguine
Spiritual Ego, "I"	Warmth	Hydrogen	Heart/Gall Bladder	Choleric

In the course of our upbringing, our constitutional temperament can be enhanced or dampened. For example, in our current school system, the choleric temperament is the model of the perfect student. Thus, there is the tendency to overemphasize one trait or aspect of the human being. Naturally, the result to society will also be imbalance. The orthodox way of schooling can be a major source of the ills in today's society—both in its pathologies (heart diseases and gall bladder dysfunction) and in its psycho-social consequences (violence, rape, war, domination, egoism).

A better alternative must be adopted to bring about the harmonious development of the temperaments. This is one of the main tasks of Waldorf (or Steiner) education, an educational system based on the expanded view of the human being discussed here. Waldorf pedagogy is the best preventive medicine in the sense that it harmonizes the temperaments, guides the timely awakening of the ego in the three-to-seven-year-old phases of the development of children, and thus avoids one-sidedness (the real cause of illnesses). Appendix 1 will elaborate more on this.

Furthermore, Steiner education harmonizes the three living systems of the human being (discussed below) using arts and artistic methods in its pedagogy.[29]

4. The Three Living Systems in a Human Being

Steiner further distinguishes three living systems in the interweaving four-fold human being. They are the *head system*, the *metabolic system*, and the *rhythmic system*. These systems are the source of activities which maintain and enliven the whole organism throughout its life.

a. The Head or Nerve Sense System

The head system is concerned with thought, consciousness, analysis, and perceptions such as light, sound, smell, and so on. It is the centripetal element in the human being, in the sense that it draws in what comes from the outside. We are most awake in the head, and the part of the body directly connected with wakefulness is the central nervous system. In the nerves and brain, there is hardly any renewal and multiplication of cells. The overuse or abuse of the nervous system culminates in stasis, and eventually physical death. In other words, to think and to be awake literally means to kill ourselves. Thinking produces sclerotic forces which dry up life in our organs. This devitalization of the life of cells and organs eventually leads to death. This is why we need sleep. Sleep is the temporary extinguishing of consciousness, allowing time for the body to repair the damage caused in waking life. It is a known fact that we can go without food for a number of weeks, but if we do not sleep for a few days, we die.

The head system and its activities are related to the ego and the sensitivity body. The ego provides the thinking activity. The nerves are the vehicle of the sensitivity body.

b. The Metabolic/Limb System

In contrast to the head pole, there is the metabolic/limb system. The metabolic/limb system is centrifugal in its tendencies, directly affecting the outside world through the action of the will. Excretion is part of this system. The formative forces here are most active in transforming inert matter into living tissues. Active cell renewal is most prominent. Within hours, the lining of the stomach is replaced by a new one, through an activity called anabolism. Thus, in the metabolic/limb system we experience anabolism (building up, regeneration) as the overall function.

Even though the whole digestive system is normally described as the metabolic system, the liver is the main anabolic organ which balances the sclerotic (devitalizing) forces produced by the head system. The anabolic (revitalizing) forces work mostly at night, when the activity of thinking ceases and the repair of tissue can go on undisturbed. We are most unconscious in this region. Even though the lining of the stomach and intestines are full of nerves, we seldom experience our digestion. When we do—such as when we have spasms—it is a painful experience.

The reproductive organs are also part of this system. Our capacity to renew life (to impart strong formative force, or life force) belongs to our reproductive system.

c. The Middle/Rhythmic System

The rhythmic system mediates the two poles of the head and metabolic/limb systems. It has the task of keeping the two opposing tendencies of a healthy organism in exact and harmonious balance. On one level, for example, the sclerotic (devitalizing) force of the head system is balanced by the anabolic (revitalizing) forces of the metabolism. On another level, thought and will are brought together in the actions of individuals on the environment infused with feelings and warmth. In both cases, the rhythmic system mediates and harmonizes the activity.

The main organ system here is the heart and lungs. The rhythmic system expresses its rhythm in two basic soul tendencies: antipathy and sympathy. These are directly related to expiration and inspiration in our breathing, expansion and contraction of our heart, and the diastole and systole of the blood pressure. When one is disgusted (antipathetic), there is forceful expiration and/or a heightened systolic blood pressure. Accenting one activity over the other disrupts the rhythm and can bring about an illness. However, if this system is rightly nurtured, it can heal almost any disease. (This will be elaborated upon in the sub-topic "Harnessing the Power of the Rhythmic System.")

The rhythmic system is described as dreamy or semi-conscious, meaning it is difficult for us to be very clear and exact about what we feel (as contrasted to what we think), but not unconscious like our metabolic system. It is indeed in between the two systems.

These three systems, by the way, are also found in every organ or sub-system of the body. In the skin, for example, we have the epidermis that is the carrier of the nerve sense system. The dermis provides the mediating rhythmic activity of the entire skin, and the hypodermis is the metabolic part that nourishes the skin. An understanding of this is important in diagnosis and therapy.

d. Neurasthenia and Hysteria: Disease Tendencies Resulting from an Imbalance of the Three Living Systems

To get an idea of how disease arises from an imbalance of the three systems, we must picture a current of forces arising from the metabolic system, carrying with it vivified substances from its digestive activity. A second current of forces coming from the head pole devitalizes and mineralizes these substances and thus makes the processes of thinking and conscious mental activity possible. What has been devitalized and mineralized by the head pole must be revitalized by the metabolic pole, and so on. The two streams of forces should work in harmony, mediated by the rhythmic systems.

There are two disease tendencies that can arise out of an imbalance in these three systems. They are called neurasthenia and hysteria. These two disease tendencies are used here not only to mean the psychic symptoms which we are familiar with, but also a whole group of illnesses that lean toward one or the other tendency.

In hysteria, the metabolic revitalizing force-system is strong, while the head pole is too weak to devitalize and mineralize it. We thus have the phenomenon of inflammation. Inflammation, with its intense vital processes, must be considered a reaction which is "hysterical" in nature.

The paralysis of thinking in the case of migraine is another indication of a disease tendency towards hysteria. To have a better picture of how migraine comes about, let me introduce the idea that the function of digestion is also to remove the foreign character (formative force and sensitivity bodies) of food substances. The head pole participates in this process by sending its forces through the digestive enzymes. (The sub-topic on "Nutrition in Health and Illness" gives a more detailed discussion of this.) Thus when food which has not been fully devitalized by the enzymes of the upper pole is absorbed by the intestinal walls, the head is forced to "digest" these substances. This situation results in migraine. Migraine, then, is the condition wherein the head devitalizing force-system has a diminished participation in the process of digestion.

In the case of neurasthenia, the reverse happens: the head devitalizing force-system is strong, while the metabolic system is too weak to revitalize it. The processes of breakdown and devitalization dominate and the organism becomes too "intellectual"—too head-centered or too nervy. The symptoms can initially be anxiety, obsession, sleeplessness, restlessness, and/or hyperactivity. There is inadequate regeneration-revitalization in the organism, which then results in the accumulation of toxins or the formation of deposits (e.g., stones). We thus have the phenomenon of the body's normal process of encapsulating toxins in the form of cysts, polyps, plaque in the arteries, tumors, and the like. Current medical terminology calls this process sclerosis. Sclerosis, then, is a typical "neurasthenic" reaction.

Paralysis of the will, an extreme form of neurasthenia, is another example. In this condition, the nerve sense system is persistently over-stimulated and overused. The person becomes completely dependent on physical sensation so that the nerve sense organs become oversensitive, and various pains come and go. Nervous exhaustion results. His body tires more easily and cannot carry through with a decision he had made because he lacks the energy to do so.

The two disease tendencies of neurasthenia and hysteria illustrate the basic disharmony that occurs in the three-fold system. The two tendencies must be seen as a unified disease syndrome. Neurasthenia and hysteria tend to overlap one another and have many variations. They are important in recognizing a patient's constitution, because every human being is inclined to one or the other. Listed below are more examples to give the reader a better appreciation of this important fundamental idea of anthroposophic medicine.

Hysteria	Neurasthenia
Hydrocephalus	Microcephalus
Large-headed Children	Small-headed Children
Extroversion	Introversion
Prolonged Youth	Premature Aging
Numbness	Pains
Female	Male

The following table outlines the functions and characteristics of the three living systems:

System	Cardinal Organ	Consciousness	Activity
Head System	Brain	Awake/ Conscious	*Thinking:* Centripetal, Sclerotic, Hardening, Catabolic
Middle/ Rhythmic System	Heart/Lungs	Dreamy/ Subconscious	*Feeling:* Antipathy/Sympathy, Expiration/ Inspiration, Diastole/ Systole
Metabolic/ Limb System	Liver/Digestion	Sleeping/ Unconscious	*Willing:* Centrifugal, Inflammatory, Anabolic

5. The Inner Relationship Between Fever/Inflammation and Sclerosis/Degenerative Illnesses

Another fundamental contribution of Steiner to the understanding of illness concerns the polarity of inflammation and fever on one hand, and sclerosis and degenerative diseases on the other. Orthodox medicine now calls them "warm" and "cold" diseases. However, orthodox scientists view these diseases as totally unrelated to each other. They have not realized that these two groups of diseases are inherently and internally related on a spectrum. This means that the suppression of "warm" illnesses will eventually lead to the development of "cold" diseases. Inducing an inflammation or a fever can heal a sclerosis or degeneration. Moreover, anthroposophic doctors know that every inflammation is the attempt of the body to heal a sclerosis. A healthy organism should be seen as having the ability to balance these two forces throughout its life.

Considering how orthodox medicine is suppressing the warm diseases of childhood, it is not surprising that younger and younger generations are suffering from a whole range of cold diseases. Today, we often hear about a thirty-year old dying of heart failure, and children developing cancer as early as three years old.

Since the end of the last century, studies have indicated the relationship between cold and warm diseases. Orthodox science has, however, failed to appreciate this relationship. Otto Wolff summarizes the various studies in Volume 1 of the *Anthroposophical Approach to Medicine*:

(T)he pathologist E. von Rindfleisch... arrived at the conclusion that "inflammations do not arise spontaneously, but they heal spontaneously; tumors arise spontaneously, but they do not heal spontaneously... Rokitansky knew about the antagonistic relationship between tuberculosis and cancer... In 1910, R. Schmidt... showed that infectious diseases, especially those of childhood, were much less common in the anamnesis of cancer patients than other patients... In avoiding the Scylla of the infectious diseases, we would steer toward the Charybdis of malignancy."

In more recent times... Engel found that of 300 cancer patients, 113 had never had an infectious disease... A low infection index is related much more to carcinoma of the rectum and colon than to stomach or breast cancer. The strict clinical investigation of Sineck led to results pointing in the same direction. Schier also confirmed Schmidt's results. In 1941, Feld reported an "empty anamnesis" in 62 per cent of cancer patients studied. According to Kurten, there is a partial weakening of the capacity for fever in cancer patients. A synopsis of these problems is given by E. Hass. Later, Feyrter and Kofler indicated the notably decreased disposition in rectal cancer patients to allergic-inflammatory diseases... Felix Ungar found, looking at 64,385 case histories, including 4,192 of cancer patients, that "on average, the number of infectious or childhood diseases was more than three times as high in the patients without cancer than those with it."

[A]llergies appear seldom or not at all with cancer. [From] Pirquet, creator of the concept of allergy... G. von Bergmann writes: "The carcinomatous metabolism appears in just those places where the body is no longer capable of an active inflammatory metabolism... Tests at my clinic show that sections of malignant tumors from rats and from human carcinomatous tissue are quickly destroyed when placed in inflammatory exudates." In 72 leukemia patients, Huth found spontaneous remission, which in more than one third of patients were connected with purulent infections or pneumonia. These are the same diseases that preceded spontaneous remission in 26 cases of sarcoma and 33 cases of carcinoma.[30]

This understanding of the relationship of the two clusters of disease is a simple yet valuable tool in diagnostic and therapeutic medicine. For example, a plant that can induce fever is very valuable in treating sclerosis or cancer. Now we can better understand why Hippocrates said, "Give me a fever and I will cure any disease." Likewise, we can understand why the suppression of warm childhood diseases by giving antipyretics at the onset of a fever, or subjecting children to indiscriminate and routine immunization, predisposes them to the earlier development of the sclerotic/cold diseases like childhood diabetes or cancer, among others.[31]

Interestingly, Hans Reckeweg, MD, in his book *Homotoxicology: Illness and Healing through Anti-homotoxic Therapy* (1980), provided additional, more comprehensive, and independent clinical evidence of this relationship of illnesses thirty years after Steiner articulated the principle. Anti-homotoxic diagnosis and therapy is guided by this relationship. For example, if tonsillitis was suppressed early in life by antibiotics, the toxins that caused the tonsillitis in the first place can emerge later as nephritis, asthma, heart muscle damage, albuminaria, or diabetes. Reckeweg found this connection when he applied his homotoxin detoxification therapy; the degenerative illness regressed back to its inflammatory stage. Thus, one of the main principles in healing degenerative conditions involves the possibility of a *healing crisis*. A healing crisis means that the toxins buried deeper in the tissues are being released from the inside out, and may possibly be expressed again as various inflammatory conditions. If this happens, we must give our interweaving body (as discussed above) time to process and excrete these toxins with some assistance from other natural therapies.[32]

6. An Overview of the Anthroposophic Approach to Therapy

Anthroposophic pharmaceuticals use a process similar to, but by no means identical with, the techniques of preparing homeopathic remedies. Anthroposophic doctors administer remedies produced from minerals, plants, and animal organs, often in *potentized* form (to be discussed in Section 2). These doctors are more concerned with the forces and the processes in the substances—which stimulate corresponding processes in the body, soul, or spirit—rather than the substance itself.

Some therapies have been adapted from other schools, such as hydrotherapy and naturopathy, and include hot and cold treatments, oil baths, herbal compresses, and plant-based diets. Antibiotics, blood transfusions, and allopathic surgery are also used, but only as a last resort. Some anthroposophical doctors do practice acupuncture and other healing modalities.

There is also a new technique developed using colors instead of needles to stimulate particular points along the acupuncture meridians. The principle behind this is that the soul (sensitivity body) actually perceives (consciously and unconsciously) the color, which in turn evokes a certain reaction in our soul. In experiments, Christel Heidemann[33] discovered that each of the twelve meridians has a color equivalent based on Goethe's theory of color.[34] To strengthen or reduce the "chi" in the meridian and/or organ system, one can use the corresponding color or its complement. This is done by placing a tiny piece of silk of the appropriate color (dyed with plant dyes) over the identified point in a specified part of the body. This is a recent example of how ancient forms of therapy are being renewed, based on the insights of Steiner's spiritual research. Other existing forms of therapy are still being studied to transform their purpose and meaning, as well as to move the practice forward whenever possible.

Anthroposophical medicine has also introduced new forms of therapy based on the indications of Steiner. They are curative eurythmy (a new form of movement), painting and color therapy, rhythmic massage, rhythmic baths using oils, and music therapy. In special hospitals, these are all integrated and prescribed along with specific diets and potentized remedies, either as injections, oral preparations, or ointments and creams. There are more than twenty companies worldwide making anthroposophic medicine under the company names WELEDA, WALA, HELIXOR, and ABNOBA in Europe, and Uriel Pharmacy and True Botanica in the United States.

B. NUTRITION IN HEALTH OR ILLNESS

Let us now look closely at how nutrition contributes to health, and becomes a factor in predisposing one to illness.

It is only recently that orthodox medical science has acknowledged the role of nutrition in the development of disease. Despite the numerous studies that prove the correlation between nutrition and particular diseases, this linkage remains controversial to many doctors. One frequently hears doctors say to their ill patients, "You can eat anything you like; the medication will provide the relief," or "Nutrition does not have anything to do with your illness!" Although experience tells us otherwise, we tend to believe our doctor, whom we look up to as the authority.

Robert Mendelsohn, MD, the "medical heretic," observed that doctors are neither trained to look at the contribution of nutrition to the genesis of a disease, nor acquainted with the latest findings in the field of nutrition.[35] Some, wittingly or unwittingly, shy away from a true and conscious understanding of nutrition in order to ensure continuous patronage of their patients—the doctor who does not discourage his patients from eating rich, good-tasting food surely maintains his following.

This attitude is another consequence of reductionist science, which points to germs and genes as the cause of disease, thus leaving out personal responsibility. The other schools of medicine cited earlier have always acknowledged the vital role of nutrition in health and illness. A review of the fundamentals of nutrition based on the findings of orthodox science is necessary to show how the anthroposophic approach to medicine has expanded this understanding.

Let me start with a quotation from Rudolf Steiner, which can be understood better when discussed in the context of the process of digestion: "One who understands nutrition correctly understands the beginning of healing."

Orthodox science has described with precision what happens to the three important life substances in nutrition, namely, carbohydrates, proteins, and fats. During the mastication of food in the mouth, the carbohydrates undergo digestion through the action of ptyalin. In the stomach, the gastric juices amylase and pepsin act on carbohydrates and protein, respectively. Carbohydrates are changed into maltose, while the proteins—which are broken down into albumin—are digested for the first time. The partially digested food moves on to the small intestines, where it is acted on by amylase, trypsin, bile, pancreatic lipase, and other intestinal juices. The partially digested carbohydrates—maltose, lactose, or sucrose—are changed into a more simple sugar called glucose. The albuminous protein is broken down further into amino acids. The fats are emulsified by the bile acids, making them available to the action of trypsin and other pancreatic juice. They are then broken down into fatty acids and glycerins. This is the only time fats are digested, while proteins undergo digestion twice and carbohydrates have a chance to undergo digestion thrice.

The broken-down substances such as glucose, amino acids, fatty acids, and glycerine are absorbed by the body and are instantaneously transformed into human starch or glycogen, human protein, and human fats, respectively.

Based on the above description, one may ask: Why do we have to break down the substances and at the same time resynthesize them? This is synonymous with buying a house, knocking it down to its basic components and rebuilding it before moving in. One may think of this as absurd, irrational, and expensive—to which orthodox science can only agree. Since orthodox scientists do not have much to say as to why this is so, let us keep this riddle in mind while we examine some new findings in science which can help shed light on this mystery.

In summary, the process of digestion is as follows:

The Three Important Life Substances	Process of Digestion	Final Product
Carbohydrates →	+ *ptyalin* (mouth) + *amylase* (stomach) + *amylase* (intestines)	*glucose* (resynthesized as glycogen or human starch in the liver)
Protein →	+ *pepsin* & *HCL* (stomach) = *albumen* + *trypsin* (pancreas) = *oligopeptides* + *peptidases* (mucosa cells)	*amino acids* (immediately resynthesized by the body into human protein for reproduction and repair of organs and tissues)
Fats →	+ *bile acids* & *lipase* (intestines)	*fatty acids* & *glycerines* (75% of this is absorbed through the lymphatic system)

1. The Biochemical Individuality and the Expanded Image of the Human Being

In 1963, Roger J. Williams, a biochemist, published his book, *Biochemical Individuality*. He elaborated on this in a later essay:

> The biochemical individuality is actually an immense and far-reaching subject, in which much remains to be discovered. The fundamental fact of the uniqueness of each individual—biochemical individuality is part of this—represents a pillar of biology... One does not usually think about the fact that each one of us has his own particular metabolism-personality, has his own unique biochemistry. We may all use the same amino acids, vitamins, and minerals, but how we use them in isolated instances, and the effects of their individual utilization, that varies infinitely in all of us.[36]

Here, then, is the reason why our digestion takes the trouble to break down food. We need to individualize it. How do we do this? The findings of Steiner's research can enlighten us on this. Bearing in mind the four-fold human being and his three living systems, this is what actually happens.

The digestive enzymes ptyalin, pepsin, trypsin, and other digestive juices are the vehicles of the higher principles in a human being, namely, the formative force body, the sensitivity body, and the ego. They have the task of removing, neutralizing, or "killing" the alien character of foods.[37] As we already know, plants have their own formative force body, and animals have the formative force body and their own sensitivity body intrinsically woven in their flesh or material substance. The action of the enzymes not only breaks down plant and animal substances to their simplest form, as described by orthodox science, but also neutralizes the forces inherent in the food so that the individual can make them his own. In other words, the process of digestion enables the biochemical individuality to fully express itself, to reassemble the substances into its own image in order that they may be used to replace and revitalize its interweaving body.

What happens when this process of digestion fully or partially fails, that is, when the alien characters of foods are not fully neutralized and are not individualized?

We have the phenomenon of allergies. The body reacts by producing histamine to neutralize the alien food or toxins that entered the body. We can therefore say that all foods are actually poisons (toxins) if our body is unable to digest and neutralize their alien forces. For example, breast milk injected into the body will create an inflammation and possibly death if given in a large quantity. But if the milk is digested through the stomach, it is nourishment to an infant. The biochemical individuality must be protected at all costs. If it is compromised, the whole organism suffers.

The pathologies which are a consequence of nutrition are clarified by more details regarding protein metabolism. Most toxins are protein— like pollens, alkaloids, peptides, and so on—causing allergic reactions such as asthma, hay fever, itchiness, and the like. Protein is the most misunderstood food substance, and many illnesses can be traced to faulty protein metabolism.[38]

2. Protein Consumption: Its Problems and Myths

What is the real function of protein? How much of it do we really need? What is the best quality of protein?

We need protein mainly for the growth, reproduction, rebuilding, and regeneration of tissues and organs of the body. Studies have calculated that the rate of renewal of organs and tissues depends on the type of protein and the organ involved. For example, protein in the ganglia in the brain is renewed every nine hours. The life of enzymes is only a few hours. The liver takes about 10 days for its protein to be renewed; muscles, 150 days; and interstitial tissue, 160 days. Thus protein is the bearer of life. Without it, we will not be able to renew our organs and tissues and thus sustain their functions. But how much protein is necessary?

Before 1971, it was believed that protein was absorbed in the intestines in large amounts. Nutritionists believed that the minimum daily requirement should be one gram of protein per kilogram of body weight. Therefore, an average person weighing about sixty kilograms would need sixty or more grams of protein daily to renew his cells and tissues.

Modern nutritionists also led us to believe that consuming more protein was beneficial to the whole body. This reinforced the protein-rich diets common in our cuisine, common at parties and special occasions. This same belief made us look down upon the predominantly low-protein, vegetarian diet in rural communities.

Careful research by K. Lang, author of the book *Biochemie der Ernaehrung* (1974) disproved this. He was able to determine that only tiny amounts of entire molecules of protein can be absorbed by the body. In his own words:

> Human beings absorb only immeasurably small traces of entire protein. This absorption is nonetheless important, as it brings about the allergic reactions that many people have to certain foods.[39]

We thus see how a person guards against every foreign protein in order to maintain his biochemical individuality, which is actually our whole immune system.

Because of this and other recent findings, enlightened nutritionists now believe that we need only 0.47 grams of protein per kilogram of body weight.[40] This is less than half the previously accepted requirement. For the average person of 60 kilos this is equivalent to about 25 grams of protein a day. How is this translated in daily nutrition?

Meat is known to be about 20% to 30% protein, fish is about 20% to 26%, legumes about 20%, rice about 7%, and wheat between 12% and 15%. One who eats an average-sized fish of about 100 grams with one cup of rice already has too much protein for the day, considering that rice also contains protein.[41] The remaining two meals are therefore superfluous with regard to the daily protein requirement.

We eat too much protein today. This is the reason why allergies in the form of asthma, hay fever, or various skin rashes are prevalent. These conditions sooner or later develop into either gout, rheumatism, arthritis, or other illnesses, depending on how the allergic reactions were treated.

Taking in too much protein overburdens the digestive system to the point that the alien character of protein is only partially neutralized. When our biochemical individuality reacts to produce allergies, these reactions are often suppressed by orthodox treatments. Their continued suppression makes our immune system lose its ability to distinguish the toxic protein, or partially individualized protein, from the body's own. In time, excess protein and toxins accumulate in the body to produce gout and arthritis.

A worse consequence of too much protein intake is when the toxic protein or partially individualized protein in the body is used to replace the worn out protein of cells and tissues. The individual organ senses that the protein is not of its own kind and thus reacts with an inflammation. Here we have the phenomenon of the inflammation of internal organs such as endocarditis, nephritis, pancretitis, hepatitis, and all the other illnesses with "itis" attached to their names. Orthodox medicine's natural reaction is to suppress this with antibiotics. This could damage the organs concerned, or inhibit further reaction. Thus the body learns to stop reacting (anergy). As a result, the health of the whole organism is undermined, and a tendency towards chronic degenerative diseases begins to dominate.

The assimilation of partially individualized protein or toxins is due to faulty nutrition and digestion. We can now see two possible strategies to heal these diseases (e.g., allergies, asthma, arthritis, gout). One is to avoid protein, and the other is to improve digestion of protein. For those who are already showing signs of improper digestion of protein, it is better to initially refrain from eating protein-rich foods—refraining for at least a month will help our metabolic organs rest and recover from the stress of digesting such foods. The digestion can be further strengthened through the use of potentized remedies. Potentized remedies are better than other types of remedies for reasons which we will explain later.

Another error in the current understanding of protein is the belief that amino acids are its building blocks. This is only partially true. Orthodox science postulated this hypothesis after seeing only the body's activity of synthesizing the human protein beyond the intestinal walls. It failed to integrate the further finding that amino acids are the product of breakdown or decay. If one has no idea of the purpose of breaking down substances as we discussed earlier—that is, to rid the protein of its alien nature—then one will consider amino acids instead of whole proteins as basic building blocks of the body.

There is danger of poisoning every time protein is ingested, because it is the nature of protein to create putrefaction products in the intestines. This is what happens in flatulence. More toxins are released in the course of putrefaction. Since they are present in the intestines, the toxins may find their way into the bloodstream, leading to further poisoning. The life-force organization of the body must fight against this putrefaction. This is one of the functions of the liver. So long as the cause of putrefaction is present, that is, over-consumption of protein and/or weak digestive system, the danger of protein poisoning cannot be avoided. According to cancer researcher W. Zabel, in his article published in *Die Interne Krebstherapie* (The Therapy of Cancer), most cancer patients "do not die from their tumors, but from protein poisoning."[42]

There are other problems related to protein over-consumption. If we give children too much protein too soon, we are predisposing them to develop arteriosclerosis at an early age.[43] Research results reveal that the body deposits excess protein in the inner peripheral layer of the capillary vessels. Here, a degenerate mucus membrane protein, insoluble in water, is formed. Research by P. Schwarz, found in the *Deutsche Aertzeblatt* (1970), states that the accumulation of amyloid (a waxy fatty protein mixture) is "the most important cause and perhaps the determining factor of decline in old age, and especially of arterioslerosis."[44] Note that amyloid is a degenerate break-down product of protein.

Another side effect of excessive protein intake is overburdening of the kidney. The kidneys eliminate uric acid and urea in the blood stream. With too much uric acid in the body, the kidneys will be overworked and eventually fail.[45]

3. The Best Sources of Protein[46]

How can we avoid consuming more protein than the required amount? The answer is: by consuming as little protein as possible, but choosing only the best quality.

The best quality protein is plant protein, especially that which comes from flowers and fruits. Quantitatively they contain very little protein— only slightly over one percent—but it is of very high quality. More importantly, fruits and flowers stimulate the dynamics (vital forces) of human metabolism, primarily by means of their own inherent dynamic forces. For example, they help regulate the construction and destruction of proteins, detoxification, and the removal of deposits.[47] Moreover, the newly discovered chemical in plants, called *phytochemicals,* destroys tumor cells. The destruction of tumor cells (or neutralizing the sclerotic forces of the head system) is one of the main functions of a healthy metabolic system.

Grains are the second best source of protein, but they must be whole grains, not over-milled rice or flour. Please see the following subtopic on devitalized food.

The third best source is milk protein. It must naturally be fresh and unsterilized or enlivened, in the form of yogurt and other fermented milk products.[48] If one arranges the kinds of milk available in the market in a spectrum, the worst quality milk is condensed milk. Condensed milk has undergone a number of processing steps that make it practically denatured and devitalized. The best is unpasteurized, unhomogenized whole milk. It should, however, come from healthy animals, preferably fed with organically grown plant materials. Powdered milk falls somewhere in between. In other words, these milk varieties may have the same amount of protein, but their ability to help revitalize the body is not the same. The next sub-topic will elaborate the reason why this is so.

Another myth with regard to protein is that the brain needs it. Current studies have concluded that the brain fulfills its needs for energy solely from glucose. The brain does not need protein; it needs carbohydrates! (However, protein is important for the brain during its formative period, i.e., in the fetal stage and the first three years of life.)

Glucose is resynthesized in the liver as glycogen, and is stored there. This happens between 3 p.m. and 3 a.m. Between 3 a.m. and 3 p.m., the liver releases the glycogen into the blood as glucose, or human sugar. About 150 grams of glycogen are stored in the liver, of which the nerve-sense system, particularly the brain, needs about 120 grams for its thinking activity. The heart and lung muscles need about 30 to 40 grams, and also provide energy for our feeling life, while the metabolic system needs 40 grams, more or less, depending upon one's activity.

Consuming as little protein as possible may go against the grain of modern thinking. However, think of the newborn human being during the first year of life, who is actively building up his body and brain. Breast milk is only 1.5% to 2% protein, depending on the diet of the mother. In this critical year of life, a child can subsist on breast milk alone without succumbing to malnutrition or brain damage. One may question why nature (or our Creator) programmed human beings to consume very little protein at the time when they seem to need it most. Can nature (or God) be wrong? Orthodox science thinks so. This is the reason why formula milk was developed. Formula milk has more protein and minerals, and is enriched with vitamins. The whole attitude of science towards nature and natural processes is revealed here. The excessive protein and mineral consumption throughout life leads to early physical maturity, arterio-sclerosis, weakening of the kidneys, and other degenerative diseases.[49]

Furthermore, the key word in the whole discussion of nutrition is *diversity*. The more diverse our food sources are, the better we can be. We must be mindful enough to eat more kinds of grains other than wheat or rice (rye, buckwheat, corn, barley, and many more). Other than eating a variety of plants, we also need the different plant parts like roots, leaf and stem, flowers, and fruits and seeds. We should also be conscious about consuming food coming from different parts of the country, and even from other parts of the world. We should be planning our meals in such a way that this principle of diversity and variety is found in our meals, day after day, month after month.

4. Devitalized and Denatured Food

Orthodox nutritional science still uses calories to measure nutrition. The human being is equated to an automobile (a mechanism) that runs on gasoline (food), where the energy spent is measured in calories. Although there is some truth to this, we may miss the whole point of why we need nourishment if we think only in terms of calories.

When we eat, what is it that we really take in with the food? To understand this, we must have the following perspective.

Carbohydrates, proteins, and fats are called life substances. There is an important distinction between the *life* and the *substance*. When we ingest food, we also ingest the life which the substances carry. One may argue that the life is neutralized by the process of digestion. Yes, this is true, as we explained earlier. But the life force of the substances, which is neutralized by digestion, is released and stimulates our own formative force body. Thus the stronger the vitality of foods, the more our formative force body is stimulated. This assertion is supported by several studies, two of which I summarize below.

The first study was conducted among prematurely born babies divided into two groups. One group was fed sterilized breast milk, and the other raw breast milk.[50] Equal weight gains were achieved only when the energy quotient of the sterile milk taken in by the first group was 135 to 150 units, compared to 80 to 120 units consumed by those who were given raw milk. Moreover, the mortality rate of those fed with raw breast milk was lower. The babies who took sterilized breast milk had to be given more to make up for the quality that is lost in the process of sterilization. But even this did not fully compensate for the quality loss, as evidenced by the higher mortality among those who took sterilized breast milk.

What is lost in the sterilizing process? Given our understanding of the four-fold human being, it is not difficult to find the appropriate answer. The study clearly points to the reality that sterilization significantly diminishes the formative force even of breast milk. This diminished force in turn reduces its capacity to stimulate the formative force bodies of the infants.

The greater quantity consumed by the first group only approximated but did not equal the quality lost through sterilization.[51]

The second study was conducted among tribal people who had never experienced the cold diseases such as cancer, heart disease, and diabetes in their community. A number of them decided to live and work in the cities, and after some time found themselves developing the said diseases. In a study by Raymond Obomsawin, "Traditional Lifestyle and Freedom from the Dark Seas of Disease," published in *Community Development Journal* (1983), he pinpointed several factors which contributed to this trend.[52] They included eating highly refined and processed foods instead of their original diet of natural, fresh, fully organic, and sometimes wild-growing food; rejection of traditional medicine in favor of synthetic drugs; and finally the loss of the traditional values, outlook on life, and security provided by their rural community.

How are foods devitalized and their quality diminished? Let us first trace where the food is grown. Today's agricultural practices depreciate the vitality of plants, as we see in their susceptibility to diseases, pest infestation, and diminishment of variety (i.e., percentage of seed unable to germinate increases as one continues to plant the variety). The main causes of these problems are the use of inorganic fertilizers and other chemicals, and the continuous planting of crops in exhausted soil. Pesticide residue makes the plants more toxic to those who consume them.[53]

It is interesting to note the experience of farmers in Holland who grew tomatoes following the principle of hydroponics. The tomatoes are planted in sand inside greenhouses. They are watered with enough chemical compounds to ensure that they receive a "balanced" supply of "nutrients." But when they bear fruit, the tomatoes are tasteless compared to those planted in the soil. What is of even greater concern is the fact that when their seeds are planted, they do not germinate.[54] What is the significance of this? A plant that cannot reproduce itself does not have enough life in it. Only life can give life to life, a basic principle of reproduction. What cannot promote life is therefore a dead chemical substance.

Orthodox science has long predicted that the day will come when human beings will need only pills to nourish themselves. Astronauts tried this, but they returned home malnourished.[55]

Devitalization of food also results when rice is polished. The best protein to rebuild our tissues is found in the bran. This is given to animals, so they are healthier than human beings. The processes of bleaching and bromating are involved in making white flour. Bleaching further devitalizes the flour, while the chemical used in bromating has now been identified as a carcinogen.[56] The flouring process in itself is already devitalizing. Bleaching makes it practically denatured.

We can go on and on with the list of how our food is devitalized today. But what is more important is to find ways to bring back the quality of what we eat. We speak here of quality in terms of the life it can provide us with, not in terms of the number of calories it contains. Thus, biodynamic, or organically grown, or wild seasonal fruits and vegetables and other pesticide-free foods are the best. They have abundant vitality to stimulate our own life body and no pesticide residue that would poison our physical body. As much as possible, they should be consumed as soon as they are peeled, cooked, milled, or harvested.

We should also avoid foods that have been treated with chemical preservatives and artificial flavors and seasonings, such as monosodium glutamate, sodium benzoate, and the like.[57] We should avoid cooking in microwave ovens or pressure cookers.[58] They deplete the life forces of foods. We should also avoid using aluminum and Teflon pans because these materials are suspected to cause senility (or Alzheimer's disease) and cancer, respectively.[59]

Thus, one who understands nutrition also understands the genesis of today's diseases. Now we understand why Rudolf Steiner said that "one who understands nutrition correctly understands the beginning of healing," and how health can be improved and maintained.

C. CHILDBIRTH AND HOW THE CONSTITUTION OF THE FUTURE GENERATION IS REMODELED BY THE MILLIONS

In the preceding discussions, we tried to understand how we make our constitution predisposed and susceptible to health or illness. Even though we do inherit from our ancestors some predisposition to a certain illness, it does not automatically follow that we will contract it. The possibility exists of neutralizing this predisposition and preventing it from fully manifesting as a dreaded disease. With our expanded and updated knowledge, we can chart our lives in order to stay healthy. Moreover, if and when we get sick, we can enhance our ability to overcome the illness. I will elaborate more on this topic towards the end of this section.

Understanding the state of wellness and health are areas of research which orthodox medicine has neglected. This is another indication that orthodox scientists are still trapped in their present one-sidedness. Orthodox medicine, with its linear thinking—limited to seeing germs, DNA, and molecules—has lost sight of the whole human being. The sad part is that the whole world has been led to believe that germs and genes determine our destiny for health or illness. This book attempts to provide you with a different way of looking at these issues.

How else are we affecting the constitution of the current and future generations by our present beliefs and practices, which arise from the authoritarian proclamations of orthodox science?

The book *Magical Child*, by Joseph Chilton Pearce, is one of the most comprehensive analyses of today's child-rearing practices,[60] including the orthodox approach to childbirth. He challenges just about every notion we have about raising children in this so-called "modern" age. One of his main points is that orthodox medicine treats childbirth as a disease,[61] making it impossible for mothers to experience a normal physiological event—the climax of the experience of womanhood. The birth practices in today's hospitals may lead to post-natal hemorrhage,[62] inability to nurse, or a modern phenomenon called post-natal depression, to name a few negative effects. Worse, babies are on the losing end. One study Pearce cites was done by a research obstetrician, William F. Windle, MD:

> Dr. Windle became concerned about childbirth practices. He made a careful analysis of hospital deliveries throughout the United States and noted, with some alarm, two questionable procedures: the widespread, automatic use of premedication and anesthetics, and the unusual practice of cutting the umbilical cord as soon as the baby's body is clear.[63]

The administration of premedication and anesthesia affects both mother and infant. This impairs the mother's ability to push, unnecessarily prolonging the passage of the baby along the birth canal, and possibly requiring forceps to bring the baby out. A baby's inability to be awake upon birth and to breathe on his own (thus the need for resuscitation after birth) can also be traced to the administration of drugs.[64]

The supine position (which benefits the attending physician more than the mother) further hinders the mother from pushing her infant out properly, and cancels out the significant aid of gravity. Furthermore, this position may tilt back the gravid uterus against the pelvis, unnecessarily suppressing the blood vessels supplying the placenta with blood.

Clamping and cutting the umbilical cord too soon deprives the infant of much blood that is still in the cord itself, as well as in the placenta.[65] This and other common practices, Windle asserted, "can be a factor in exacerbating an incipient hypoxemia and can thus contribute to the danger of asphyxial brain damage." Brain damage at birth is the leading cause of mental retardation, with cerebral palsy as its extreme manifestation. Other lesser cases of suspected brain damage at birth result in a whole spectrum of learning disabilities, behavioral problems, and possibly a tendency to addiction. To apply what we have learned from the expanded image of the human being, the "I" or ego of the organism cannot fully incarnate in a defective brain. Learning disabilities or behavioral problems are mere symptoms of the ego's inability to dominate the lower bodies. Thus the baser passions, emotions, and temperament dominate the lives of these human beings.

Dr. Windle made a simple test to prove his point. He induced a condition in infant monkeys whereby they had to be artificially resuscitated at birth. He divided them into groups and subjected them to different periods of asphyxiation (from four to twenty-one minutes) before resuscitating them.

Those that underwent eight or more minutes of asphyxiation immediately showed signs of behavioral abnormalities. They could not walk on their four limbs and could not even cling to their mother, unlike their normal counterparts. Windle examined the brains of these monkeys and found lesions, or damage to the brain. Those who had a longer asphyxiated time died, in spite of mechanical assistance from oxygenated tents and other apparatus. The others eventually appeared normal after two to three weeks of medical assistance.

Windle then wanted to determine if any sign of damage remained even after the monkeys appeared to have grown normally. After three, six, twelve, and twenty-four months he examined each of the brains of the monkeys and found the same pattern of lesions. The damage to the brain was permanent.

Windle worked further (whenever possible) with autopsied deceased human infants who had known birth histories citing the use of anesthetics, low Apgar scoring,[66] premature cutting of the umbilical cord, and so on. His investigation showed that the brains of these infants harbored exactly the same lesions he found in the brains of his monkeys. He also studied three- and four-year olds who died and had similar birth histories, and found the same lesions in their brains. Dr. Windle concluded:

[Our experiments] have taught us that birth asphyxia lasting long enough to make resuscitation necessary *always damages the brain* (emphasis added)... A great many human infants have to be resuscitated at birth. We assume that their brains, too, have been damaged. There is reason to believe that the number of human beings in the US with minimal brain damage due to asphyxia at birth is much larger than has been thought. Need this continue to be so? Perhaps it is time to reexamine current practices of childbirth with a view to avoiding conditions that give rise to asphyxia.[67]

This is concrete proof of the weakening of the constitution of human beings on a massive scale. Orthodox medical science has again almost completely misunderstood the natural processes in childbirth and intervened counterproductively.[68] It has induced complications at birth, endangering the health and lives of mothers and infants. We have been unwitting accessories to this crime. We have succumbed to the threats of obstetricians (nocebo effect) regarding the pain and risk of childbirth.[69] This indoctrination of the parents takes place during the regular pre-natal check-ups.

Before the widespread use of hospitalization in childbirth, birth complications occurred in less than 5% of total births involved. Today, this rate has gone up to more than 15%. I can appreciate Dr. Mendelsohn's claim in his two other books, *Mal(e) Practice: How Doctors Manipulate Women* and *How to Raise a Healthy Child In Spite of Your Doctor*, that obstetrics and pediatrics are two professions that are superfluous in today's practice of medicine, if they continue to practice the way they do now. These professions can be renewed if physicians themselves adopt an expanded image of the human being and start perceiving an incarnating individuality, as described in Appendix 1 of this book.

D. SELF-INFLICTED NATURE OF DISEASES

Our look into the constitution of human beings, and their disposition and susceptibility to illness, leads us to conclude that the tendency to health or illness is always within us, and is man-made. All diseases have a self-inflicted nature. The way we think, feel,[70] and act affects our constitution for health or illness.[71] What we eat, how we eat,[72] and when we eat[73] have their repercussions which manifest in time. What we believe,[74] and what other people (like doctors and advertisements) lead us to believe, can affect our constitution for better or for worse.

For example, mothers condition their children to fear being wet with perspiration, or walking in the rain, or even a drizzle. The hysterical mother makes negative statements about this and suggests that the child may get sick. This prevents the development of the child's inner strength to resist the elements. A time comes when the child automatically gets sick after failing to instantly dry the perspiration or getting caught in the rain. While many may outgrow it when the "I" becomes capable of seeing through the folly, others retain it for the rest of their lives.

Adding support to this assertion is a study done by a research psychiatrist, Dr. Bennet Braun, on multiple-personality cases. He observed that when the patient's different personalities alternate, warts, scars, and rashes appear and disappear, along with hypertension and epilepsy. In adopting one personality, the patient can immediately become color-blind, but return to normal upon shifting to the next personality. One patient may not be allergic to orange juice when possessing a certain personality, but when the personality shifts—even while the orange juice is still being drunk—the new personality realizes it is allergic to it, and the allergic reaction is immediately evoked by this same individual.[75] The personalities have identified themselves with the particular diseases. They become sick because they need to be.

Similarly, many of our illnesses are actually self-inflicted. We over-work or over-relax ourselves into an illness. We anger or disappoint ourselves to death. We can also eat ourselves into an illness—we can develop diabetes or a heart ailment if we are not able to control our appetite for sweets or animal flesh.[76]

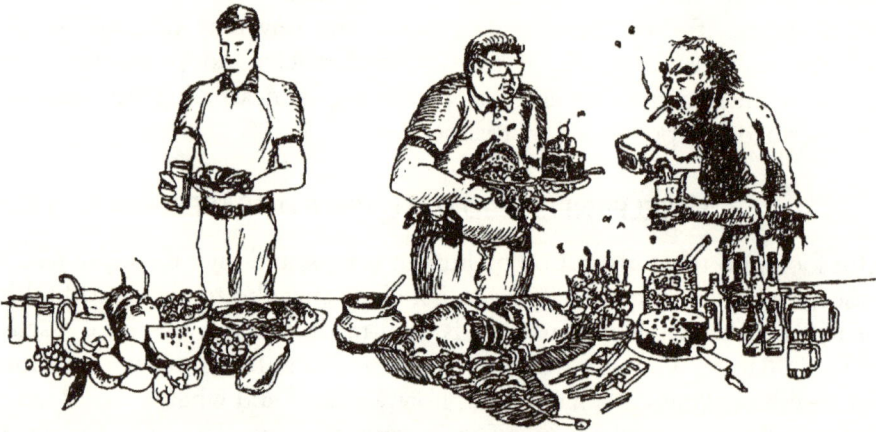

Almost always we tend to blame others for our misfortunes. In an illness, orthodox medical science conditions us to blame germs and our genes. When suffering becomes intense, we even blame God (or rationalize that it is our karma, whatever this may mean). After having read this book this far, I hope you will stop doing so, and instead take charge of your own life and accept the responsibility for all your actions. Ultimately, what is crucial in this earth life is how we confront and grapple with our troubles/illnesses, and how many insights we have gained from them.

E. THE MEANING OF ILLNESS

An illness can have multi-level meanings. On one level, illnesses (including childhood diseases) are like mathematical problems. The individual must learn to grapple with them on his own. Once the illness is overcome through natural means (the full effort of one's inner being), a capacity is born. The organism not only learns to tackle the same illness later, but a new aspect of his personality, character, or spiritual intention is able to be expressed. On another level, illnesses may be the effort of the incarnating child to remold the inherited physical body[77] into a body that can genuinely express the full intentions and purposes of the "I" or individuality on earth.[78] Illness may also be telling us to slow down, rest, or think things over. A good rest during an illness may provide one with a new perspective on life. Some may need to take a closer look at themselves, their lifestyle, attitudes, and beliefs. An illness may be telling us something that has been overlooked for a long time and which now needs some attention.

This brings us to another study involving four hundred cases of spontaneous remission of cancer. Elmer and Alyce Green of the Menninger Clinic in the United States pointed out that all the patients concerned had only one thing in common—they all changed their attitude before remission occurred, finding some new way to become hopeful, courageous, and positive.[79] There were also reported cases of spontaneous remission of cancer among members of tribal communities. After adopting an urban lifestyle, some developed cancer. When they returned to their rural home to die (readapting to their original culture and environment), they fully recovered after only a few months.[80]

This quest for meaning in illness is not found in orthodox medicine. As I pointed out earlier, meaning, mind, soul, and purpose are not quantifiable and therefore have no part in "scientific" medicine.[81] We are all conditioned by today's society to measure success and meaning using the amount of accumulated wealth as the gauge. Today, especially in the more affluent parts of the world, people possess wealth in abundance—beautiful cars, expensive houses, social security, and the like—but most still find themselves empty inside. Depression, mental diseases, and their consequent effects on constitution and disposition are reaching epidemic proportions.[82] Most of us have adapted this worldview and its tacit attitudes. The accompanying diseases cannot be far behind.

Sadly, the whole world has a one-track mind toward a mode of development that looks only at the economic aspects as its goal. All of us are continually being conditioned to think that progress means material success and development. There are, however, efforts and initiatives of non-governmental organizations (NGOs) and civil society organizations (CSOs) that try to counteract this trend.[83] Most of those involved in these groups have abandoned material pursuits as the basis of their life quest. They are working out the foundation for the new premises that would guide the reorganization of society. Some have shown concrete proofs that new thinking in economics, politics, agriculture, education, medicine, culture, and other fields of life is realizable. Nonetheless, far more people are required to spare time and resources in order to intensively and extensively address this reorientation and reorganization of society.[84]

F. MID-LIFE CRISIS, PURPOSE, AND THE MEANING OF LIFE

It is appropriate to discuss the phenomenon of mid-life crisis at this point.[85] During middle age, many of us are confronted with a certain uneasiness about life. Some are fortunate to be able to articulate this feeling into life questions such as: Who am I? Am I doing what I really should? What is the meaning of my work, my family situation? But for many people, this unsettled feeling remains unarticulated and could lead to depression and extreme emptiness. This feeling can take its toll on the entire family. Either spouse may take on another partner, or develop extramarital relationships in the hope that the uneasy feeling can be resolved by others. Some may attempt to overcome this feeling by re-living their youthful days, indulging in activities such as drinking and dancing.

Whence comes this feeling which leads to the mid-life crisis? One explanation lies in the fact that every individual or "I" incarnates in a specific place and time to perform deeds—deeds to gain experiences that are worthy of such a time; deeds that would change the world usually for the better and not for the worse; deeds that would mend or amend relationships with other people and the environment. If one's purpose in incarnating remains unfulfilled at the mid-point of life (which coincides with the beginning of the decline of physical prowess), an internal alarm is triggered to warn of an impending failure.

Those who choose to confront this crisis in full consciousness gain strength to undertake a search for meaning in their work by either accepting or changing (reinventing) their work situation, or seeking a spiritual path. Thus we witness certain individuals resigning from prestigious positions to take on new socially responsible careers and adjustments in their lifestyle. Some join a spiritual renewal movement or a meditation group in the hope of finding meaning in life. Still others affirm their materialistic and sensual pursuits. Each path has its own consequences for health or illness. On one hand, we often hear of miraculous healing taking place in an extra-religious celebration, or a blooming of the person's vitality. On the other hand, hard-line materialists may eventually develop the sclerotic, cold, and hardening diseases.[86]

For severe depression, the true remedy is not Valium, Prozac, or similar drugs. They are mere palliatives and make the situation worse by their cumulative effect. True healing will only be achieved if the individual goes through a quest for the meaning of his life—his real purpose for being on earth.[87] Being consistent with one's purpose in life is a strong healing force. To seek the meaning of one's life is in itself a healing process. But getting to the point of recognizing the emptiness in the soul is a long, drawn-out process for many people. This is where the individual will be met and tested by various situations in the form of illness, accidents,[88] or other difficulties which require confronting oneself and creatively working things out.[89] For many, the realization of emptiness comes only when it is filled with the meaning of these experiences. Thus, to leave meaning out would likewise be setting true healing aside.

It is safe to say then that *true healing is self-healing*. Doctors, family, and friends are there to mirror to us what we need to heal in ourselves, and in our environment—that is, to reflect back to us or affirm our intention or purpose in this lifetime. In this sense, *self-healing is also self-transformation*. Without transformation in one's habits, work, lifestyle, or attitudes, there can be no true healing.[90] There is a large kernel of truth in what Aristotle once said: "The self-indulgent man is of necessity unlikely to repent and therefore incurable, since a man who cannot repent cannot be cured."

On another level, self-healing can be enhanced if we are also involved in social reorganization and transformation. The environment we find ourselves in reflects and radiates the habits, lifestyle, attitudes, and beliefs that make us sick. Believing that we can remain healthy without changing our environment is another illusion we must eliminate.[91]

Notes

1   For example, Mann F. *Acupuncture: The Ancient Chinese Art of Healing.* London: William Heinemann Medical Books Ltd.; 1971; and Ulett GA. *Principles and Practice of Physiologic Acupuncture.* Warren Green Inc.; 1982.

2   At this point, it is important to distinguish anthroposophy from spiritual science. Spiritual science is the *methodology* for the study of the spiritual processes and phenomena in human life and in the universe, while anthroposophy is the *body of knowledge* or wisdom that arises out of spiritual science. Anthroposophy is a non-sectarian spirituality. Those who study it experience a fructification and greater understanding of their religions. Thus, among those who study anthroposophy are Buddhists, Muslims, Jews, Christians (Catholics, Protestants, Orthodox, and other sects), and many more. Anthroposophy provides a perspective to situate the teachings of the various religions and their role in the evolution of human consciousness.

3   Steiner education started in 1919 in Stuttgart, Germany. Today, there are over 800 Waldorf schools worldwide. There are more than a hundred books written on Waldorf education. For an overview of this pedagogical system see Childs G. *Steiner Education in Theory and Practice*. Edinburgh: Floris Books; 1991.

4   There are close to 600,000 hectares all over the world using this system of agriculture. In Europe, North America, Australia, and New Zealand the produce is marketed under the label Demeter. In the Philippines, Ikapati Farm pioneered biodynamic agriculture in 1988. After only three years, it became the largest producer of pesticide-free vegetables, servicing thousands of consumers in metro Manila. Another group, Don Bosco Sustainable Development Foundation in Mindanao, is currently servicing close to three thousand hectares of farmland with an equal number of farmers. For an overview of biodynamic agriculture see Koepf H et al. *Bio Dynamic Agriculture*. Spring Valley, New York: Anthroposophic Press Inc.; 1976.

5   There are now close to a hundred communities in more than fifteen countries that are following Steiner's indication for handicapped children. For many parents who have felt rejected by society and at times burdened by having a child with a handicap, the experiences of the Camphill movement give a heartwarming message. There are many books written about this special pedagogy. For an overview see Hansmann H. *Education for Special Needs: Principles and Practice in Camphill Schools*. Edinburgh: Floris Books; 1992.

6   For an overview of Steiner's architectural impulse see Bresantz H, Klingborg A. The *Goetheanum: Rudolf Steiner's Architectural Impulse*. London: Rudolf Steiner Press; 1979.

7   See Steiner R. *The Arts and Their Mission*. Spring Valley, New York: Anthroposophic Press; 1964.

8   This new form of movement particularly stimulates the formative force, or life body. Through definite gestures of and around the life body, eurythmy activates healing and strengthens and regulates the forces right down to the physical body. How is this possible? Our capacity to speak results from the joint action of the speech organ and

the life body. One can observe how the strength of a sick person's speech diminishes. Steiner's research showed that in this joint action, rhythmical movements occur when we speak. Thus in speech eurythmy, the movement reveals the rhythmical gestures which are concealed in living languages and activates healing. This finding also paved the way for the inclusion of speech in therapy. See Steiner R. *A Lecture in Eurythmy.* London: Rudolf Steiner Press; 1967.

9   The logical-analytical capacity of thinking includes the ability to integrate and synthesize into a whole that which has been separated and analyzed through our perceiving. The science of neurophysiology refers to this as the full use of our brain's left and right hemispheres. However, the willful thinking with the heart advocated in this book involves thinking with the whole body (thinking, feeling, and willing) and therefore it activates, integrates, and brings coherence to the whole of the brain.

10 A common belief of orthodox science is that our ancestors learned the use of medicinal plants through trial and error. However, more recent anthropological findings reveal that shamans or "witch doctors" gain their wisdom through apprenticeship training—a procedure that ensures the proper understanding of healing. During the training, the apprentice is guided to reach a higher state of consciousness that enables him to communicate to spiritual beings who possess knowledge of particular plants or treatments for a particular illness. This was personally communicated by Robert Kasberg during a visit to the Hanunuo Mangyan community. See also Hungry Wolf A. *The Good Medicine Book.* Warner Communications Company, 1973. This book describes how American Indians learn their medicines. See also Castaneda C. *The Teachings of Don Juan: A Yaqui Way of Knowledge.* New York: Pocket Books; 1971.

11 This new technology is called "cryogenic charge-coupled device (CCD) camera." The intensity of the light emitted by the body is 1000 times lower than the sensitivity of our naked eyes. See *sciencelinks.jp/j-east/article/.../000020000599A1042823.php.* Today, the acupuncture points are measured using an electromagnetic field device. The biophotons, just like the electromagnetic field, are physical expression of the light or energy emitted by our life body.

12 Ritcher G. *Art and Human Consciousness.* Spring Valley, New York: Anthroposophical Press; 1985. Art is the process of making something (invisible) visible. The history of art then can be the expression of the innermost biography of humanity. Richter went through the various art forms found in the different periods of human history and discerned how the people of those periods were expressing their corresponding changes in consciousness.

13 Imagination, inspiration, and intuition are described by Steiner as the states of higher

human consciousness through which the "I" (or ego) can perceive the three levels of the supersensible or spiritual world—namely, the etheric-astral, the lower devachan, and the higher devachan. The meanings of these terms should not be confused with their everyday use. Steiner very specifically characterized each of them. For a thorough discussion of these states of higher cognition, please see Steiner's *Knowledge of Higher Worlds and Its Attainment.*

14 For the anthroposophic view of the evolution of the earth, humanity, and the cosmos, see Steiner R. *An Outline of Esoteric Science.* Spring Valley, New York: Anthroposophic Press Inc; 1972.

15 The pioneering book in nutrition was written by Rudolf Hauschka (*Nutrition.* London: Rudolf Steiner Press; 1967).

16 Steiner's best work in epistemology is found in his book *Philosophy of Spiritual Activity: Basic Features of a Modern World View.* New York: Anthroposophic Press; 1986.

17 After describing and elaborating the various aspects of the soul in books and lectures, Rudolf Steiner's indication for psychology was pursued further by his pupils. For some samples see Treichler R. *Soulways: The Developing Soul-Life Phases, Thresholds and Biography.* Hawthorn Press; 1989; and Lievegoed B. *Phases: Crisis and Development in the Individual.* London: Rudolf Steiner Press; 1979. Sardello R. *Freeing the Soul from Fear.* New York: Riverhead Books; 2001; and Sardello R. *The Power of the Soul: Living the Twelve Virtues.* Charlottesville, Va: Hampton Roads Publishing; 2002.

18 For a sample of an enriched approach to natural science see Schad W. *Man and Mammals: Towards a Biology of Form.* New York: The Waldorf Press; 1977.

19 See Steiner R. *Towards Social Renewal: Basic Issues of the Social Question.* Smith FT, trans. London: Rudolf Steiner Press; 1977.

20 The other initiatives are on organizational development, ethical banking, and rural development. See also Davy J. *Work Arising from the Life of Rudolf Steiner.* London: Rudolf Steiner Press; 1975.

21 Steiner R. *Goethe the Scientist: A Theory of Knowledge Implicit in Goethe's World Conception.* Spring Valley, New York: Anthroposophic Press; 1986.

22 Steiner R. *Spiritual Science and Medicine.* London: Rudolf Steiner Press; 1948.

23 I have read many writings by clairvoyants attempting to communicate their insights to the public. Besides my Benedictine school training, I have gone into hypnotism, Buddhism, traditional Jewish Kaballah, ritual magic, mediumism, various forms of healing in the Philippines, and Alice Bailey's Tibetan Master's revelations. From them, I have learned to open myself to the idea of the spirit and the possibility to know it.

After reading Rudolf Steiner's spiritual research, which I consider to be much more thorough, consistent, and coherent, works of other clairvoyants seem limited and focused only on certain facets of life. Steiner, on the other hand, delves into specific topics but at the same time did not lose his overall perspective. His insights can be concretized into practical activities which lead towards self- and social transformation. Being involved in the work for social transformation since 1970 during my student activism days, I find this aspect of Steiner's work most appealing.

24 Quoted in King F. *Rudolf Steiner and Holistic Medicine.* Maine: Nicolas-Hays Inc.; 1986:15.

25 At this point, I would like to caution the reader that the following discussion may demand a little more patience and imagination to understand the meaning behind the words. I suggest that you read through the rest of the section first before making a judgment of its parts.

26 From here on the description given is based on my own understanding and synthesis of the subject. They have been discussed in almost all of the books on anthroposophy written by Steiner or by others who articulate anthroposophy through medicine, art, education, and other disciplines. This indicates how Steiner's framework or system of thinking is so well integrated, coherent, and consistent, such that it can be applied in almost any field of life.

27 Alternative health practitioners in the US call this "body" ELF, or extremely low-frequency electromagnetic field. Like a magnet, its field is revealed when one scatters iron filings on a paper and underneath the paper one places a magnet. The iron filings align in a particular way. Similarly, the way the minerals are made to align to produce the human form is like a field created by the north and south poles of a magnet.

28 See *www.plosone.org/.../info:doi%2F10.1371%2Fjournal.pone.0006256.* These scientists have photographed the light that is emitted by a human body. This light is not visible to the normal human eye. However, this is still not what I mean by the "astral body." The light I mean here is more akin to our inner light of consciousness, as it is visible to someone who can see with the spiritual eyes.

29 The negative effects of this one-sided development can no longer be ignored. One of the main factors that bring about this one-sidedness is today's education. The major issue is early intellectualization (nerve sense system) at the expense of both the willing (metabolic/limb system) and the feeling life (rhythmic system). In Waldorf education, the specific curriculum and method at each grade level ensures harmonious and integrated development of the child's aesthetic feeling life, intellect, and will. This holistic development has a tremendous impact on the constitution and disposition to health or illness. For example, the obsessive-compulsive behavior of modern youth is a result of an unbalanced development in childhood. The will does something

(compulsion) and clings to it (obsession) without the head being fully conscious of it. The reverse can also happen. The young adult who is obsessed with something will do anything, even resort to force and violence, to acquire it (irrationality). The middle system that has definitely been paralyzed is unable to link or balance the two other systems together.

These negative effects can be redeemed by nurturing the spiritual "I." Please see the succeeding discussion in Section 1, Chapter 4: *Harnessing the Power of the Spiritual "I."* But as a preventive measure (medicine) for a better future and a better society, a balanced, good quality education and upbringing of children must be an important concern in social transformation. See Appendix 1 for a more extensive discussion of this matter.

30 Husemann F, Wolff O. *The Anthroposophical Approach to Medicine* (3 vols). Anthroposophical Press Inc.; vol 1:187-189.

31 After researching the arguments against immunization, I consciously decided not to let my two children be immunized, but rather to face the disease if it comes. My position vis-a-vis the immunization program of the government is that parents must be informed of all the possible effects of immunization—meaning its alleged benefits as well as risks and dangers. Moreover, emphasis must be given to the importance of proper nutrition; adequate and appropriate time to sleep; emotional, psychological, and spiritual security; and sanitation and hygiene in strengthening the general vitality of the child. For studies on the adverse effects of immunization see Benjamin CM et al. Joint and limb symptoms in children after immunization with measles, mumps and rubella vaccines. *British Medical Journal* 1992(April);304:1075-1078; Miller E et al. Risk of asceptic meningitis after measles, mumps and rubella vaccines in UK children. *Lancet* 1993(April);341:979-981; Hall A. Lessons from measles vaccination in developing countries. *British Medical Journal* 1993(November);307:1294-1295 ("Vaccination should be introduced only after rigorous trials with mortality as an end product..."); Herroben L et al. Central nervous system demyelination after immunization with recombinant hepatitis B vaccine. *Lancet* 1991(November;338:1174-1175; Garenne M et al. Child mortality after high titre measle vaccine: prospect study in Senegal. *Lancet* 1991(October);338:903-907 ("Higher risk death in the two high titre vaccine groups remain significant"); Hassan W, Oldham R. Reiter's syndrome and reactive arthritis in health care workers after vaccination. *British Medical Journal* 1994(July);309:94.

Moreover, some vaccines are not even effective, i.e., they do not confer immunity and unnecessarily expose the healthy individual to their adverse effects. See Sutter RW et al. Outbreak of paralytic poliomyelitis in Oman: evidence for widespread transmission among fully vaccinated children. *Lancet* 1991(September);338:715-720 (This study cites recent outbreaks in Gambia, Brazil, and Taiwan and points to the ineffectivity of oral polio vaccine); van Niekerk ABW et al. Outbreak of poliomyelitis in Namibia. *Lancet* 1994(July);344:661-664; Ponninghaus JM et al. Efficacy of BCG against leprosy and tuberculosis in Northern Malawi. *Lancet* 1992(March);339;636-639 ("there was no statistical significant protection by BCG against tuberculosis in this population"); Typhoid vaccines: weighing the option. *Lancet* 1992(August);340:341-342 ("...that of three available vaccines, none has proven any ability to confer protection against typhoid"); Christie CDC et al The 1993 epidemic of pertusis in Cincinnati: resurgence of disease in a highly immunized population of children. *New England Journal of Medicine* 1994;33:16-21; Hersh BS et al. A measle outbreak at a college with prematriculation immunization requirement. *American Journal of Public Health* 1991;81:360-364; Gustafson TL et al. Measle outbreak in a fully immunized secondary-school population. *New England Journal of Medicine* 1987;316:771-774.

I could cite more studies on epidemics affecting fully immunized children but that would take perhaps another volume. Why is this happening? Is it time to question the herd theory (scientists think humans are mere herds of animals) behind immunization itself? What is the real meaning of natural human immunity? (See note 77 for some indications of the meaning of natural immunization.) Orthodox medical science's greatest mistake is to believe that vaccination and medical intervention were responsible for the decline of infectious diseases, even though the statistical evidence says otherwise. As mentioned in the Introduction, the studies done by John and Sonja McKinley (McKinley J, McKinley S. The questionable contribution of medical measures to the decline of mortality in the United States in the twentieth century. *Milbank Memorial Fund* 1977;405-430) and T. McKeown (McKeown T. *The Role of Medicine: Dream, Mirage, or Nemesis*. Princeton, New Jersey: Princeton University Press; 1979) with data coming from England and Wales, are very revealing: the death rates from all diseases were already in decline when medical interventions like vaccines or drugs were introduced to control the diseases.

More recently, Robert F. Kennedy, Jr., exposed and pointed to the thimerosal (a preservative containing mercury) in the vaccine as the possible culprit in the sharp rise of autism, ADHD, and other neurological disorders in children. You can download his article "Deadly Immunity" from *www.salon.com*. A website dedicated to the education of parents on this matter is *www.thinktwice.com*. For a more comprehensive discussion on immunization please see Murphy J. *What Every Parent Should Know About Childhood Immunization*. Boston: Earth Healing Products; 1994.

32 Other examples of illnesses in inflammatory stage if suppressed by chemical drugs are the following: eczema can become asthma, liver damage, angina pectoris, hypertension, pylorospasmus, or cancer; flu can emerge sooner or later as nephritis, pleuritis, gastric ulcer, asthma, liver damage, psychosis, or endocarditis; ulcus cruris can become Hodgkin's disease; gonorrhea becomes sarcoma; furuncle transforms into diabetes; suppressed menstruation into sciatica. For degenerative diseases that have been

reversed by homotoxic detoxification therapy, Hans-Heinrich Reckeweg's research revealed the following: hypertension can lead to carbuncle inflammation; sciatica to diarrhea; uteri cancer to phlebitis; catatony to flu; dorsal tabes paralysis to malaria; sarcoma to sepsis; most cancers may turn into erysipelas, gall bladder pistula, malaria, and other inflammatory conditions; breast cancer into cellulitis; and many more. Once the toxins are in the skin or are excreted by the body—for example in the sputum—this German scientist and his cohorts made chemical analysis of the toxin, and the analysis revealed that the original toxin came from the suppressed inflammatory illnesses. I suggest you read this book: Reckeweg Hans-Heinrich. *Homotoxicology: Illness and Healing Through Anti-homotoxic Therapy.* Albuquerque, NM: Menaco Publishing Company; 1980. You will need it to guide you in the processes of healing your degenerative conditions if and when you develop a healing crisis.

33 Heidemann C. Meridien Therapie: Die Wiederherstellung der Ordnung Lebendiger Prozesse (Bands 2 and 3). Unveranderte Auflage; 1988. See also *www. meridiaankleurentherapie.nl/pags/info*

34 Schindler M. *Goethe's Theory of Colour.* Sussex: New Knowledge Books; 1964. Just type *Goethe's theory of color* in your internet search engine for more information.

35 Mendelsohn R. *Mal(e) Practice: How Doctors Manipulate Women*, pp 131-132. The lack of understanding of the significant role of nutrition on health is reflected in the way food is served in hospitals. Patients who are supposed to avoid fats are served oily foods, or those with diabetes, sugary foods. The latest call to recognize nutrition in healing comes from Garrow J. *Starvation in Hospitals*, p 934; and Mc Whirter J et al. Incidence and recognition of malnutrition in hospitals. *British Medical Journal* 1994(February);308:945-948. They reiterated that nutrition is given too little attention by doctors, nurses, and managers. They also highlighted the need for education on clinical nutrition.

36 Quoted in Schmidt G. *Dynamic of Nutrition.* Wyoming, Rhode Island: Biodynamic Literature; 1980:24.

37 Ibid, p 32. See also Husemann F, Wolff O. *The Anthroposophical Approach to Medicine* (3 vols). New York: Anthroposophical Press Inc.; vol 1:209-301.

38 I cannot go into a discussion on the role of fat in nutrition in the main text. To help you evaluate fats, consider the chart at the end of this footnote. (There are two types of fatty acids: saturated and unsaturated.) It seems that from the data in the chart that the consumption of more saturated fatty acids in a predominantly meat diet may lead to early sclerosis or even cancer. A 12-year study has indicated that those with high intake of vegetables, fruits, cereals, pulses, and nuts (i.e., a minimum of saturated fats and a relatively high amount of unsaturated fats) are 40% less likely to die of heart

disease and cancer. See Thorogood M et al. Risk of death from cancer and Ischaemic heart disease in meat and non-meat eaters. *British Medical Journal* 1994(June);308:1667-1670. A National Cancer Institute study revealed that those who consume 15% or more saturated fat are about six times more likely to develop lung cancer than those whose meals have 10% or less fat. See Fat diet raises risk of lung cancer among non-smokers, study says. *The Philippine Star*, July 2, 1994; Hunter D. Breast cancer: nutritional factors. *Lancet* 1992(October);340:905; Otani H et al. Long term effects of a cholesterol free diet on serum cholesterol levels of Zen monks. *New England Journal of Medicine* 1992(February);326:416; Lee HP et al. Dietary effects of breast cancer risk in Singapore. *Lancet* 1991(May);337:1197-2000. Soya products are rich in phyto-oestrogen and may protect against breast cancer in younger women.

Saturated	Unsaturated
33% of fat in body	67% of fat in body
Found mainly in the nerves sense system	Found mainly in the metabolic system
More intense connection with carbon e.g., stearic acid C18 H36 O2	More intensive connection with hydrogen (good for warmth dev't), e.g., oleic acid C16 H34 O2
Tendency towards rigidity, fixation, hardening, and sclerosis	Tendency towards warmth and inflammation
High melting point, e.g., 69.6 C stearic acid	Low melting point, e.g., 2 C olive oil
Predominant in animals	Predominant in plants

39 Quoted in Schmidt G. *Dynamics of Nutrition*. Wyoming, Rhode Island: Biodynamic Literature;1980:50.

40 Lappe FM. *Diet for a Small Planet*. New York: Ballantine Books;1975:72. An amount of 0.47 grams of protein per kilogram body weight may still be too much, according to Rudolf Steiner. He warns us that "The greatest imaginable care must be taken, that neither too little nor too much protein is taken into the body. Just the right amount absolutely must be found." Proteins in the digestion correspond to the production of mental pictures in the thought activity. If we burden our metabolic system with consumption of too much protein, the higher activities "which make for effective thinking" will correspondingly suffer. Quoted in Schmidt G. *Dynamics of Nutrition*. Wyoming, Rhode Island: Biodynamic Literature;1980:53.

41 This is a simplified example. Modern nutritionists talk about the net protein utilization (NPU) of every food, meaning even though meat has 20% protein its NPU is only 67%; soy beans and whole rice approach the NPU of meat. The highest NPU yields among the different sources of protein are milk (82%), eggs (94%), and fish (80%). If you wish to follow this theory of protein utilization and the combination of plant proteins to fulfill the daily requirements of ingesting the so-called 8 essential amino acids (the amino acid which nutritionist believe the human body cannot produce) please see Lappe FM. *Diet for a Small Planet.* New York: Ballantine Books;1980. Another view of protein is called the "amino acid pool." From the digestion of food and from the recycling of proteinaceous waste, the body has all the different amino acids circulating in the blood and lymph. The liver and cells are continually making deposits and withdrawals of amino acids, depending upon the concentration of amino acids in the blood. Thus we do not need to ingest all the 8 essential amino acids every day, contrary to today's nutritional gospel. Moreover, most fruits and vegetables (though only about 1% protein) have all the 8 essential amino acids human beings need. This is one reason why fruitarians do not succumb to lack of protein. For more discussion on the protein pool see Diamond H, Diamond M. *Fit For Life.* New York: Warner Books;1985:88-101. Type *amino acid pool* in your internet search engine. However, anthroposophical nutritionists have another idea of how we nourish ourselves, as will be discussed in the succeeding pages. This is more related to the formative forces behind food—how they stimulate our protein-forming forces in our metabolic system, and the effect of protein on the production of mental pictures in the thought activity, as stated in the previous note.

42 Op cit; quoted in Schmidt G. *Dynamics of Nutrition.* Wyoming, Rhode Island: Biodynamic Literature;1980:93.

43 Children's bodily organs for digestion are still young and unable to properly digest protein (the way adults do), especially protein coming from animals. If your child is showing signs of improper digestion of protein such as eczema, asthma, and various forms of allergic reaction, please remove animal protein from the diet (to let the organs rest) and redirect the child's diet to more plant-based sources. Among the vegetables, we should avoid giving children eggplant, unripe tomatoes, okra, potatoes, and pepper. They come from the nightshade family and have a toxin called solanin. Children and adults with problems in protein digestion (arthritis and gout) should avoid these vegetables.

44 Ibid, p 92. The amyloid degenerate protein is being suspected for other denegerative diseases. See Yankner BA. B Amyloid and the pathogenesis of Alzheimer disease. *New England Journal of Medicine* 1991;325:1849-1857. Other degenerated protein is responsible for new diseases. See Pablos-Mendez A et al. Infectious prions or cytotoxic

metabolites? *Lancet* 1993 (January);341:159-161. Prions are protein structures devoid of nucleic acids and are the cause of a new class of diseases. This study opines that prions are "toxic proteins that accumulate (rather than replicate) by deranging the normal processing of a metabolite in the central nervous system." How do they accumulate? By having too much protein in the diet and our interweaving bodies are not able to handle them. They concluded that "the host, more so than the inoculum, seems to determine the form of the toxic product." See also Solomon A et al. Nephrotoxic potential of Bence Jones proteins. *New England Journal of Medicine* 1991 (June);324:1845-1851. See Wikipedia by just typing *amyloid protein*.

45 For a more recent study about excess protein and its toxic effect on the kidney, Combe C, Aparicio M. Body building, high protein diet and progressive renal failures in chronic glomerulonephritis. *Lancet* 1993 (Februrary);341:380; High protein diet may promote kidney cancer. *The Philippine Star.* August 4, 1994:21. The report was based on a study published in the *Journal of the National Cancer Institute*, August 3, 1994.

46 The current theory on protein in nutrition science says that among the many amino acids that constitute whole proteins, a minimum of 8 amino acids are not produced by the human organism, and thus they should come from animals or a combination of plant protein. I used to subscribe to this way of thinking until I encountered studies and first-hand accounts of people who ate just fruits for more than 10 years and did not succumb to protein deficiency. Please type in your internet search engine *fruitarian nutrition* and *raw food vegans* and you will find a small but significant number of people subscribing to these diets. Others do not even have to eat at all. See Jasmuheen. *Living on Light: the Source of Nourishment for the New Millenium.* Koha Publishing; 1997. Certain individuals have developed themselves to the point that their only intake is water, and they do not need any solid food at all to remain alive and well—they rely on sunlight, our primary form of energy. Wouldn't you be curious as to how they can maintain being healthy? Are there ways to maintain our physical health other than taking food? This is what science should be investigating as a research question so we can learn from them.

47 *Newsweek,* April 25, 1994, reported the discoveries of phytochemicals found in fruits and vegetables. Phytochemicals detoxify cancer-causing chemicals. This verifies Steiner's own findings through spiritual research 80 years ago.

48 As a word of caution, David Rowland, author of *Milk - Healthy or Hazardous* (see *rowlandpub.com*) revealed that most human beings are actually lactose intolerant. Normal human beings stop producing lactase after the first year of life. Allergies to cow's milk protein are often overlooked by doctors. Vomiting, diarrhea, runny nose, nasal congestion, excessive mucus, bronchial infection, asthma, ear infections, dermatitis, eczema, hives, pallor, gastrointestinal tract problems, insomnia, headache,

tension, fatigue, hyperactivity, and bed-wetting are all symptoms of cow's milk allergies. Milk companies have been successful (through their half-truth advertising) in making most people of the world drink milk. Thus, we have an ongoing epidemic of diseases, especially among children, connected to over-consumption of milk. In suggesting that milk is the third best source of protein, I do not mean to recommend consuming it by the liter a day. Small quantities will be enough, eaten together with other foods. Moreover, it should be from healthy cows eating grass grown organically, and unpasteurized and unhomogenized.

49 Recent studies indicate that the difference between breast-fed and infant formula-fed children is more significant than is currently believed. The first is Farquharson, Cockburn F et al. Infant cerebral cortex phospolipids fatty acid composition and diet. *Lancet* 1992;340:810-813. Their investigation revealed that infants fed with infant formula develop a brain with a different composition of cortex gray matter. They traced this to the lower amounts of unsaturated fatty acids in cow's milk. The second study (Pisacane A, Impagliazzo N et al. Breast feeding and multiple sclerosis. *British Medical Journal* 1994(May);308:1411-14122) followed the lead of the first one. The authors studied 300 cases of multiple sclerosis (MS), and their "data indicated that patients with multiple sclerosis were less likely than controls to have been breast-fed for a prolonged period of time." Several reasons were put forward why prolonged breast-feeding may be associated with a decreased risk of MS. MS is the accelerated degradation of the myelin sheath (a membrane supplying nutrients to nerve cells in the brain). In the first year of life, a child's brain is still developing and diet is most important. Thus the different composition of cortex gray matter of those fed with infant formula facilitated the entry of an infective agent across the blood-brain barrier and accelerates the degradation of the myelin itself. Just type *multiple sclerosis and infant formula* in your internet search engine to read more studies on this.

50 Husemann F, Wolff O. *The Anthroposophical Approach to Medicine* (3 vols). Anthroposophical Press Inc.; vol 3:95. Studies reveal that exclusive formula-fed preterm babies tend to develop neocrotising enterocolitis 6 to 10 times more than breast-fed infants, while breast milk has a beneficial effect on neurodevelopment. See Lucas A, Cole TJ. Breast milk and neonatal necrotising enterocolitis. *Lancet* 1990(December);336:1519-1523; Lucas A et al. Breast milk and subsequent intelligence quotient in children born preterm. *Lancet* 1992(February);339:261-264.

51 Orthodox science explains this phenomenon by stating that sterilization destroys the essential vitamins in the milk. This reveals the essential character of vitamins as carriers of formative forces. If this is the case, then vitamins cannot be captured in a chemical retort nor synthesized! However, orthodox science has conditioned us to think that there is no significant difference between the synthetic vitamins and those

which fruits and vegetables contain. This may be another illusion. See Schmidt G. The so-called vitamins: the necessity of correcting our current viewpoint. In *Dynamics of Nutrition*. Wyoming, Rhode Island: Biodynamic Literature; 1987:275 281.

52 Obomsawin R. Traditional life style and freedom from the dark seas of disease. *Community Development Journal* 1983(18, issue 2).

53 Those who are not convinced that pesticides can harm the body would have probably stopped reading this book by now. I purposely did not discuss this subject in the main text for obvious reasons. (A common attitude among people these days is not to believe until they see or directly experience, rather than critically learn or know that the effects of these chemicals are cumulative, that is, it may take some time for the full impact to be felt). The recent banning of a number of pesticides by the US Food and Drug Administration was due in part to the adverse effects on the users and the residual effect to the consumers. In any case, those who still need to be fully convinced should see Davis DLF, Blair A, Hoel DG. Agricultural exposure and cancer trends in developed countries. *Environmental Health Perspectives* 1992. They have noted that agricultural chemicals have been linked to increased mortality for melanoma, multiple myeloma, non-Hodgkin's lymphoma; and breast, prostate, brain, and kidney cancers. Wilkensen CF. In Wilkinson CF, ed. *Insecticide Interaction in Insecticide Biochemistry and Physiology*. New York: Plenum Press: 1976. "Chemicals appear to have synergistic effects... The induction or stimulation of mixed function oxidases can enhance or inhibit metabolism and, depending on whether the metabolic product or the precursor is the active agent, decreases or increases toxicity." Quoted in Kilbrun KH. *Epidemics Then and Now: Chemicals Replace Microbes and Degeneration Oust Infection*. p 4; Carpenter L. Cancer in laboratory workers. *Lancet* 1991(October);338:1080-1081; Saracci R et al. Cancer mortality in workers exposed to chlorophenoxy: herbicides and chlorophenols. *Lancet* 1991(October);338:1027-1032; Breast Cancer Collaborative Group. Breast cancer: environmental factors. *Lancet* (October);340:904. Frances Moore Lappe (in *Diet for a Small Planet*, pp. 31-35) warns that foods of animal origin continue to be a major source of chlorinated organic pesticide residue in the diet due to bioaccumulation. Worse, meat, poultry, or pork may have residue of chemical drugs. She recommends eating low in the food chain. Just type *pesticides and health* in your internet search engine.

54 Narrated to the author by a colleague at the training in the WALA Heilmittel GMBH, Ekwaelden, Germany, April to October 1992.

55 Taken from the Seminar on Anthroposophic Medicine attended by the author on October 15 to November 14, 1992, in Arlesheim, Switzerland.

56 Ban on flour improver hailed. *Bulletin Today*. February 8, 1994:B19.

57 Chemical food additives contain free radicals. Free radicals can penetrate into the

DNA of a cell and change its "blueprint," resulting in altered cells. The mutated cells are the main factor in the formation of the composite substance known as plaque. Plaque is deposited in the arterial walls and is the major cause of arteriosclerosis. For a more detailed discussion see Rowland D. *Vascular Cleansing: A New Hope for Heart Disease.* Uxbridge, Ontario: Canadian Nutrition Institution Inc.; 1986:L9p, 1T2; and Halliwell B. Free radicals and vascular disease: how much do we know. *British Medical Journal* 1993(October);307:885-886. See also Hans Reckeweg (in *Homotoxicology,* p. 124) for a discussion on the mutation of cells due to the use of chemical drugs.

58 A study conducted in Germany, reported by a class teacher in Heidenheim Waldorf School while my wife was there for observation and training in Waldorf education from April to June 1991. Mice fed with food cooked from microwave ovens resulted in deformed offspring at the third generation.

59 Birchall JD, Chappell JS. Aluminum, chemical physiology and Alzheimer's disease. *Lancet* 1988(October);1008-1010; Neri LC. Aluminum, Alzheimer's Disease and drinking water. *Lancet* 1991(August);337:390; Dudley N. *Good Health on a Polluted Planet.* London: Thorsons; 1991:71. This is one of first comprehensive guides to environmental hazards, with over 80 entries conveniently divided into food and drink, home and office, outdoor hazards, pesticides, transport, and other hazards. Another book, by Jennifer Meek, is *Sick Earth Syndrome and How to Survive It.* London: Optima Book;1992.

60 An example is when parents minimize direct contact with their offspring through the use of the crib. Pearce cited several studies to illustrate that our current way of child rearing is inimical to the child's development of intelligence. The most startling evidence is a study done by Marcelle Geber: Geber M. The psycho-motor development of African children in the first year, and the influence of maternal behavior. *Journal of Social Psychology* 1958;47:185-195. She studied children in Kampala, and Dakar, Uganda, and found them to be more advanced in their psychomotor and intelligence development than the European children.

   Ms. Geber hypothesized that the attitude of mothers towards children seems to be largely responsible for the differences. The arrival of a baby is not a source of anxiety for the future, but rather is always looked forward to with great pleasure. "Before the child is weaned, the mother's whole interest is centered on him. She never leaves him, carries him on her back—often skin-to-skin contact—wherever she goes, sleeps with him, feeds him on demand at all hours of the day and night, forbids him nothing, and never chides him. He lives in complete satisfaction and security, always under her protection. He is, moreover, continually being stimulated by seeing her at her various occupations and hearing her interminable conversations, and because he is always with her, his world is relatively extensive... Weaning makes a sudden change in the child's life. The mother does not only stop giving him the breast, but oftentimes behaves as though she is deliberately trying to effect a separation... Sometimes the separation is geographical, with the child sent for many months to his grandparents and seldom visited... Children for whom weaning had not caused a sudden break in the way of life retained their liveliness after weaning, and developed without interruption."

The table below gives the comparison.

Activity/Description	African Children within...	European Children after...
1. Can be drawn up in a sitting position, back straight and able to prevent head from falling backwards	9 hours	6 weeks
2. Able to focus their eyes	1 day	8 weeks
3. With head held firmly, looking at face of examiner	2 days	8 weeks
4. Supporting herself in a sitting position and watching her reflection in the mirror	7 weeks	20 weeks
5. Holding herself upright	5 months	9 months
6. Taking the round block out of its hole in the form-board	5 months	11 months
7. Standing against the mirror	5 months	9 months
8. Walking to the Gesell box and doing the test	7 months	15 months
9. Climbing the steps alone	11 months	15 months

Most of what the African mothers (for that matter child-rearing customs of indigenous peoples of the world) do for their children has been abandoned today. We may conclude that the child's ability to fully develop his capacities has been negatively affected. Then, we are surprised at how different the children of today are. Is this the price of "progress," of "individual freedom"? Or is it due to the loss of genuine love of our humanity? My intention in raising this issue is for everyone to appreciate the wisdom of the old practices and retrieve the essential ones relevant to our times. This should not be misconstrued as a call to return to the past.

See also Gantley M et al. Sudden infant death syndrome: links with infant care practices. *British Medical Journal* 1993(January);306:16-20. Lack of rich sensory environment (e.g., tactile) and long periods of lone quiet sleep are some factors that contribute to a higher sudden infant death rate among whites than among Asian infants.

61 Arms S. *Immaculate Deception: A Look at Women and Childbirth.* Bantam Books; 1975.
    Sousa M. *Child Birth At Home.* Bantam Books; 1977. They have extensively documented
    the adverse effects of hospital births. For an alternative way of childbirth, see Bing E.
    Six Practical Lessons for an Easier Childbirth. Bantam Books; 1977; and La Maze F. *Painless
    Childbirth: The La Maze Method.* New York: Pocket Books; 1972.

62 Pearce mentioned in his notes that a fine MD friend of his "pointed out that every
    obstetrical text emphasized leaving the cord strictly alone until all activity in it ceased.
    He could not believe doctors had abandoned such a commonplace and obvious
    necessity." A young doctor, however, told him that in his internship, "he had delivered
    ten babies under his supervision and that he had been instructed not only to cut the
    umbilical cord immediately after it was available, but also to jerk the cord [a reason
    for hemorrhage to occur] to dislodge the placenta—the quicker to get the delivery
    room cleared. Two obstetrical nurses testified that my [Mr. Pearce's] evidence was,
    if anything, understated, that the actual situation was far more grim." Pearce, *Magical
    Child*, p. 276.

    In 1985, when the author's daughter was born by La Maze method, he tried to
    convince the doctor not to cut the umbilical cord until the placenta was delivered. Still
    the doctor proceeded with his usual routine, asserting that he was in control, and did
    not follow the father's suggestion. Considering the grave consequences arising from
    ignorance of these important details of childbirth, there should be a law against such
    a crime.

63 Quoted from Pearce, *Magical Child*, p. 54.

64 Most orthodox doctors believe that the drugs taken by the mother during pregnancy
    as well as during labor do not penetrate the placenta barrier, and therefore in no
    way affect the fetus. This is absolutely untrue. Barbiturates cross the placenta in all
    stages of gestation. All narcotics, as well as inhalation and regional anesthetics, can
    depress the newborn. Thiazide diuretics, coumarin anticoagulants, and antithyroid
    medication have their specific ill effects. For example, Dr. Brackbill, in studying the
    effects of meperidine (popularly known as Demerol and the most commonly used
    drug during labor) on newborn infants found that infants of mothers who have been
    pre-medicated performed less capably and less efficiently on many Neonatal Behavior
    Assessment scale items than did infants who had not been pre-medicated. Dr. Brackbill
    concluded that there is clear evidence that meperidine produces outstanding neonatal
    differences in ability to process information. Should we then wonder why children do
    not perform as well in school today? See Arms S. *Immaculate Deception: A Look at Women
    and Childbirth.* Bantam Books; 1975:79-87.

65 Human beings start life on earth with their first breath. Prior to this and while still in the womb, the circulatory system remains partially differentiated. With the first breath, the system fully divides into arteries and veins. The infant itself shuts off the umbilicus. Life permeates the infant's body and is now in control. The common fear of obstetricians that blood would flow out of the umbilicus is "utter nonsense!"—so exclaimed Otto Wolff after narrating the above facts in his lecture during the seminar on anthroposophic medicine in Arlesheim, Switzerland, which the author attended. Flowing out of the blood is possible only if the infant has not yet taken the first breath. Since most obstetricians clamp the umbilical cord and cut it as soon as the baby's body is clear, it is highly probable that the first breath has not yet been taken by the newly born. The danger of lack of blood and oxygen depletion is then more likely. This is another example of orthodox medicine's inability to understand life. Superstitions and fears dominate, leading to interventions detrimental to the incarnating life on earth. See also Kimmond S et al. Umbilical cord clamping and preterm infants: a randomized trial. *British Medical Journal* 1993(January);306:172-175. In this study the delay of just 30 seconds in cord clamping gave pre-term infants a higher initial pack cell volume and higher arterial alveolar oxygen tension ratio in the first day. If only obstetricians give these pre-term babies (and normal babies, too) more time to breathe by themselves before clamping and cutting the umbilical cord, there would probably be fewer complications and higher survival rates. Please note that it takes an average of three minutes to complete blood infusion from the placenta to the infant. See Yao AC et al. Distribution of blood between infant and placenta after birth. *Lancet* 1969;ii:871-873; Yao AC et al. Effect of gravity on placental transfusion. *Lancet* 1969;ii:505-508. The baby must be placed lower than the mother to effect blood infusion. Type in your internet search engine *umbilical cord clamping* for more updated information on this issue.

66 Apgar score is used as a general measure of the infant's post-delivery health. The baby's heart rate, respiration, muscle tone, color, and reflexes are scored accordingly: 0-2 points at one minute and five minutes after birth. A score of 10 points, doctors say, indicates "perfect" health; 7-9 points is considered normal; 5-6 indicates some kind of distress; 4 or below is poor and indicates a need for treatment. Like all tests it has its limitations. However, orthodox doctors use it to defend hospital procedures, making them oblivious and blind to the adverse effects of drugs and their interventions which may manifest later in a child's life.

67 Quoted from Windle W. Brain damage by asphyxia at birth. *Scientific American*. October 1969:84.

68 Other useless interventions by the obstetrician on the mother about to deliver an infant are: multiple vaginal examinations, administration of an enema, shaving of the

pubic hair, performance of an episiotomy, and giving an oxytocic drug to expedite placenta delivery. All of these have been proven to be of no benefit and give more risk and discomfort to the mother in the process of childbirth. As far as the infant is concerned, one should object to the use of fetal monitoring machines, fetal blood sampling through the amniotic sac and scalp, x-ray, ultrasound, and dropping silver nitrate on the eyes of the newborn—all of which may prove harmful later on. On the whole, any artificial intervention in this natural process should be frowned upon.

69 How should one handle childbirth? A homebirth is preferable, but that alone is not sufficient. One should view pregnancy and childhood as a whole process of preparing the body, soul, and spirit. Complete acceptance of pregnancy is ideally the best starting point. The mother's diet should include plenty of uncontaminated fruits and vegetables with the living forces intact. Protein should come from the best sources as described in this chapter. Any fear related to childbirth must be confronted and overcome. Humming tunes daily to the unborn child would increase bonding. The pregnant woman should avoid stress, tension, and extreme bouts of emotion; she should practice equanimity. Most importantly, she should avoid exposure to chemicals and cigarette smoke, and the intake of caffeine. For those who want to prepare for childbirth and need assistance, get in touch with trained individuals who offer the course on prepared childbirth using the La Maze method or Bradly method.

70 Caroline Myss, PhD (in *Why People Don't Heal and How They Can*, London: Bantam Books, 1999) gives us a profound insight as to how "fear and other negative emotions adversely affect healing, you may more easily identify how you are interfering, consciously or unconsciously, with your own healing process." Years before this, Louise L. Hay (in *You Can Heal Your Life*, Santa Monica, CA: Hay House, 1987, p. 6) stated, "We are each 100% responsible for all our experiences. Every thought we think is creating our future... Everyone suffers from self-hatred and guilt—'I'm not good enough.' It's only a thought, and a thought can be changed. Resentment, criticism, and guilt are the most damaging patterns... Self-approval and self-acceptance in the now are the key to positive changes... We create every so-called 'illness' in our body."

71 Acknowledging the contribution of psychosocial factors in the disease process is another area where orthodox science is too cautious and is thus lagging behind. In spite of our common experience and the numerous reports and books that have come out from other fields, e.g., psychology, and personal and accumulated accounts showing that psychosocial factors do matter and in many cases are even a crucial ingredient, orthodox science hesitates to look into this causal relationship. It could be that their simple minds are unable to grasp the complexities of human life and disease processes. They would rather limit themselves to a single cause than complicate and confuse their thought processes by assuming that a disease is multifactorial.

In any case, some bolder scientists have come up with studies which occasionally get published in medical journals showing the relationship of belief, disease, and survival, and attempt to wake up these narrow-minded geniuses. See Philips DP et al. Psychology and survival. *Lancet* 1993(November);342:1142-1145. They studied the death of 412,632 adults, with 28,169 of them Chinese American. They found that Chinese-Americans die younger if they have a combination of disease and birth year which Chinese astrology considers ill-fated, and that more years are lost by groups strongly attached to Chinese tradition. See also Eysenck HJ. Psychosocial factors, cancer, and ischaemic heart disease. *British Medical Journal* 1992(August);305:457-459. This article cited the studies of Grossarth-Maticek wherein the relationship of psychosocial factors (i.e., personality, behavior, stress) was clearly linked. For example, coronary heart disease personality is characterized by strong reactions of anger, hostility, and aggression; or the cancer-prone personality is characterized by suppression of emotion and an inability to cope with interpersonal stress, leading to feelings of hopelessness, helplessness, and finally depression. Appropriate behavior therapy (e.g., stress management) then can act prophylactically to make disease-prone people less likely to get sick. Other risk factors were mentioned, such as smoking and diet, that act synergistically—not additionally—in developing health or illness. See also Spiegel D et al. Effects of psychosocial treatment on sample patients with metastatic breast cancer. *Lancet* 1989(October);888-889. Patients who underwent psychosocial treatment lived significantly longer than did controls by an average of eighteen months; Boyle CAO. Disease with passion. *Lancet* 1993(November);342:1126·1127; Philips D, King EW. Death takes a holiday: mortality surrounding major social occasions. *Lancet* 1988;ii:728-732; Goodwin JS et al. The effect of marital status on stage treatment, and survival of cancer patients. *Journal of the American Medical Association* 1987(December);258:3125-3130.

These sample studies refute the assumption in the standard medical training that diseases are either wholly organic or wholly psychological. This conditioning can be traced back to the philosopher Descartes (350 years ago), who propounded the rigid separation of the mind and body. If doctors still believe in this assumption, then a void will definitely be created in their understanding of health and illness. See also Hodgkinson N. *Will to Be Well: The Real Alternative Medicine*. London: Hutchinson Ltd.; 1984. It is the mind that makes us ill, and can make us well too, given the knowledge of how to do so. Type into your internet search engine *mind body medicine* for more discussion.

72 For example, not chewing our food long enough can have repercussions in our capacity to digest sooner or later and/or promote the growth of pathogenic bacteria (and their toxic metabolites) in our gut. Studies suggest that every mouthful of food should be chewed at least 30 or more times depending on the type of food. See *www.whfoods.org*.

73 Recently compiled studies presented at an international conference held at Norwich, United Kingdom, September 13-16, 1992, address the role of food in the prevention or genesis of cancer. Mutagens and carcinogens in foods as well as diets that inhibit or suppress tumor development are discussed. For example, there are anti-tumorgenic substances in rice bran found by some Japanese scientists. Here, the mere consumption of polished rice provides the consumer less material substances in preventing the occurrence of tumors. See Waldron KW, Johnson LT, Fenwick GR, eds. *Food and Cancer Prevention: Chemical and Biological Aspects.* Cambridge: The Royal Society of Chemistry; 1993. See also Renzenbrink U. *Diet and Cancer. An Anthroposophical Contribution to Cancer Prevention.* London: Rudolf Steiner Press, Medical Press Center; 1988. He brings in new dimensions in the understanding of food quality, such as light and warmth in foods, as specific characteristics of the vitality of edible plants.

74 A belief among most human beings that may induce untimely death is that when it is time to die or when God says "your time is up," there is no way to avoid it. Studies have shown this to be one major reason why patients hesitate to change their diets, lifestyle, or attitudes in spite of the efforts of their enlightened doctors to convince them that doing so may alter the situation. This is not viewed so much as a fatalistic attitude if one is really on the verge of death, i.e., no other lifesaving devices can hold back the dying process. However, when one is still quite well and able, every decision he makes may either be for better health or a step closer to death. The discussion in Section 1 brings to our mind the possibility that we can lead life the way we want it to be. A closely related belief is to "drink, eat, and be merry, for tomorrow we die." This could be self-fulfilling, especially for those who think that all there is to life is material and sensual enjoyment. The succeeding discussion and notes shed more light on this.

75 Chopra D. *Quantum Healing: Exploring the Frontiers of Mind/Body Medicine.* New York: Bantam Books; 1989:122-125.

76 The uncontrolled consumption of meat not only leads to heart ailments but may also increase the risk of prostate cancer, colon cancer, and many other diseases. See Cowley G. Medicine: red meat and prostate cancer. *Newsweek.* September 25, 1993:48B. He reported a study by Dr. Eduard Giovannucci of the Harvard School of Public Health involving 51,000 American men, and found that the men eating the most red meat suffer 2.6 times more illnesses that those eating the least. See also Ulbricht TLV, Southgate DAT. Coronary heart disease: seven dietary factors. *Lancet* 1991(October);338:985-992; Hunter D. Breast cancer: nutritional factors. *Lancet* 1992(October);340:905. The United Kingdom is moving towards instituting diet as part of cancer prevention in primary care. See Austoker J. Diet and cancer. *British Medical Journal* 1994(June);308:1610-1614.

77 Salter J. *The Incarnating Child.* Gloucestershire: Hawthorn Prelis; 1985:112-117. She

writes that "perceptive parents often notice a marked change in their children after childhood disease, for example, measles or mumps. A child weak in will and rather pale and withdrawn may emerge from such a disease with greater inner strength, enhanced vitality and better all-round health. It is the experience of the disease process and the struggle to overcome the sickness that is strengthening the soul. This could be of great benefit to the child's destiny well into the future... Vaccines deny the child this experience and so the chance of significant development is lost. Therefore, the vaccine does not confer true 'good health,' but rather, prevents its development." For more discussion on the problems of immunization see link to websites in previous note 31.

78 If only parents will find the courage not to have their children immunized and let them go through their fever without suppressing them with antipyretics, inherited predispositions to certain diseases can be prevented from being expressed. Most children also inherit the lifestyle of their parents, and all the possible consequences to either prevent or (mostly) promote inherited diseases.

79 Chopra D. *Quantum Healing: Exploring the Frontiers of Mind/Body Medicine.* New York: Bantam Books; 1989:162. See also Fawcett A, Smith C. *Cancer Free: 30 Who Triumph Over Cancer Naturally.* Compiled by East West Foundation. New York: Japan Publication Inc.

80 When I conducted a workshop in May 1993 in Tabuk, Kalinga Apayao, Philippines (a province of an indigenous people), one participant narrated exactly the same phenomenon I described. He originally could not understand how the remission happened, but upon hearing the above discussion, the "miracle" was demystified.

81 One book I came across after writing this section, edited by Mark Kidel and Susan Rowe-Ieete, is *The Meaning of Illness* (London: Routledge; 1988). The authors likewise challenge the mechanistic medical model and redeem illness from its exclusively negative connotations. Illness is not a curse but a potential gift. See also Mees LFC. *Blessed by Illness.* Anthroposophic Press; 1990, which asserts that illness may be instrumental in solving life problems. Doctors can assist through understanding this view and adopting a new approach to therapy.

82 My nine-month stay in Australia in 1989 with my family, and my seven-month stay in Germany in 1992, gave me this impression. In Germany, I met certain men and women who went from one new doctor to the next in search of relief from their illnesses. Some came to me for treatment after learning that I did acupuncture; I tried to do what I could to help. By treating them I gained the insight that what I did to them was merely palliative. True healing can only come from their quest for meaning in their lives.

83 Notable among the international NGOs are Amnesty International, Green Peace

International, and Global Network 3, to name only a few. Many local NGOs and CSOs are found in most countries advocating issues of equity in the social, cultural, economic, and political spheres of life, working mostly with the victims of our current inequitable and one-sided economic relationship. If you want to get in touch with the latest amalgamated report on alternative development programs, please subscribe to *truthforce.info.ph*. This is an alternative news website that features efforts of individuals and organizations trying to realize a more just, equitable, and sustainable world.

84 A pioneering work on this subject comes from Nicanor Perlas (*Shaping Globalization: Civil Society, Cultural Power, and Threefolding.* Manila: Center for Alternative Development Initiatives, 1999). His main thesis is that the dominant forces behind globalization are economics and politics. Many of our modern societal ills (poverty, loss of culture, among others) have emerged because of this lopsided development. The emergence of NGOs and CSOs in most countries, advocating alternative views on sustainable development, is a symptom that a third aspect of society is being extricated and disentangled from the dominance of our current bi-polar power struggle between business or the private sector and the governments of nation states. This third system is the cultural sphere of society: "a third global force has emerged with elemental strength to contest the monopoly of the two other powers (economics and politics) over the fate of the earth… [I]t is part of a massive cultural revolution going on around the world. It is a revolution that involves tens of millions of so-called 'cultural creatives,' individuals who are challenging the materialistic and hedonistic assumptions behind elite globalization… one that is potent enough to transform elite globalization into comprehensive sustainable development."

85 The works of Bernard Lievegoed (*Phase, Crisis and Development in the Individual* and *Man on the Threshold: The Challenge of Inner Development,* Rudolf Steiner Press and Hawthorn Press, respectively) are important breakthroughs in understanding the phenomenon of mid-life crisis. He brings out the real issues behind many contemporary problems of life.

86 Worse, some consciously or unconsciously realize the futility of changing their lifestyle, attitudes, or relationship and make an inner decision to end their life. Thus, in the highly urbanized centers of the world, suicide, fatal accidents, and heart attacks occur most during this period of crisis. In the US, heart attacks occur most frequently between 8 a.m. and 9 a.m. on Monday mornings. This indicates that human souls refuse to go back to a work situation that is monotonous, humdrum, and meaningless. They would rather abort their existence.

87 The pioneering work of Viktor E. Frankl, *Man's Search for Meaning,* is important to mention here. Even in the most absurd, painful, and dehumanized situation, life has potential meaning and therefore even suffering is meaningful. This conclusion served

as a strong basis for Frankl's "logotherapy." An example of Frankl's idea of finding meaning in the midst of extreme suffering is found in his account of an experience he had while working in the harsh conditions of the Auschwitz concentration camp. He survived the condition of the Nazi camp along with several others in his barracks because they never lost hope and meaning in what they were experiencing. Those who did not find meaning or hope beyond their current state died early. He discovered that without hope, meaning, and other intangibles (which are all aspect of realizing the spiritual essence of life), we would easily fall prey to disease and then death.

88 Thus, accidents in one's life are not really accidents—rather they are telling us something because we have not been listening, looking, paying attention, or discerning. It is a way for our spiritual "I" to redirect us to potentially "see" our original intention.

89 One way of processing our life experiences is called the "biography workshop." Here one consciously looks at the events and encounters in one's life and discerns patterns and recurring themes. Sickness, accidents, successes and failures, ideas which influenced one's way of thinking, and other variables are chronologically identified. From this panoramic view, one trains his thinking to recognize what these facts may be saying regarding one's original intention in life (that is, the intention we took upon ourselves before incarnating on this earth life). See also Schottelndreier J. *Life Patterns Responding to Life's Questions, Crises and Challenges.* Cornelis JM, trans. UK: Hawthorn Press; 1989.

90 A good book I found after writing the main text is Neville Hodgkinson's *Will to be Well: The Real Alternative Medicine.* London: Hutchinson Ltd., 1984. This book is a guide for patients to the inner dynamics which create habitual and often addictive patterns of behavior and feeling that lead to many illnesses. It seeks to show how we may become more able to steer ourselves back into an acceptable and sustainable level of health without running into the hazards of medical treatment.

91 One's environment can be seen materialistically, or with an eye for what is inherently spiritual, woven into nature. The work of Robert Sardello, *Love and the Soul: Creating a Future for Earth,* gives us a different picture of the world/environment and our relationship to her. The world has soul, and the way to connect with her soul is our activity of love. Thus, without changing our views of the earth and then transforming our way of treating her, we will not invoke enough healing response and support from her, whether for oneself or for others.

Chapter Four

✤

Harnessing the Power Within

*"Maintaining order rather than correcting disorder
is the ultimate principle of wisdom. To cure disease after it has
appeared is like digging a well when one already feels
thirsty or forging weapons after the
war has already begun."*
– Yellow Prince Classic[1]

The quotation above expresses succinctly an overall theme of our discussion: to learn how to correct disorder in our systems before the disorder turns pathological or the organ involved starts to degenerate. To maintain order in our whole being, we should learn more about tapping the healing power within us. Health here does not mean the absence of disease, but rather the capacity to overcome any illness. In many ways we are overcoming illness daily. How to realize this capacity to the fullest will be our focus in the succeeding pages.

A. HARNESSING THE POWER OF THE LIVER AS THE MAIN ANABOLIC ORGAN

As said earlier, the liver is the main anabolic organ.[2] *Anabolism* means the rejuvenation and repair of tissues that were devitalized or damaged while one was awake and active in the world. Quality sleep is therefore important. Sleep temporarily extinguishes the activity of consciousness and allows the complete force of anabolism to unfold. If we go without sleep for a few days we die.

In the figure below, the brain wave patterns of persons who are asleep are compared with the brain wave patterns of those who are awake. The left picture depicts a smooth and harmonious wave pattern, while the right one has a sharp, pointed, disharmonious, and depolarizing pattern. Being awake means destroying the harmony of the life force that flows through our body. We learned from our previous discussion that the action of the two higher bodies, that is, the emotional life of our sensitivity body and the thinking activity of our ego, has a catabolic and devitalizing effect on the two other bodies, namely, the formative force body and the material or physical body. They exhaust the life forces in cells, organs, and tissues. In sleep, the activities of these two bodies are temporarily extinguished. Steiner's research clearly revealed that during sleep the ego and sensitivity bodies actually withdraw from the formative force and physical bodies.[3] With the extinction of consciousness, full anabolism can proceed.

Brain Wave Patterns

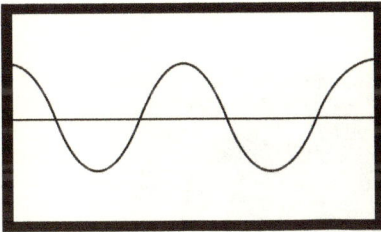   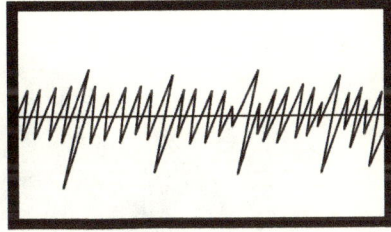

Asleep   Awake

For this knowledge to be useful in maintaining health or promoting healing, more information about the rhythm of the liver is required. Orthodox medical science has identified 3:00 a.m. as the physiological midnight. This is very much connected to the shifting function of the liver and the gall bladder. That is, from 3:00 a.m. to 3:00 p.m. the liver releases glycogen in the form of glucose in the blood, while the gall bladder is ready to release the bile acids (if there are fats in the food to emulsify). During this period, the liver constricts and diminishes in size. The gall bladder empties its contents and supports the liver in bile production. From 3:00 p.m. to 3:00 a.m. the liver regenerates.[4] It stores glycogen (human carbohydrates) and rebuilds itself, while the gall bladder recycles bile from the intestines and stores them in its bladder. This is the wisdom behind the Greek legend of Prometheus, who is chained to the rock of calculus. Every day a vulture (representing human thinking and feeling activities) comes to gnaw his liver, which then regenerates during the night. The Greeks were actually aware of what was happening to the liver every day and night, depicting the knowledge in pictures.

Now, how can we harness to the fullest the power of the liver as the main anabolic organ? Getting enough sleep that coincides with the liver's period of regeneration is very important. This means that sleeping early promotes a fuller anabolic activity than sleeping and waking up late. It is the quality and timing, not necessarily the number of hours, that is attuned to the rhythm of the liver, which would matter most in sleep. If someone were to conduct a statistical survey of workers on the night shift, or graveyard shift (the term speaks for itself), I believe the results would show that they are poorer in health than those who can sleep at night.[5] Moreover, sleeping early is a must if one is ill and/or recuperating. For workaholics to stay healthy, the recommendation is that they sleep early and start working early, too. This way, the stressful and catabolic life of the day can be better balanced by the harmonious, anabolic phase of sleep.

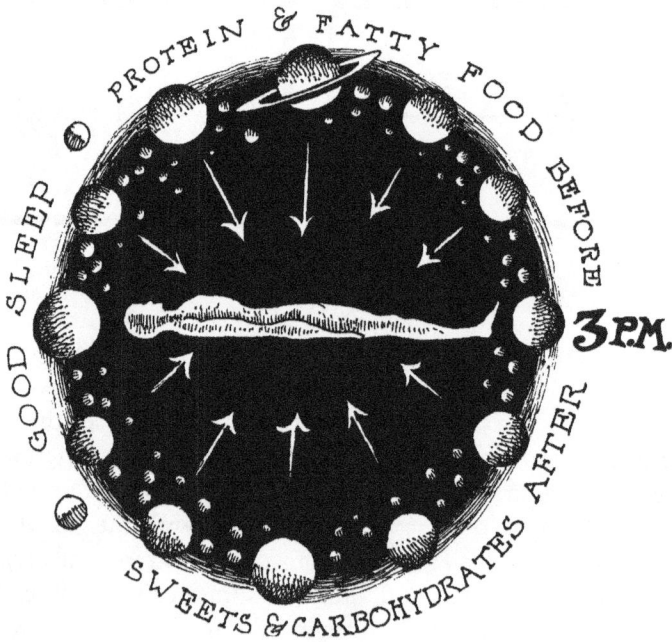

We should be more cautious with children regarding sleep. Children are still developing and building up their bodies (in an anabolic building-up phase). They certainly need more sleep than adults. Thus, children from 0 to 7 years of age need 11 to 12 hours of *night sleep*. As they grow older, this can be reduced to 10, then 9 hours when they are in their teens. A lot of accidents, irritability, lack of focus and attentiveness, tantrums, and the like may be avoided if we let children sleep more, so that they can have better control of their bodies.[6]

The same idea can also be applied to nutrition. It is healthier to eat fatty and protein-rich foods in the morning than in the evening. The gall bladder is ready to release its bile acids, which would emulsify these fats. Eating sweetened foods (like marmalade or jams) in the morning disturbs the function of the liver, which is already releasing glucose in the blood. On the other hand, after 3:00 p.m. eating carbohydrates and sweetened foods will actually help the liver rebuild itself. The liver needs carbohydrates in order to synthesize glycogen.

At this point let me differentiate between simple sugar (that is, table sugar) and complex sugar, which includes carbohydrates like whole rice, corn, wheat, rye, barley, potatoes, taro, yam and other root crops, and fresh and naturally dried fruits. What I advocate is eating complex sugar and not simple sugar contained in soda drinks, marmalade, chocolates, and the like, where either white sugar or high fructose sugar is used. High consumption of simple sugar tends to overwork the pancreas and may lead to dental caries and diabetes.[7]

Alcohol is poison to the liver. We all know that cirrhosis is sclerosis (hardening) of the liver. Alcohol has been identified as the leading cause of the hardening of connective tissues found in cirrhosis. Thus to protect the liver, it is best to avoid the intake of any alcohol.[8]

The liver should be protected as much as possible. However, today's norms promote a lifestyle that is harmful to the liver. We disregard the rhythms of our body. We sleep late, work late, eat rich and devitalized food any time of the day and night, and indulge in perceptual (TV, video)[9] and sensual pleasures, ignoring the deteriorating effects they have on our health. It is true that our bodies can take much abuse and misuse, especially in our younger years. But they have their limits. Judging from the gravity of today's illnesses, this notion of freedom (oblivious or ignorant of responsibilities) has very severe consequences for our generation, and more so for future ones. Should we not then rethink how we exercise our freedom?[10] Each individual has to answer this question on his own, come to a personal conclusion, and accept the consequences or reap the benefits.

Certainly, it is best to have a full breakfast where one would experience moderate fullness. As the word denotes, we need to "break the fast." This meal wakes up our digestive system.[11] Corollarily, eating too much in the evening will be injurious to the liver. The forces of the liver, which is regenerating at that time, are exhausted in the process of digesting a big meal. In addition, a heavy meal inhibits sleep. The higher aspects of the human being are not able to fully excarnate because the physical body needs their forces to digest and neutralize the alien forces of the food. Without good sleep, full anabolism cannot be accomplished.[12]

B. HARNESSING THE HEALING POWER OF OUR RHYTHMIC SYSTEM

From the discussion of the three systems in the human being, we learned that the rhythmic system is the mediator and balancer between the nerve sense system and the metabolic/limb system. Disease arises when there is an imbalance in this system.

The rhythmic system is directly related to the heart and lungs. Here we find the two fundamental gestures of our feeling life: sympathy and antipathy. The heart and lungs mirror these two gestures, respectively, in inspiration and expiration in our breathing, and the systole and diastole of the blood pressure. If nurtured well, the rhythmic system should be able to hold the two other polar systems in balance. In our daily life, however, we favor one over the other. In an emotion-filled argument, we tend to take one side. In a party, we tend to eat what is appetizing rather than what is properly nourishing. In facing an archrival, we tend to disagree with everything he says or condemn everything he does. All of these actions make our rhythmic system imbalanced.

What can we do to maintain a balanced rhythmic system?[13]

We can try to develop the capacity to rise above the feelings of sympathy and antipathy.[14] Start with this simple exercise a few minutes each day. Listen to two people arguing. Withhold your immediate judgment (i.e., your sympathy or antipathy) and try to hear what each one is really saying. Trying to understand where each one is coming from develops in us a "higher" sympathy that enables us to understand the point of view of each person. We are also able to discern and understand the situation from a broader perspective. With practice and perseverance we will notice a change for the better in how we approach similar situations.

A follow-up exercise is to listen to someone we totally dislike, distrust, or always argue with. Attempt to understand what he really wants to say without getting affected by his manner of speaking or interrupting with a rebuttal. If you are able to do this, you will develop your capacity for equanimity. This will then result in a healthier rhythmic system capable of balancing the head and metabolic poles.

A genuine inner life is likewise fundamental to the development of a healthy rhythmic system. Most people generally have a poor inner life. Upon waking up in the morning, they turn on the radio or television set full blast. Many keep them on the whole day, and even the whole night. This habit overloads the nerve sense system and produces strong sclerotic forces. It also hinders the individual processing of inner experiences and inhibits the possibility of the individual coming to himself.

For a genuine inner life, one should remain comfortable in silence. In this silence one can process feelings, thoughts, and past actions, trying to discern what they are as well as their real meaning. If we are always distracted by so many stimuli from the outside, we are in fact letting them take over our feeling life. We will find it extremely difficult to distinguish them from our own. Not having our own inner life makes us susceptible to being easily swayed by whoever wants to control us, for example, advertisements, ideologies, or religious dogmas.

Engaging in artistic activity fosters the development of the rhythmic system. Thus, painting and experiencing colors can be highly therapeutic. Playing a musical instrument[15] or singing exalted songs[16] can harmonize our feeling life. Moving with balance and grace cultivates our sense for beauty and life.

This brings me to the most important healing force which we can harness: *love*. Unfortunately, most of what is considered love today is actually selfish love. To illustrate: most parents want to give their children the "best." But what is "best" for them is often measured in terms of material goods and physical development, while the emotional, psychological, and spiritual nourishment is overlooked. Parents no longer spend quality time with their children because they are too preoccupied with material pursuits.[17] The situation can swing to the other extreme, that is, too much attention is given to the child to the point that the latter's own individuality cannot grow. The child becomes an alter ego of the parents and fails to have a life of his own. Love here is one-sided, and the child learns to view this kind of love as the most desirable.

A narrow type of love is one that does not go beyond the self and the family. Much of societal strife, and even illnesses, can be directly traced to this confining, selfish love. What we must also learn to develop is a higher expression of love, that is, love informed by reason and knowledge stemming from the spiritual activity of the "I." For example, as an expression of love, parents should control their children's intake of soft drinks or chocolates.[18] They contain caffeine which can lead to addiction in children and make them hyperactive. Sugar corrupts the taste buds, deters proper nutrition, and later on damages their overall capacity to properly digest food.[19] The decision to control the intake should be based on reason and knowledge, not just succumbing to the mere wishes of the child, to the influence of advertisements, or to social convention. The parents and caregivers have the moral responsibility to properly guide and direct the likes or dislikes of the child. If they are always satisfied regardless of consequences, the child may grow up believing that he should and can always get what he desires. With this one seemingly trivial decision, we can expect far-ranging effects on the constitution and disposition of children well beyond what we can imagine (like avoiding the current modern epidemics such as obesity,[20] and learning difficulties like attention-deficit-hyperactive disorders[21]).

Finally, this higher Love[22] which we need to develop transcends family, tribe, nation, race, or even religion. This Love should develop in us the capacity to concretely realize unity in diversity: enhancing individuality while promoting unity in a collective, and advocating nationalism while at the same time working for planetary synthesis and the planet's sustainable future. Its most exalted personal expression is to be able to love one's enemy. If we can develop and promote this kind of love, then literally, illness may vanish in the future. This may seem far off from our time, but we have to start somehow, somewhere, sometime so that the succeeding generations may benefit from our efforts. This is the best gift we can offer our children and the rest of humanity, the true meaning of progress in human evolution.[23]

C. NURTURING THE SPIRITUAL "I"

Where will we get the power to develop all of the above? We have already given some indications. The spiritual "I" should always be aware and in command of the natural tendencies of our lower bodies—the sensitivity body, the formative force body, and physical body.[24] The "I" is like the charioteer who tames the horses and directs their course. Through the cultivation of healthy common sense, this "I" discerns the truth, acquires knowledge, and eventually attains wisdom. Our "I" is purposeful, and in this world intends to perform deeds that will contribute to the progressive evolution of earth and humanity. This higher "I" does not succumb to its lower counterpart, the small "i." The small "i" lives in the individual's likes and dislikes, is easily swayed by advertisements or outside opinions, and is a slave of one's constitution and temperament. The small "i" is conditioned to live in order to eat, and desires to survive mainly to pursue sensual pleasure. Moreover, the small "i" lives solely for one's self and usually acts for personal benefit.

The spiritual "I" is the true "I," while the small "i" is the false one. Most of us live in varying degrees between these two, or oscillate from one to the other. The ideal is to strive for the full transformation of the small "i" into the greater "I."[25]

Once in the state of the spiritual "I" awareness, one can go in and out of any situation. He can fully experience his emotions and not be possessed by them. He can approach any system of thought and assess its strengths, limitations, and meaning. He can examine almost anything and find out its value for the understanding of the world, or for transforming himself and the environment for the better. More importantly, he is able to free himself from cravings, sentimentalism, one-sidedness, prejudice, and bias.

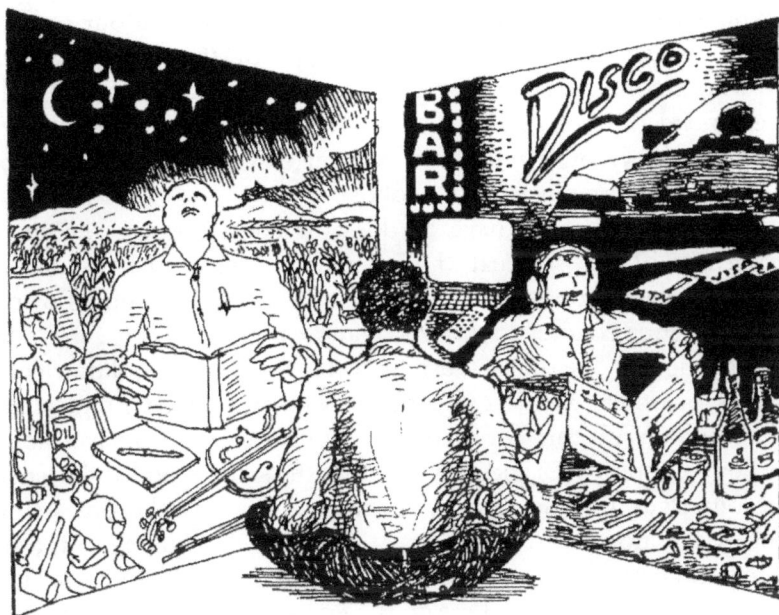

Today's culture favors the development of the small "i." Egotism, prejudice, sensual pleasure, and unconscious consumerism are found everywhere. We have to double our efforts to develop our spiritual "I" and begin to remold our lives and our environment.

In the previous discussions, I have already given some exercises to strengthen the spiritual "I." We start by being comfortable in silence in order to nurture a genuine inner life. Equanimity in any situation will eventually develop our cognitive feeling, which is a higher form of perception. It is a feeling capable of properly discerning what has been perceived and at the same time reaching out to the deepest core of the other. Cognitive feeling is the step towards developing a new clairvoyance, that is, a capacity to see how the spirit weaves into matter and material events.[26]

Another preliminary exercise for strengthening the spiritual "I" is this: every time we feel pain or anger, get sick or meet an accident, we ask ourselves how this pain or illness speaks or what it is telling us. Cognitive feeling can be enhanced by merely asking this question. And if the question is sincerely asked in a consistently living way, we can get insights about ourselves and the situation we are in. Continuous practice allows us to think with our whole being and not just with our head.[27]

There are other preliminary exercises which involve cultivating the capacity for pure thinking, an outlook of positivity, and openness to every life experience, as well as recognizing the newness in all our encounters in life. However, they are beyond the scope of this present work. For those who are interested and ready to embark on such spiritual training, I recommend the book *From Normal to Healthy: Paths to the Liberation of Consciousness,* by Georg Kuhlewind, as a starter. For other materials, please consult the bibliography of this book.

Obviously, all these have to do with consciousness training. The development of the spiritual "I" can only be achieved consciously and through one's inward effort. To think that it will happen on its own is an illusion and runs counter to the whole idea of the "I."

Training of the consciousness brings about true knowledge of ourselves, of others, and of our experiences—and a greater understanding of the world. With this knowledge, we will begin to perceive more and more how the spirit lives and moves within the sense world and events, and within ourselves. Our perception or sense of the spirit becomes tangible, practical, and non-abstract. The way we used the findings of Steiner's research in the preceding discussion is a case in point. If a spiritual path or meditation technique fails to create the environment for these insights to arise, then it may no longer be relevant to our modern times. Its practice will not allow our spiritual "I" to fully develop capacities necessary to progress and evolve further. Moreover, consciousness training should give us the possibility to find creative solutions to the world's problems and help the rest of civilization move forward.

At first glance, the requirements stipulated above may seem to be unreachable. It is noteworthy that in the past only the so-called initiates had the possibility of aspiring for such a spiritual path.[28] The time has come when everyone can attain this goal, but it must be done consciously. Each of us is in varying degrees of spiritual evolution, struggling with certain ideals one way or the other. In many ways, what is important is the striving itself. The effort of sincerely trying is the actual path which develops the capacities. Just as a healthy individual is one who struggles to maintain order and balance out the disease tendencies in his being, the individual who is struggling and striving towards his spiritual "I" is also the healthy one.

A last quotation from Steiner may give us a further indication of the basic mood or attitude we need to develop so that we will be capable of transforming ourselves.

> If we wish for health, then as a preliminary condition we must accept illness into the bargain. If we want to be strong, we must arm ourselves against weakness by taking weakness into us and transforming it into strength.

D. OTHER FUNDAMENTAL INGREDIENTS TO SELF-HELP MEDICINE

Faith in authority has become the rule nowadays, and has resulted in the feeling of helplessness to form judgments for oneself. People tend to declare themselves unqualified to comprehend matters regarding various fields in life, and simply accept what orthodox science (and any other field of expertise) has to say. We must consciously fight against this tendency. The first step is to educate ourselves. We must be inquisitive. We must think things through. We must learn lessons from our individual experiences as well as from the experiences of others.

To develop the capacity to heal ourselves using natural remedies, we should first learn more about other schools of medicine. Many books are available on this subject. If you have a degenerative form of illness, please be aware of a possible healing crisis that you may encounter in the process of healing.[29] To improve our skill in diagnostics, *we need a conventional book which discusses the various symptoms associated with particular diseases.* We must recognize that one of the best contributions of orthodox medicine is in the field of diagnostics.[30] A certified doctor (as long as he has not become a mere prescription-dispensing machine)[31] may be consulted to verify one's own diagnosis. If your doctor says you need to undergo some laboratory examinations, you can tell him that you prefer to have an iris analysis or a pulse reading from an acupuncturist.[32] Their diagnostic processes are non-invasive and respect your dignity. Several opinions can be solicited from a number of doctors.

The discussion in Chapter 3 about the three systems of the human body can also be used in diagnosis. If one has a history of inflammation in the upper parts of the body, then our metabolic system is unnecessarily hyperactive and needs to be toned down, or we need to heighten our thinking activity to counteract our metabolic system.[33] Numbing, hardening, deposits of some kind in the gall bladder, kidney, or other parts of the body indicate that our nerve sense system is overworked or too active and may require adjustment in our lifestyle.[34] We achieve this by lessening nerve sense impressions, stress, and other anxiety-stimulating activities to give the metabolism more time to enliven what has been devitalized and damaged by excessive wakefulness. Some changes such as in sleep, diet, and harmony of daily activities may first be resorted to before any form of medication is taken.

If symptoms persist, then we can embark on a search for remedies. A set of Bach Flower remedies[35] or a homeopathic kit[36] may be worthwhile to have at home. Nowadays, with an explosion of information on the internet, one can surf through it to find various natural alternatives to address one's illness. One must, however, learn to firmly discern what is appropriate for one's condition. I hope that reading this book will provide you an anchor for your judgments.[37]

To develop your own skill of diagnosis, you may want to learn about traditional Chinese medicine's way of diagnosis. Chinese medicine has a very elaborate field of diagnostics using the acupuncture points, the points in the ear, the color of the tongue, the lines in the face, the moods and emotions of the individual, and the odor of the body.[38] Every time one gets sick or encounters a sick individual, one can take this as an opportunity to develop one's capacity to diagnose and think of the possible strategy for treatment.

Each one of us has the power to comprehend and make a judgment through the spiritual "I." We can be our own authority with regard to our own health. As we gain experience through time, we can be our own doctor. When we are able to realize and understand the totality of our being, we will know where the illness is coming from and what it is telling us. Knowing this, we can start working also on ourselves. Plant, mineral, and animal remedies such as the ones presented here are the major sources of forces that aid us in healing. We know that fever and inflammations are natural processes of the body and therefore they should not be suppressed. These reactions should be guided by the remedies listed here.

In advocating an attitude of self-reliance, I do not mean that we should absolutely do away with doctors. Their skill is still important for those who cannot help themselves and those who require special help in addressing specific illnesses. The point is that we need to change our relationship with our doctors. We should change from being merely dumb and mute patients to being actively participative ones. We may then get doctors to change from near-dictators to genuinely concerned and accommodating guides and helpers in evoking the healing power within each patient and complementing this with remedies from nature.

On the societal level, we should advocate a pluralistic practice of medicine.[39] Each school of medical thought has its way of viewing the human being and many different ways of addressing an illness. Thus, each one should be given a chance to present an appropriate viewpoint and therapy. The patients will then have a wide range of alternatives leading to a well-informed choice. Pluralism in medicine is one way to avoid one-sidedness and monopoly of viewpoint. The governments in every country around the world should be the leading force in ensuring that the various novel and ancient therapies found in the world are represented in every country.[40] Moreover, in this way, we help begin to redeem the practice of medicine itself by making diverse human knowledge and experience the basis of healing the whole human being.

Notes

1   Quoted in Beinfield H, Korngold E. *Between Heaven and Earth: A Guide to Chinese Medicine.* New York: Ballantine Books; 1991:7.

2   The liver is one of the most important organs in our body that sustains life. Consider its following functions. 1) The liver is the central organ for the fluid metabolism which includes the absorption, excretion, and distribution of water. It manages five fluid movements: the arterial blood, the venous blood, the lymph that streams through all the organs; it receives the blood from the portal veins, and the bile flows from it. The diuretic and anti-diuretic substances are found here. It regulates the water content of the blood and serves as an essential blood storage organ. Edema is a liver dysfunction. To treat edema, one must stimulate the liver to enliven the fluids. Thirst is also connected with the liver. 2) The liver acts as the chemist of the body in a) mineral metabolism, especially that of potassium and sodium. Though mineral metabolism is primarily subject to the adrenal cortex, the triggering organ is the liver. Potassium helps the liver in the control of fluid metabolism. Thus too much sodium in the diet tends to displace potassium in the liver and impair this function. b) the liver synthesizes glycogen (human starch) in the process of carbohydrate metabolism. c) the liver plays a special role in protein metabolism. The integration of the process through which the nitrogen fraction is eliminated is an essential function of the liver. d) detoxification is another important function. This is intimately connected with the problem of deamination (the removal of the amino group NII2 from a molecule, usually by hydrolysis, oxidation, or reduction with the accompanying formation of ammonia) and transamination (the transfer of an amino group from one molecule

to another, usually by the action of a transaminase) in protein metabolism. Thus, this function plays a significant role in the establishment of an allergy. Allergy, as has already been pointed out in the discussion on nutrition, is the body's reaction to toxins. Hypoalbuminaria indicates a weakness of the formative force body in the liver. Several dermatological problems are also connected with the proper protein formation by the liver and can occur together with liver disorders. e) The liver produces enzymes to detoxify chemical pollutants, e.g., cytochrome P450 [Purdey]. f) The liver is important in lipoid metabolism, renewal of cholesterol (about 2 % a day), and the formation of bile acids. (Bile acids should be seen in conjunction with the gall bladder.) 3) The liver mediates and transforms intended ideas into deeds. If the organic basis is incompletely developed due to upbringing and schooling, it is possible that the person will remain inactive despite his best intention. The individual is unable to will because the organic basis, the liver, does not provide the "material." In other words, the person is stuck in thinking.

On the whole, one should see the liver as a sense organ. It perceives everything that enters the body as nutriment. If the liver is healthy, it allows useful substances to enter the body and excludes those that are detrimental. For further discussion on the importance of the liver, see Husemann F, Wolff O. Liver-gall system and its diseases in *The Anthroposophical Approach to Medicine* (3 vols). Vol 2.

3   The reader may wonder where the sensitivity body and ego go during sleep. Steiner's research revealed that they return to what can be termed as the spirit world. There they rest from being in a dense material body and receive inspiration from the spirit. Thus when they re-unite with the physical and formative force bodies, the different members of the human being are revitalized, and the individual is ready to face the world again. For those without any genuine inner life, the inspiration carried back from the spirit world is not retained in the consciousness. Impressions from the surrounding material world immediately dominate their waking consciousness at the expense of the inspiration. Others may wake up and instantly change or adjust their lives to suit the new inspiration. For more details see Steiner R. Sleep and death, in *Occult Science: An Outline*. Spring Valley, NY: Anthroposophic Press; 1972.

4   For a more extensive discussion on the liver's 24-hour rhythm, see also Schmidt. *Dynamic of Nutrition*. pp 95-96.

5   Kubo T, Ozasa K et al. Prospective cohort study of the risk of prostate cancer among rotating-shift workers: findings from the Japan Collaborative Cohort Study. *American Journal of Epidemiology* 2006;164(6):549-555. The researchers found that men who worked fixed night shifts had slightly elevated prostate cancer risk, compared to men who worked fixed day shifts. They believe lower levels of melatonin, a hormone which regulates sleep patterns and has been shown to protect people from cancer, may be

an important factor. Previous studies have indicated a higher risk of breast and bowel cancer for shift workers.

6 Moreover, total darkness must accompany sleep. More melatonin, a hormone produced by our brain's pineal gland, is secreted when our eyes (whole body) experience total darkness: "Melatonin gets made during the dark period," studies say; "If you get light exposure during the normal dark period, it severely reduces the amount of melatonin that is made." See LeVert S. *Melatonin: The Anti-Aging Hormone.* New York: Avon Books; 1995. Search the internet for *sleep and immune system* to know more about their relationship.

7 See Gloeckler M, Goebel W. *A Guide to Child's Health.* Edingburgh: Floris Books. 2003:247. See also note 20 on sugar consumption.

8 See *www.liverdisease.com* for updates on alcoholic drinks and painkillers like acetaminophen and paracetamol in inducing liver damage and failure. You can also type *pain killers and liver damage* in your internet search engine. See also FDA eyes painkillers warning for heavy drinkers. *The Philippine Star,* July 8, 1993. In this report the advisory panel of the US Food and Drug Administration warns that painkillers and alcohol may produce fatal liver damage. How is this possible? The liver produces the enzymes to detoxify chemical pollutants. The intake of alcohol weakens the liver which becomes unable to produce the said enzymes. The painkillers then being chemicals, damage the liver and can produce instant death. See also Bray GP. Liver failure induced by paracetamol. *British Medical Journal* 1993(January);306:157-158.

9 In the last three decades, a number of issues have surfaced against television viewing. The more familiar one is the content of the shows, for example, violence and sex which are definitely inappropriate, especially for children. The less known issue is the negative effect of the medium itself. Television passively glues the viewer in front of it. This in itself goes against the innate nature of children, which is to do, move, and physically interact with the environment. Children addicted to TV may end up paralyzing their will in adulthood. A more immediate effect is for the unused will forces to burst forth in the form of tantrums or even hysteria. Another ill effect is the suppression of creative imagination due to the projected fixed images which destroy the child's capacity for creative fantasy. This capacity is the basis of creative intelligence later in life. With television, we may be developing more and more uncreative individuals who no longer possess the ability to act positively in this world. For a more comprehensive analysis of TV viewing and the medium of television, computer, and videos see Mander J. *Four Arguments for the Elimination of Television.* New York: Quill; 1977; Large M. *Who's Bringing Them Up? Television and Child Development: How to Break the T.V. Habit.* Hawthorn Press, 1980; Winn M. *The Plug-In Drug.* Penguin Books, 1977. In a more recent book by psychiatrist Aric Sigman (Sigman A. *Remotely*

Controlled: How Television Is Damaging Our Lives and What We Can Do About It. London: Vermillion; 2005), he states: "…the new generation of very recent medical studies has caused me to see television as a major health issue." In brief, TV viewing slows the body's metabolic rate, stunts the development of children's brains, may permanently hinder children's educational progress, increases the likelihood of children developing ADHD, is a leading cause of half of all violence-related crimes, lowers adult libido, and is a major cause of depression. See *www.qoulkids.com* for a more comprehensive discussion.

10 Only in our spiritual activity of thinking and conscious willing can we be truly free, that is, thinking which is thoroughly willed and will which is thoroughly thought out. Freedom results from the first and Love results from the second. Those who claim to be free to do whatever they wish may actually be victims of or possessed by their sensual habits, instincts, or bodily sensations. This may neither be a true "I" experience nor genuine freedom, as will be discussed later.

11 See *www.nutrition.about.com* for the importance of breakfast in our daily life. Studies show that children who eat breakfast do better in school. It doesn't take much further thought to realize adults will feel better and perform better at work as well. Whether you work at home, on the farm, at the office, at school, or on the road, it is not a good idea to skip breakfast. Eating a good breakfast sets the tone for the rest of the day.

12 What then can one do if sleep is already a big obstacle? Insomnia is now an epidemic. We should then try to rehabilitate our metabolism, particularly the health of the liver. Taking a lot of fruit juices from organically grown fruits will be a good start. Doing a liver cleanse will be essential to help the liver resume its multifaceted function. Just type *liver gall bladder flush* in your internet search engine to get instruction on how to do a liver cleanse. After the liver cleanse one should take a probiotic food supplement to replenish the population of good bacteria in our intestines. From the description of the plants in Section 2, I found Coffea D30 to be good in putting one to sleep if the above procedure still does not work.

13 The eightfold path as reconceptualized by Rudolf Steiner for the modern time is most appropriate in developing the rhythmic system. It consists of a focused practice of one "fold" each day of the week: Monday is right speech; Tuesday, right deed or action; Wednesday, right human standpoint; Thursday, right effort; Friday, right memory; Saturday, right opinion or thought; Sunday, right judgment. The eighth fold, right synopsis or contemplation, is practiced every day to review the day rightly. One should do the exercises daily until they become second nature. Rudolf Steiner added six supplementary exercises in order to create the mood to develop further the eightfold path. They are: controlled (concentrated) thinking, will initiative, equanimity, positivity, freedom from prejudice, and forgiving. See Kuhlewind G. *From Normal to*

Healthy. Great Barrington, MA: Lindisfarne Press; 1988.

14 Normally, our feeling life is entangled with our emotions. We should start differentiating between feeling (the act of perception) and emotion (like fear, anger, disgust, joy, satisfaction) that is triggered by our perception. Thus, the succeeding discussion and exercises are meant to make this possible for us and begin the development of a conscious faculty of cognitive feeling.

15 It is important to distinguish between music produced by electronic instruments and that of using classical and traditional instruments. Electronic instruments produce a metallic sound which may adversely affect the feeling life. Try to experience the two sounds and find out the difference.

16 Metallic music and songs tend to unbalance rather than harmonize the feeling life. It is important to expose children to Renaissance, folk, classical, and old church music to teach them to discern the emptiness of metallic music.

17 For example, obesity in today's young adults is clearly linked to parental neglect. See Lissau I, Thorkild, Sorensen LA. Parental neglect during childhood and increased risk of obesity in young adulthood. *Lancet* 1994(February);343:324-326. Just type *obesity and parental neglect* in your internet search engine to read more studies.

18 The president of the Philippine Pediatrics Society and associate dean for academic affairs of the University of the Philippines College of Medicine, Dr. Amelia Fernandez, explained that "soft drinks merely fill up the stomach, usually preventing those addicted to it—the children, especially—from taking in healthy foods, like milk and juices… soft drinks also contain from 31 to 65 milligrams of caffeine in every 12-ounce bottle, providing an addictive 'kick' to soft drink 'addicts'." See Pediatrician warns vs. habitual soft drinks consumption. *The Philippine Star*, November 9, 1993. Just type *soft drinks and health* in your internet search engine for more discussion.

19 See Matsen J. *The Mysterious Causes of Illness: and How to Overcome Every Disease From Constipation to Cancer.* Canfield, Ohio: Fischer Publishing Corporation; 1986. "Disease is a result of inefficient digestion due to nutritional and/or emotional stress."

20 See Bhattacharya S. Cut sugar to battle obesity. *New Scientist* 2003(March);15:8. "The call for a drastic reduction in sugar consumption comes in an expert report issued jointly by the World Health Organization and the Food and Agriculture Organization. It warns that in 2001, chronic diseases resulting from poor diet contributed to 60 per cent of the 56 million reported deaths worldwide and nearly half the global burden of disease." To update yourself on the link between sugar consumption and obesity, just type *sugar and obesity* in your internet search engine.

21 See *www.newideas.net/adhd* to get a sample of a dietary plan for children with this

new neurological illness. The internet is full of articles on the link between diet and common neurological illness. Search for *adhd and diet* and *autism and diet*.

22 A number of individuals today have reached this stage of Love for humanity. They are living and promoting it through the peace movement; international non-governmental organizations involved in the issues on ecology, sustainable development, upholding various aspects of human rights, new system of governance; and many other efforts which attempt to resolve the various inequities in the world. They are aware of their work towards a common goal of planetary synthesis. See Institute of Planetary Synthesis, *www.ipsgeneva.com*. Another world organization advocating socially engaged spirituality is the General Anthroposophical Society founded by Rudolf Steiner in 1923. This society continues to propagate, elaborate, and find practical application to daily life of the body of knowledge left behind by Rudolf Steiner, called anthroposophy. This is done by organizing conferences of practitioners (doctors, nurses, farmers, artists, eurythmists, teachers, and other professionals) to exchange ideas and deepen their professional practice and understanding of anthroposophy. To find out more about this organization, see *www.goetheanum.org.ch*.

23 The work of Robert Sardello (see Sardello R. *Love and the Soul*. Berkeley, CA: North Atlantic Books; 2008) is important to mention at this point. "Humanity is now approaching a new sense of love—the capacity to create love as a world-forming force." This book teaches us how the soul can be properly engaged with the outer world. By acquiring a conscious awareness of inner purpose and beauty, by developing a true sense of individual imagination, we bring what is inside us out into the world and help the world evolve (in Love).

24 There are new findings of science which support this role of the ego or "I" in affecting our immune system. Twenty years ago, molecular biology discovered a new class of minute chemicals called neuro-peptides, neuro-transmitters, and monocytes. Neuro-peptides are secretions of the brain. For every thought we have, a chemical counterpart is simultaneously created and secreted. Neuro-transmitters are runners that race to and from the brain telling every organ inside us of our emotions, desires, memories, intuitions, and dreams. Wherever a thought wants to go, these chemicals must go too, and without them, no thoughts can exist. Monocytes are receptor cells for neuro-peptides and neuro-transmitters in the immune system. They travel to the bloodstream, giving free access to every cell of the body. Whenever we feel or think, are sad, happy, or excited about an idea, or blissful because of a realization, our immune system experiences it, too (Chopra, pp. 58, 67). This means that whatever we think or feel predisposes us either to a certain illness or continued health. We can even think ourselves into an illness. One who feels deprived, envious, or oppressed would be predisposing himself to all sorts of illnesses. We can then ask: Who is doing the

thinking? What is this being like? The capacity to transform the "I" from the small "i" to the true "I" determines our ability to ward off or produce illnesses.

25 Currently, technology caters too much to the comfort (or sentient life) of humanity. It does not only condition man to be complacent but also inhibits the development of one's natural capacities. For example, calculators replace our capacity to do mathematics mentally. Cars have replaced our legs. The telephone system eliminated the possibility of using other means of communication. (Eskimos used to know whether a relative or a foe was coming by the howling of the wolves.) Technology, as it is used widely now, must be viewed critically. It has its place in modern life, but we need to beware that it does not lead us to become mere automatons at the service of negative forces seeking to dominate an unfree society.

26 Why a new clairvoyance? The old clairvoyance of our fore-parents enabled them to perceive the spirit weaving in matter and material events. However, they expressed their vision in myths and legends—a language no longer suitable to our age. Moreover, the old clairvoyance can be characterized as spontaneous, compulsive, and unable to give human beings their freedom. This was necessary at that stage of human evolution. Then came the period of materialism with the mission of totally cutting off humanity from any notion of the spirit and the spiritual world. Materialistic science's view of "matter as the only reality" successfully inculcated this attitude. Thus, human beings must acquire the new clairvoyance in freedom (find their way back to the spirit as a free choice and effort). They need their logical/analytical thinking (coupled with the development of the intelligence of the heart) in discerning as well as in expressing what they see. They must be fired by the mood of scientific investigation, but using their own soul/spirit (experiences) as the instrument for investigation. Those who still possess the old clairvoyance must develop also their logical/analytical thinking. This faculty is crucial in grounding oneself in the world. Those who are unable to develop their logical/analytical thinking may run the risk of being diagnosed as schizophrenics. Their vision due to clairvoyant faculties will be irrelevant to the present age because it cannot be translated in humanity's everyday language. For the steps in the process of developing the new clairvoyance see Steiner R. *Knowledge of Higher Worlds and How It Is Attained.*

27 We must always extract our lessons and insights from our "good" and "bad" experiences, either immediately or through time. Through the accumulated insights along with their interrelationships, we develop wisdom. Wisdom helps us live through the second half of our life and aids us in warding off sclerotic illnesses. Wisdom is the fruit we will carry with us at the portal of death. It will metamorphose into capacities of our immortal "I" to do more creative deeds, mend or amend relationships, and fire the progressive evolution of the world and humanity. For more details regarding how capacities are

born in specific individuals see Steiner R. *Theosophy: An Introduction to the Supersensible Knowledge of the World and the Destination of Man.* New York: Anthroposophical Press; 1971.

28 In the ancient schools of initiation—during the Indian, Persian, Egyptian, Babylonian and Chaldean, and Greek and Roman periods, or Chinese, Mayan, and Aztec ancient civilizations, or among indigenous peoples all over the world—apprentices/students were chosen. Thus there was strict secrecy in the knowledge and processes imparted. The masses were scorned as ineligible.

29 Healing crisis is one possible path your interweaving bodies will resort to in the process of healing a degenerative condition. Toxins will be excreted from the inside out (skin, sputum) and from top to bottom. You may relive your old inflammatory illness or develop new ones as part of the healing process. See Chapter 3, note 32.

30 Let me qualify this statement. Orthodox medicine is very precise when the disease has already reached its pathological state, that is, something is already wrong with the organ or tissue involved. Thus it has various names for illnesses coming from different layers of the tissues or organs. This diagnostic system lacks an early warning system. I discussed earlier that most doctors think that fever, inflammation, and allergies are diseases and treat (suppress) them accordingly. However, they fail to treat the underlying weakness of the organs concerned. The Chinese way of diagnosis can indicate certain organ dysfunctions even before the organ starts becoming physically diseased. Type *Traditional Chinese Medicine* (or *TCM*) *diagnosis* in your internet search engine.

31 Most doctors spend an average of seven minutes attending to each patient and proudly present their prescription. How could one fully diagnose someone's condition in just seven minutes? If your doctor does the same, consider looking for another one. Practitioners of other schools of medicine allow more time to fully understand the patient's situation within the context of a very specific view of the nature of the human being. They try to see the ailment from as many points of view as possible—attitudes, emotions, family, work situation, past experiences, fear of the future, diet, and many others.

32 More and more physicians are using iridology for diagnosis. Orthodox science is suspicious of it because it cannot understand the principle behind iris analysis. But a new science called holographic science provides an explanation. One of holography's basic axioms is that the part mirrors the whole. Thus in the iris, the condition of the whole body is imprinted. The same applies in ear acupuncture and reflexology, both for diagnosis and treatment. See also Schjelderup W. The principle of holography: a key to a holistic approach in medicine. *American Journal of Acupuncture* 1982 (April-

June);10:167-171.

33 Wetting the head with cold water every morning can stimulate more nerve activities, especially for children with a large head. This is another way to stimulate the head pole to balance the excessive activity of the metabolic pole.

34 We can also use warm compresses after evening meals or before going to bed (for 20 minutes) to activate more metabolic activity and counteract too much nerve activity of the day.

35 See Scheffer M. *Bach Flower Therapy: Theory and Practice.* Wellingborough, UK: Thorsans Publishers, Inc.; 1993. Bach flower remedies are very simple to use and tailor-made for readers not trained in medicine. There should be a practitioner in your city.

36 Homeopathic home kits are available in the US, UK, Europe, India, New Zealand, and Australia. Just type *homeopathic home kits* in your internet search engine. I suggest you begin with 6X or D6 potencies (for reasons which will be discussed in Section 2) if you decide to get one. As you begin to use them, you will eventually master the remedies in the kits and begin to help others help themselves.

37 At the beginning of the book I mentioned in the notes about ear acupressure or auricular therapy. Using the points in the ear for diagnosis and treatment is actually simpler. Ear acupressure is also complementary to Bach Flower or homeopathic remedies. Doing both will speed up the healing process and perhaps avoid a healing crisis.

38 See Porkert M. *The Essentials of Chinese Diagnosis.* Zurich: Chinese Medicine Publications Ltd.; 1983.

39 There is a trend towards complementary medicine in the developed countries. In the US, the Center for Complementary and Alternative Medicine intends to bring together new and old therapies with allopathic practices. In England, dialogues on very new and exciting developments have been going on among the Royal College of General Practitioners, the Royal Society of Medicine, and the British Medical Association. Some of these developments are described in detail in Pietroni P. *The Greening of Medicine.* London: Gollanez Paperbacks; 1991. See also Fischer P, Ward A. Complementary medicine in Europe. *British Medical Journal* 1994(July);309:107-110. Public demand is strong and growing for acupuncture, homeopathy, manipulation therapy, herbal medicine, and other forms of alternative medicine.

However, much remains to be done to fully achieve the goal of complementation. Orthodox doctors will hardly give up the position of power and authority. Transnational companies will not simply abandon their multibillion-dollar profits. Lay people should assert their participation. Fence-sitters are not allowed in this affair. Orthodox medicines with their adverse effects continue to claim their victims. Every time you take a pill to eliminate a headache or fever, you start becoming a victim. Each one of us is called upon to actively think about this issue. We should not leave the "experts" to define what complementary medicine is, but rather we as ordinary folks must come together and propose our own definition.

40 See Ted Kaptchuk and Michael Croucher (*The Healing Arts: A Journey to the Faces of Medicine*, British Broadcasting Corporation, 1986). They have embarked on an approach called multi-dimensional, pluralistic, or integrated medicine. In their open clinic, practitioners of various healing arts are brought together, allowing each to be distinct and recognizing their inherent limitations. Consequently, patients have a wide range of choices in their therapy. Unlike in complementary medicine, this model does not work towards integrating other healing arts into the mainstream, but rather the mainstream is formed by all the tributaries. In suggesting that the governments of our societies encourage the presence of practitioners of various healing arts and medical systems found in the world, I mean to enlarge the number of tributaries to create a true mainstream. This diversity and possible synergy of principles and skills are our hope to eliminate the one-sidedness and fragmented medicine that dominate the lives of human beings. Search the internet for *complementary medicine, alternative medicine,* and *integrative medicine.*

Chapter Five

🌿

Model of a Healthy or Disease Process: Summing Up and Conclusion

A. THE ORIGIN OF ILLNESSES

The illustration on the following page is my attempt to sum up what has been discussed in this section and postulate a broad model of a disease process. By knowing what makes us ill, we will be able to know how to prevent it from happening.

My theory of illness posits two fundamentals sources: Firstly, a weakened, underdeveloped, or misdirected "I,"[1] and secondly, a weakening vitality or formative force body. They are mutually and internally related, as I will try to show in this discussion.

Let me first discuss the second fundamental source of illnesses—weakening vitality. Focus your attention on the illustration from the encircled phrase "weakening vitality" downwards. Weakened vitality in certain areas of the body brings about a dysfunction of the tissues and organs involved. This weakened vitality is expressed in homeopathy as the derangement of the vital body, and in traditional Chinese medicine as insufficiency of the "chi." (Appendix 1 is a picture as to how current notions of bringing up children can weaken their vitality, develop new illnesses such as various kinds of neurological disorders, or predispose them to degenerative illnesses sooner or later in life.)

How does this translate to the level of biophysical and chemical processes? I must first introduce some new information. Our body has approximately 75 to 100 trillion cells. Every day, about 300 billion cells die in the body and must be replaced by an equal number. About 70% of the material is recycled[2] by the body, while the rest is eliminated in the form of urine, sweat, breath, etc. Nutrition and other forms of nourishment replace the eliminated materials. This is what we discussed earlier as the process of catabolism (breaking down, devitalization, dying process) and

PAST

1. Meaning of the past (nature, nations, civilizations, regions, kinship, personal)

2. Predisposition of geography (nation, tribe, family, individuality)

3. Conditioning by family, social status, others
   a. Preconception factors (drugs, alcohol, tobacco, emotional security, others)
   b. Prenatal environment (diet, well-being, reverence, others)
   c. Childbirth method & environment (premature cutting of umbilicus, medical drug use, etc.)
   d. Upbringing (0-21 years)
      1) Devitalized/imbalanced diet
      2) Inappropriate school methods & content
         a) early intellectualization, "carrot/stick"
         b) inartistic & abstract, one-sided development
      3) Inadequate psycho-social nurturing
      4) Lack of spiritual nourishment, e.g., value modeling
      5) Misdirected purpose & meaning of life (material wealth as measure of success)
      6) Mishandling of childhood diseases (vaccines, antipyretics, others)

4. Other factors
   a. Capacities not nurtured
   b. Unprocessed, dis-integrated, or incoherent experiences
   c. Guilts, fears, limited and/or distorted beliefs

PRESENT

SENSORY OVERLOAD
1. Visual, tactile, audible, stimulants
2. Unprocessed experiences
3. Devitalized/denatured food
4. Ingestion of synthetic chemicals

ARYHTHMIC LIFESTYLE
1. Sleeping/waking
2. Introversion/extroversion
3. Rest/stress
4. Inner/outer life
5. Thinking/doing
6. Eating

1. Inadequate sense of, or misdirected individuality
2. Extreme sympathies & antipathies
3. Inability to handle or resolve conflicts
4. Moral degradation
5. Rigid habits, attitudes, & beliefs
6. Narrow-mindedness & perspectives

1. Environmental degradation & pollution
2. Exposure to radiation (x-rays, electromagnetic)
3. Decadent political life
4. Distorted economic system
5. Inadequate cultural life
6. Loss of purpose & meaning of life
7. Old age

ALIENATION FROM ONE'S NEIGHBOR & NATURE

FUTURE

1. Perception of the challenges of the future
   a. World trends
   b. Regional & national trends
   c. Individual's role, mission, to bring the future

KEYS TO WELLNESS & HEALING

1. Accepting the givens (inner peace, intuiting insights, developing transcendence)
2. Self-transformation, e.g., raising personal experiences to level of eternally true & good
3. Detoxifying body, soul, & spirit (food, feeling life, attitudes, ideals, beliefs)
4. Developing rhythm, equanimity, balance, positivity
5. Cultivating living thinking, right actions
6. Conscious nourishing of the Spiritual "I" (Higher Self)
7. Rediscovering one's original intention & purpose in life
8. Consuming living foods
9. Working for a healthy environment
10. Using natural therapies (naturopathy, acupuncture, homeopathy, massage, herbal medicine, anthroposophic medicine, ayurveda)
11. Working for the reorganization of structures & relationships in society (local & international whenever possible)
12. Fructifying & renewing of professions
13. Business activities, careers on a more ethical/moral basis.
14. Educating children towards freedom
15. Evolving a broad, holistic & dynamic perspective & comprehension of life, humanity, & the universe

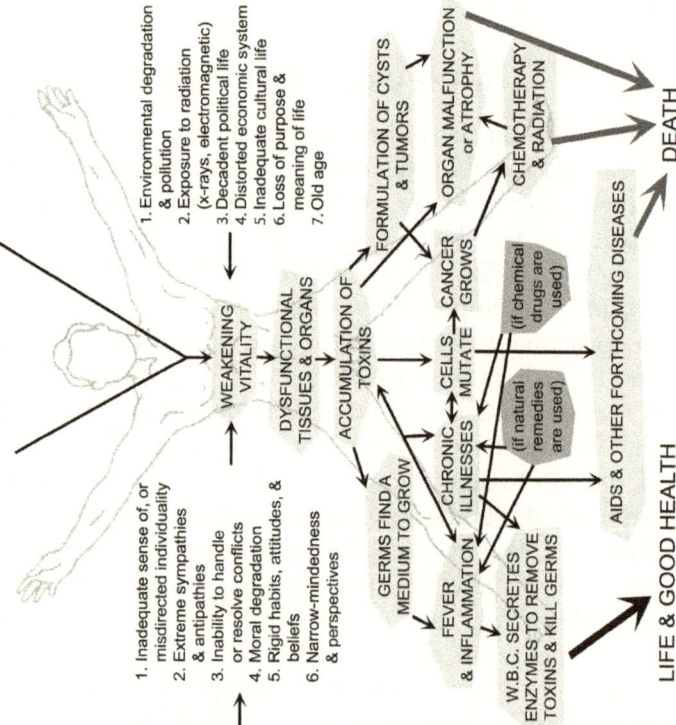

WEAKENING VITALITY

DYSFUNCTIONAL TISSUES & ORGANS

ACCUMULATION OF TOXINS

GERMS FIND A MEDIUM TO GROW

FEVER & INFLAMMATION

W.B.C. SECRETES ENZYMES TO REMOVE TOXINS & KILL GERMS

CHRONIC ILLNESSES

CELLS MUTATE

CANCER GROWS

(if natural remedies are used)

(if chemical drugs are used)

FORMULATION OF CYSTS & TUMORS

ORGAN MALFUNCTION OR ATROPHY

CHEMOTHERAPY & RADIATION

AIDS & OTHER FORTHCOMING DISEASES

DEATH

LIFE & GOOD HEALTH

Illustration 1: Model of a Healthy or Disease Process

anabolism (building up, revitalization, enlivening process). Any weakening of the vitality in any part of the body brought about by a host of factors (indicated by the numerous arrows) may inhibit the full catabolic and/ or anabolic processes. If catabolism is impaired, a dysfunction of the tissue or organ ensues, i.e., the tissue or organ is unable to, or only partially secretes the enzymes, hormones, or chemicals needed to break down the dead cells, bring the recyclable parts into readily usable form, and have the rest excreted through the normal eliminating channels. The result of a slight or severe dysfunction is an accumulation of toxins: dead cells, waste products of the catabolic process, and other toxic materials.[3] With the continued presence of the toxins, germs may find a medium to grow or feed on.

In certain situations, our wise immune system encircles and isolates the toxins into styes, boils, cysts, polyps, myomas, and other tissue outgrowth to prevent damage to the surrounding organ and avoid the growth of germs. In certain cases, our interweaving bodies react with a fever or an inflammation in any stage of the above-described process to remove toxins, kill germs (if germs are already proliferating) by secreting interferon and other enzymes through the white blood cells, and revitalize the weakened tissue or organ. If a chemical drug is used to suppress the fever or kill the germs, the toxins are pushed deeper into the tissues and more toxins accumulate. This may lead to a relapse, a reinfection, a new disease, or to chronic diseases. In other words, allopathic chemical drugs do not address the underlying weakness that brought about the proliferation of germs in the first place.

As a curative strategy, we should appreciate and work with our normal four-fold bodily reactions and not suppress them. A heightened temperature means our "I" is actively engaging the body to "burn" the germs and toxins. If we experience pain, then our sensitivity body is penetrating further into the surrounding tissue, inducing it to secrete the appropriate enzyme to catabolize the toxins and kill the germs. Our white blood cells and other body fluids circulate twice as fast for every degree centigrade rise in temperature for the same purposes. Our heart beats faster or lessens the desire for food to support the heightened activity of our interweaving bodies, and to concentrate its whole effort in healing itself. In the first place, we should give time for this healing activity to express itself.

We can resort to anthroposophic medicine, homeopathic preparations, acupuncture, and other therapies that can help our body revitalize the weakened vitality of a particular organ or tissue. With a stronger vitality (the "chi" restored) tissue function resumes, and normal catabolic and anabolic processes take over. We should also try detoxification therapy in combination with the above, such as enemas, herbal teas, sitz baths, linen wraps, and hot and cold baths to help our system remove the toxins as soon as possible.

Antibiotics should be resorted to only when all these measures seem "not enough" and when natural body reactions seem to be "failing" or "over-reacting." In the thirty years since I started to fully manage the illnesses of my family, I have not had reason to give an antibiotic or an antipyretic.[4] Those who may need antibiotic therapy are those whose vitality has been so weakened by a host of factors that they have an overload of toxins in many parts of the body, and germs proliferate uncontrollably in these various parts. The use of antibiotics then would be justified. This is their rightful place: during emergencies, or life-and-death situations. This seems to be where allopathic medicine is at its best. I hope you will learn enough from this book so that you will never find yourself in this particular situation.

As we continue following the arrows in the diagram, we see that chronic illnesses can lead to tumors, cell mutation, degenerative and cancerous diseases, and eventually the atrophy of the tissue and organ, and then death—especially if chemical drugs are indiscriminately resorted to. Our broad lines of natural therapies can still address these illnesses, but may take a longer time to detoxify cysts, tumors, or cancer and revitalize the tissue or organ to induce it to perform its normal function. Acquired Immunodeficiency Syndrome (AIDS) is the weakening of vitality in many parts of the body resulting in an almost simultaneous infection. (The causes of AIDS are multifactorial, as we have already discussed in note 76, Ch. 2.)

If the trend of therapy in orthodox medicine continues the way it is today and people continue to be mesmerized by its "scientific declarations," we can expect more serious diseases or debilitating epidemics to come.

Orthodox science only sees germs, tumors, and cell mutations. These are already the last stages of the disease process. Obviously when an illness becomes pathological (i.e., the organ or tissue is already damaged), it will be harder to achieve a cure. Our body's attempt to heal itself may no longer suffice, because it has been weakened by the regular use of chemical drugs, among other things. Other allopathic therapy then becomes like a patch-up job: incise a tissue here or remove and replace an organ there, substitute a product here, do dialysis or a transfusion there. This is neither an art nor a science, but the work of a mechanic or a technician, as I have pointed out. The true art and science of healing is to correct the disorder before its pathological manifestation occurs. If we train ourselves in recognizing disease at its early stages, i.e., weakened vitality, then we can avoid much of the illness, suffering, and premature death we find all around us. The way the remedies are described in Part 2 of this book will help you develop this capacity to recognize an imbalance at its early stage.

Now let us look at the genesis of diseases from the other pole I mentioned—the weakened, underdeveloped, or misdirected "I," or individuality. Why would this condition predispose us to illness? As we already learned, the spiritual "I" manages the three other bodily sheaths like a charioteer directing the horses. If we have a weak sense of individuality, we can be easily swayed by our sympathies and antipathies, in other words, by our emotions. How many of you have experienced losing yourself in an emotional outburst? What did you feel afterwards? Exhausted, right? If this goes on frequently in your life, then it would weaken your vitality. The kidney and liver may first be involved, and then accumulation of toxins in various parts of the body can ensue. On a societal level, a weakened "I" or individuality manifests as masses of people that are swayed easily by opinions, advertisements, idols (like movie stars), dogmas, or even ideologies. They are candidates for fanaticism, if not fanatic themselves already. Their judgment of other people and situations will be colored by this imbalance in their sympathies and antipathies. One consequence is the inability to handle conflicts, thus resorting to violence, cheating, corruption, or enslavement of others. With this tendency towards one-sidedness, their moral sense can easily be subverted by anyone who has any sort of control over their life. If each individual is unable to strengthen his weakened "I" or straighten out his misdirected "I" (by giving his spiritual "I" a chance to express itself or be in control), all the implications of disease tendencies brought about by this imbalance will manifest in his body, soul, and spirit, as well as in his environment.

In other words, if the "I" is not in command of our lives, now, the consequences will be great. The situation around us speaks for itself: unconscious consumerism, obsessive/compulsive behavior, lust for power, sex, and material possession, egotism, fanaticism, racism, prejudice, drug abuse, cancer, violent crimes, and more. Worse still, we are conditioned to think that this is the normal way of life.

How can the past weaken us? Unresolved experiences, for example, may linger on in the present, haunting us in the form of guilt, fears, and erroneous beliefs.[5] If the past still flashes back and gains control over our present, it diverts our attention, distorts our perception of the present, and in the process weakens us in fulfilling our true goals in life. In some, guilt, fears, traumas, and repressed desires (individually or collectively) can manifest as physical and "mental" illnesses in various forms. We must then learn to accept the past, forgive ourselves and others, extract insights that can teach us, and move on. Once we have an objective relationship to our past experiences, we are in fact transcending them and transforming them into capacities, knowledge, and later on, wisdom.

How can the future weaken us? Whether we know it or not, our everyday decisions are also influenced by our perception of the trend we see in the future.[6] If we see a dim future like orthodox science envisions— extinction, destruction, and death of even the fittest—then what is there to live for? With no meaning to live for, disease and death find a space within us and weaken our vitality. In every situation we find ourselves feeling helpless; when we continue saying, "that is very difficult or impossible to do," or "I cannot change myself, my lifestyle, and my behavior," this means that we are suppressing the creative energies of our "I." As we discussed earlier, our "I" works in a very creative way. It can work through any situation. There may be difficulty but not impossibility. There is always another way, if there is the will to address the difficult or the impossible (though this may take a little longer than we would like).

One should then cultivate the attitude of positivity in every situation. Positivity is seeing the good and true in the worst situation, and working with what is good and true in every experience. This way everything is possible.

The question of karma can now come into the picture. What really is karma? The idea of karma is usually attached to negative incidents in one's life. Thus every time one encounters difficulties, accidents, illnesses (especially seemingly incurable ones), or situations which we term as unfortunate, we commonly hear people say that karma has caught up with the person or family. One seldom hears well-being, wealth, capacities, and talents referred to as part of karma.[7]

Karma is everything we set before us in our life that will help us develop ourselves (i.e., to make the spiritual "I" shine through all our thoughts, feelings, and actions) and our relationships with others and with the world. We should then ask these simple questions: What did we do with the situations we met in our lives? Did we grapple with the difficulties and exhaust the learning we could get from them, or did we avoid them? Did we delude ourselves of our "good" fortune, or use this good fortune in pollutive and oppressive enterprises? Did we use our talents and wealth to improve our relationships and make the world a better place to live in? In other words, accidents, difficulties, good fortune, illnesses, or wealth are set before us as challenges to grapple with and learn from, developing ourselves and others for the better expression of our spiritual intentions.

Whether we believe that karma comes from previous lives or not is not initially important.[8] What is foremost is whether we face it squarely, or succumb to the temptation of easy wealth and easy living and back off from the difficulties. Whatever are the answers to the above questions will determine our next challenges, i.e., if we have grappled well, exhausted the learning, and developed the capacities, then greater challenges (opportunity to develop) will come. If we avoided them, challenges will be compounded and may come all together (for example, fatal accidents, cancer, or environmental destruction).[9] If our spiritual "I" is awake and in control of our lives, then we need not fear whatever challenges are brought before us. We will face them with open arms.

Cultivating the spiritual "I," then, is the best preventive medicine. For us adults, contemplation, meditation, and consciousness training are the positive ways to experience the true nature of this spiritual "I" and let it slowly take over our everyday life.[10] Once any karma comes our way, we will be able to face it for what it can mean and do for us.

To ensure then that the young generation will not have difficulty in experiencing their true "I," an overhaul of the educational system and child-rearing practices must be done. We should educate a child not for competition or to be a mere hub in the wheels of economic machinery, but towards freedom (as explained in Appendix 1).

B. THE CHALLENGE FOR THE 21ST CENTURY

The monopoly of orthodox science and medicine in our lives has brought about a monocropping of mindset regarding the image of the human being and the genesis of diseases. Up until today, orthodox science has not understood what life is. It treats the human being and all life merely as chemicals and physical processes. This way of thinking likewise dominates political decision-making, media, and the scientific and academic educational system. Whether we are aware of it or not, that point of view conditions not only our thinking, but that of the future generation. For example, a February 21, 1988, New York Times editorial about "Life, Industrialized" reported the successful cloning of seven prized bulls and the awarding of patents for genetically improved animals. It was also then that the National Academy of Sciences advocated a $3 billion project to work out the full chemical database of human genes, now known as the Human Genome Project. The editorial ended with the statement:

> Life is special, and humans even more so, but biological machines
> are still machines that now can be altered, cloned, and patented.
> The consequences will be profound, but taken a step at a time, they
> can be managed. Though science fiction has prepared everyone for
> the worst, lawmaking that is steady and careful can create a path
> towards the best the new technology can offer.

Thousands of miles away from New York City, local politicians, media men, and scientists (or anyone who is able to read the latest "scientific" pronouncements) reflect their blind faith in what orthodox science claims to be the truth. We are made to believe that out of this alleged truth, biotechnology (and other technologies) will only bring good for the vast majority of people.

The crusader-scientists, uncritical politicians, and media men—of any country whatsoever—are oblivious to the fact that the science is flawed, extremely one-sided, and limited. A flawed science can only result in a product or service that can be dangerous to human health.[11]

The root problem orthodox medical science faces is directly connected with this reduced image of the human being. Since we are all affected by this reductionist and materialistic view, we must think through and take a stand on what kind of a being we truly are—a biochemical one, or the four-fold interweaving being which we characterized earlier. The first image cannot heal, and will ultimately reduce the human being into its limited chemical/material image. The battle for the 21st century is then a battle for the true image of the human being. Medicine is only one arena of human life where this battle is raging. In agriculture, psychology, sociology, and other sciences involving life, a revolution in thinking and practice is underway. Whatever we imagine ourselves to be will determine not only our disease or health tendencies, and the kind and conduct of therapy, but also the way we will bring the rest of humanity towards a certain direction in evolution. Clearly, the biochemical image of the human being (if we allow it to continue as the leading concept of development, particularly in medicine) will bring humanity towards self-mutilation and self-destruction. Thus this identity crisis is critical, and each one's stance is equally crucial.[12] Once this question is resolved in each individual, he or she must militantly stand by it and live it, or else others will push for their own version, consciously or unconsciously, with all their wealth, power, and might.

For those who have the will to take a stand, this true image must then guide them towards adjusting their lifestyle, work situation, and relationships to be worthy of such an image. It should give one the insight to help others get rid of their blinders and together work in dismantling the illusion/delusion-making structures that exist. We should replace them with new structures and relationships worthy of the true human being.

In the preceding discussion, I sought to empower us ordinary folk to find a point (the spiritual "I") where one can dismiss illusions, recognize delusions, and integrate and synthesize details and points of view into a coherent whole.[13] From such understanding and profound comprehension, we can transform ourselves and our environment. I also tried to show that a technological solution is at most palliative, a patch-up job. True healing arises through learning to tap and creatively work with the power within, the true inner doctor.

I sincerely hope that with the above discussion as a structure of premises, and the remedies described in the next section, a true source of healing power can be nurtured to create a healthy society, and in the process, save the world.

Notes

1   The weakened, underdeveloped, or misdirected "I" is not prominently found in the drawing. One must visualize the "I" in the third dimension, i.e., behind all thoughts, feelings, and actions of the individual trying to assert greater influence through time. The younger one is, the less the influence of the spiritual "I" can be discerned in terms of consciously thought-out decisions or taming excessive emotionalism. The older one gets, the more the spiritual "I" should be in command, taming the excessive sympathies and antipathies and achieving equanimity, positivity, and right thoughts and actions.

2   For example, from dead blood cells comes colic acid, an ingredient in the production of bile acids.

3   Orthodox science has only recently looked into dead cells and their elimination as a possible cause of disease. This cell death and elimination process is termed *apoptosis*. However, orthodox scientists are investigating cell death within the framework of molecular biology. They speculate how genes or tissue chemistry can be altered to inhibit premature cell death or break the cells down and eliminate the toxins sooner. Without considering the role of the subtle bodies and how they interact, orthodox scientists will continually be blind to the real cause of apoptosis.

4 The decision to take these drugs as a last resort depends upon your ability to work with fear. Fear is always trying to possess us and often we adopt the most convenient and speedy way out, like taking drugs or running to a doctor. Courage must always be called upon to keep fear at a distance. Be cautious. However, don't be overconfident to the point of recklessness. It keeps one from perceiving the true progress of the illness. To know more about how to work with your fear, please see Sardello R. *Freeing the Soul from Fear.* New York: Riverhead Books; 2001.

5 We could also avoid the consequences of a revengeful spirit on health and illness.

6 The uncertainty of the survival of our individual consciousness after death can bring anxiety, depression, and fear in our earthly life. People react to this uncertainty by clinging to their physical existence. They surround themselves with unnecessary material possessions, keep themselves busy with certain tasks and activities that prevent them from thinking about this uncertainty, or they totally immerse themselves in a sensual life of sex, liquor, cigarettes, drugs, and similar pursuits. To have a clear idea of how our individual consciousness can survive after death is as important as knowing that the sun will rise again tomorrow. Without this certainty, disease and premature death find a space in our soul.

7 Those who have an inkling about repeated earth lives and how karma is woven into the lives of people may read Rudolf Steiner's *Manifestations of Karma* (Spring Valley, New York, 1975). Here the author's presentation is quite understandable to the present consciousness. He also debunks a number of misconceptions about it. It may be an aid in understanding and connecting many experiences outside the mainstream of everyday life.

8 In the long run, it may be important to know that what we have sown in previous lives, we reap in this lifetime. Thinking this through may give us many insights about our true immortal self or spiritual "I." We should not, however, fall into the trap of trying to know who we were then, i.e., our personality or small "i," or we may be caught in all sorts of delusions.

9 Cancer and AIDS are in many ways karmic diseases of the individual and of the whole of humanity. They are due primarily to the delusion of materialism—our inability to discern the intrinsic spirit in matter and material events. Seeing only calories in food results in diets that have no more life in them. This has been an underlying theme of our discussions all along. Orthodox science will continually fail to find a genuine cure for cancer or AIDS without considering self- and social transformation as necessary ingredients to the healing process. See also notes to the Introduction.

10 Once the spiritual "I" is fully in control of our lives, the Christian saying, "not 'I' but the Christ in me" becomes very meaningful and concrete. It also indicates the original

substance where our "I" comes from: a spark or "drop of the divine." Thus, it is understandable why the Christ is the universal healer once He is found living in our heart and directs our whole being. Other religions or spiritual paths may have their own version of this phrase.

11 See Hubbard R, Wald E. The eugenics of normalcy. *The Ecologist* 1993(Sept-Oct);23:185-191; Coghlan A. Biotechnology faces trial by jury. *New Scientist* 1994(Nov 19):5; "the jury condemned the industry for not producing anything of substantial benefit to society... called for labels to allow consumers to identify genetically engineered products... expressed worries about the escape of 'foreign' genes from crops into wild plants... questioned the role of the Advisory Committee on Releases to the Environment [pointing out that]... '[t]his committee has not stopped a single experiment going ahead and does not monitor releases once they have started.'" Gene test: the parents' dilemma. *New Scientist* 1994(Nov 12):40-44. "We are in danger of slipping into a eugenic system by default... the greatest problem of population screening would appear to be one of false reassurance... a 'cheap and cheerful' approach to genetic testing may create more problems than it solves." Duesberg PH, Schwartz JR. Latent viruses and mutated oncogenes: no evidence for pathogenicity. *Progress in Nucleic Acid Research and Molecular Biology* 1992;43:135-204. The website *www. humancloning.org/* is promoting human cloning and the main enticing argument for it is: to improve your health. Someone who has not thought the issue through regarding the genesis of illnesses will easily succumb to the enticement of cloning to improve one's health. Thus billions of dollars are now being donated by super-rich individuals to research in biotechnology, nanotechnology, and artificial intelligence, thinking (believing) that the solution to humanity's woes will be addressed by technology, instead of self-development.

12 There are no fence-sitters in this battle. Not taking a stand means supporting the biochemical image of the human being and all of its consequences. If you think you already take a stand because you are religious or are involved in some spiritual path, then it may be worthwhile to think this through again. Our conditioning has been quite thorough, and this conditioning continues through the media and the very structures of society (religion is not spared from this), so that most often what we think and believe does not conform to what we do. For example, I know of priests and religious leaders who blindly adhere to their materialistic science. Once I asked a scientist/priest to comment on the possibility of tapping the force of antigravity (the formative force field). He said that would violate the law of thermodynamics; it would create matter/energy out of nothing. The priest/scientist would not even speculate on the possibility. Clearly, the way he answered is typical of a materialistic scientist. He is blinded by his own scientific discipline, and his thinking is not fructified by his religion. Another example is from an observation made by a foreign friend whom I brought

to an Earth Day celebration. She could not help noticing that people kept throwing things around in spite of the presence of waste cans. In this case, what one believed was not translated into practice and our deeply ingrained conditioning dominated. Truly, our conditioning has been thorough, and it would take a tremendous amount of soul-searching and willful rethinking to get out of the maze and consciously unify our thinking and our actions.

13 The study of anthroposophy is one of the first steps one can take to bring one's consciousness to a coherent and even greater whole. Spiritual science and anthroposophy, given to us by Rudolf Steiner, are the spiritual impulses for modern times. Learning and understanding anthroposophy is in itself healing. In this light, I invite each and every one who has read this far to be students of anthroposophy.

Appendix 1

Illustration 2: Two Streams of Bodies Converging at Birth

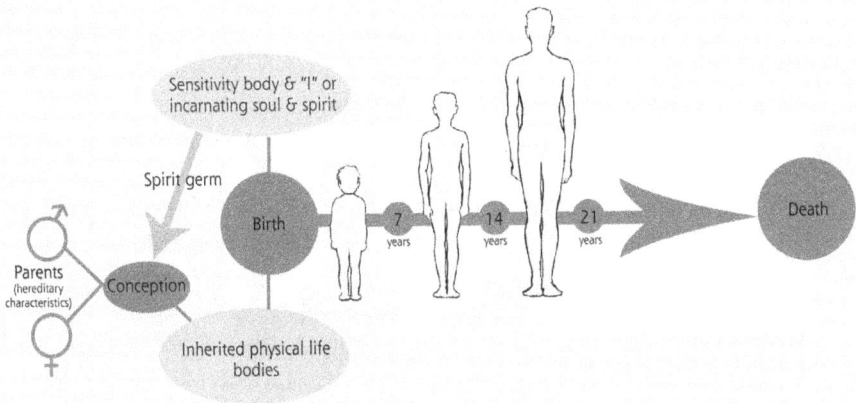

Illustration 2: Two Streams of Bodies Converging at Birth

A DESCRIPTION OF A CHILD'S INCARNATION PROCESS AND HOW MODERN DAY BELIEFS AND PRACTICES FOSTER THE DEVELOPMENT OF NEW DISEASES AND HEREDITARY ILLNESSES

In this appendix I would like to give a more comprehensive discussion of child development, because many of the neurological illnesses experienced today can be traced not only to the way the child is delivered (as discussed in Chapter 3), but from the moment of conception till 20 to 21 years of age as well. The methods of child rearing, schooling, and treatment of illnesses may actually be behind these new diseases, for example Attention Deficit Disorder (ADD), childhood cancer, and others.

This appendix is also an elaboration of Illustration 1 in Chapter 5 ("Model of a Healthy or Disease Process," p. 126), explaining why young adults today have an inadequate or misdirected sense of individuality that is contributing to their weakened vitality, and vice versa.

Please note Illustration 2 above: "Two Streams of Bodies Converging at Birth." We normally associate the birth of a child (when he takes his first breath) as the beginning of life on earth. The breathing indicates life ("The child is alive!") and the possibility to continue this life outside the womb of the mother, provided appropriate care is given.

The child's physical body and initial formative force body—coming from the parents—possess hereditary characteristics, like predisposition to certain illnesses, possibility for certain talents (for example music) to be expressed, among others. Since the turn of the 21st century, a number of studies have been made public linking certain genes to possible causes of illnesses. It is now common belief that if certain diseases are found along any of the family lines, it is almost certain that the offspring will develop the disease. If my child develops asthma early in life, and someone in our family line has a history of asthma, the child's illness is conveniently explained as "hereditary." No mystery; no questions asked. Most parents are resigned to simply alleviate the symptoms and not work for a possible cure. Worse, the medical establishment now uses genetic compatibility test to find out if potential couples are genetically compatible to produce healthy offspring, or to ensure neither spouse will cheat on the other.[1] An attitude of genetic determinism is dawning on us.

How can we explain the rise of hereditary illnesses? Chapter 2 of Section 1 on the gene theory of disease explains that only 2% of humanity's disease load can be considered hereditary, thus 98% is preventable. We may have the predisposition to the illness, but its expression sooner, later, or not at all can be determined by the continuous stimuli one receives or perceives from the environment. How can we better understand our surroundings so that we will be able to give the children a different atmosphere so that their predisposition to illnesses may not be expressed?

At conception, the development of the embryo is greatly influenced by the state of health of both parents. Getting pregnant when one is too young (below 18) or too old (above 35) increases the risk of underdevelopment, deformity, or abnormality of a part of the body, expressed in varying degrees.[2] The pregnant mother's exposure to alcohol, prohibited drugs, chemical drugs and other synthetic chemicals like nicotine and dioxin (as discussed in Chapter 2 of Section 1) contributes to this risk. Usually, a woman learns that she is pregnant when the fetus is already about 6 to 8 weeks old. If she is in the habit of taking alcohol (socially or otherwise), the fetus would already have been subjected to whatever negative influences the alcohol or artificial chemicals may have.[3]

The emotional life of the mother also affects the development of the fetus. Insecurity or emotional trauma, for example, cause the pregnant mother to secrete a hormone called testosterone. Excess testosterone can inhibit the proper development of the brain, particularly the left hemisphere[4] of the neocortex, predisposing the child to left-handedness and possibly less ability to use the left brain.[5] During pregnancy, the mother needs the support of the husband with regard to her emotional and physical well-being in order to ensure the full development of the physical apparatus of the child.

At birth, with the first breath, the infant's sensitivity body and "I" incarnate into his inherited physical and formative force bodies, like an awakening from a deep sleep. The sensitivity body and "I" rouse into consciousness the physical and life bodies. But the child's consciousness is not the same as the adult's. The child must gradually penetrate/incarnate into these inherited bodies until its individuality takes full control of all faculties and becomes effective and responsible on earth. This is the reason why childhood is a 20 to 21-year-long process. It takes this much time for human beings to evolve into responsible adults able to direct themselves in life with purpose and meaning. Age 21 years is recognized across cultures throughout the world as the child's coming of age.

Rudolf Steiner's research reveals that at conception, the "I" from the spiritual world sends a spirit seed to the embryo, influencing its development. Thus, if one looks at the developing embryo, the primitive streak (attributed to the activity of the sensitivity body) suddenly appears at around day 16 - 18. From here, the embryo begins to turn into a fetus, i.e., differentiating cells to become the nerves, bones, tissues, organs, and the like. The "I" of the child works on the fetus by orchestrating this differentiation process, organizing the whole body into the archetypal image of the human being, and stamping its individuality into the child's physical body to the point that the child has his own unique fingerprint, among other individualized features.

Once born, the tasks of the incarnating child consist of the following: 1) continue to remold the inherited body to make it his own, be comfortable in it, and let its individuality interpenetrate this developing body to be in command of all cellular, tissue, and organ secretions and functions; 2) differentiate his soul capacities of willing, feeling, and thinking and eventually integrate and harmonize them into a coherent whole; and 3) develop, integrate, and sharpen his senses to perceive himself, other human beings, and the world to be able to gain a true and unified conception, sooner or later, of himself, others, and the world.

If these three main tasks are only partially fulfilled, we then witness the genesis of disease tendencies, expression of hereditary illnesses, behavioral and neurological problems, and social inequity in both children and adults in the world today.

1. Remolding the Inherited Physical/Life Bodies

If one observes the whole of human life, childhood is the time when most illnesses of an inflammatory nature happen. Childhood diseases are characterized by high fever, and at times skin rashes appear as in measles, chicken pox, roseola infantum, and the like. Children can easily develop high fever even up to 41 degrees centigrade (106 degrees Fahrenheit). How do we explain this phenomenon?

When the incarnating sensitivity body and "I" of the child penetrates his inherited physical/life bodies at birth, there is not always a perfect match. There can be rough edges or cases of mismatch. The incarnating "I" brings intentions, talents, and capacities which have to be expressed in a vessel. This initial vessel is the inherited physical/life bodies which serve as the instrument to perceive and act in the world. An imperfect or defective instrument bars the full expression of a talent or intention.

Fever (the "I" working in warmth) and childhood diseases are specific means of the incarnating child to remold (by burning away inherited proteins) and recast his inherited physical body to allow the individuality to become comfortable and eventually be in total control of its instrument. Thus, fever and childhood diseases should not be suppressed by chemical drugs or vaccination. These modern measures may inhibit the full transformation of the inherited body and, among other things, promote the expression of inherited predispositions to illnesses. The untransformed inherited proteins can also distort the individual's perception of his original intentions and unnecessarily divert the direction of one's life. Thus, we witness many young and middle-aged people drifting in sensual pleasure and addiction to alcohol and drugs, unable to discover what they need to do in life.[6] Others get on with life but take on their parent's wishes. Still others conform to the current society's materialistic goals and missions (oblivious to their real intentions in life) and suffer the consequence to their health and to society (as explained in Section 1).

At around 6 or 7 years of age, the milk teeth of children everywhere in the world start to fall and are replaced by the permanent teeth. This indicates that the formative growth forces (belonging to the child's individuality) have essentially finished the task of transforming the inherited physical body. These partially released growth forces then become available for memory and thinking. Thus the child is ready to go to school. Prior to this period, however, reading, writing, memorizing, and learning about the world in an abstract way must not be the activity of the child.[7] The formative growth forces are still busy transforming the inherited physical/life bodies and bodily organs. If these forces are diverted into early academics, memorizing, and abstract thinking, then the health of the bodily organs may suffer, since the work of transforming the inherited body remains incomplete.[8]

The child continues to grow thereafter, occasionally having a fever or an inflammation to adjust one or the other functions of the body. For example, when a child begins to menstruate, the period may be irregular for some time. Then the child may go into a fever, and thereafter the menstrual period becomes regular. A shy child unable to interact with other children can become quite social after a fever. In these two examples, fever adjusts and fine-tunes a bodily function (menstruation) in the former, while in the latter case a fever helps the child express his soul capacities better. Imagine if this process is partially obstructed by the suppression of the fever. We now have epidemics of young women with painful menstruation (dysmenorrhea), ovarian cysts, myoma (benign tumors of the uterus), and even endometriosis (hardening of the uterus). We encounter and hear about young adults unable to express their social capacities and other talents, thus resorting to violence, cheating, or withdrawing from life altogether. This is typical "fight or flight" mentality we see in normal people nowadays.

Puberty, approximately around 12 to 14 years of age, is another milepost in child development. Girls and boys truly change, and not only sexually. The voice of males becomes one octave lower, while girls only a note. Normally, young children have lower hemoglobin content in the blood, then it gradually increases until puberty. For females, hemoglobin content plateaus at 14 gm per 100 ml of blood, while that of the boys continues to rise to 16 gm. This difference has a particular meaning in itself, which I cannot go into in this appendix.[9]

The growth forces continue to differentiate the three living systems of the human body in order for them to be used as instruments for thinking, feeling, and willing,

The 21st birthday of the child is the moment every parent is waiting for. The young adult is now ideally a responsible member of society, able to give direction and purpose to his life. The "I" of this individual should now be more firmly incarnated in the body and in control of all his faculties and bodily functions.

2. Differentiating Soul Capacities of Willing, Feeling, and Thinking

Upon birth, the most obvious and seemingly developed part of the body is the head. The child's head is about 1/4 of the body, while in the adult the head is about 1/7 or 1/8 of the overall body proportion. The formative growth forces then work on the child's body downwards, differentiating the neck, the torso, and then the limbs. It is thus more appropriate to say that the child grows downwards (not "grows up" as we normally exclaim). (See Illustration 3, p. 143.)

a. Educating the Will

In the first seven years of life, the limbs of a young child are the most active: grasping, holding, kicking, tasting, among others. A baby slowly learns to manipulate his body from the head downwards: raising and turning the neck, lifting the shoulders, crawling, turning the trunk left to right, turning over from back to its tummy, sitting down with an erect spine, struggling to stand up and gain balance, and finally taking the first step. What one sees is pure *will*. Thus in this first seven years, one can characterize the soul life of a child as all *will*. Though this will is not conscious, it is nevertheless the most awake at this time (a paradox), as contrasted to the life of feeling and thinking. Willing, feeling, and thinking have not yet differentiated. In other words, the child thinks and feels with the will and whole body. Thus, when the child starts to speak and says, "hand," the hand is raised together with the word. When a child feels pain, he cannot pinpoint exactly which part of the body aches. The child is still in the process of differentiating his "thinking, feeling, and willing."

From birth to 7 years, the child is a total sense organ. He perceives everything in his environment, from the gestures and deeds of the adults, to their feelings, attitudes, intentions, and thoughts. What the child experiences around him, he imitates—whether socially appropriate or not. Adults surrounding the child should then be worthy models of imitation. Children will copy everything, trusting that the adults know what they are doing, and that it is always good. Parenting and teaching in nurseries and kindergartens must begin with the self-education of the adults involved. Thus, when a child is unruly, the adult must first ask: how am I today? Is there something I have not resolved within myself or with other important persons in my life? Children's initial misbehavior can truly just reflect one's environment. After clarifying the adult's condition, investigating other possible causes of misbehavior can be considered, such as the child's lifestyle, diet, electronic media exposure, lack of sleep, and the side-effects of medicine, as discussed in Chapters 2 and 3 of Section 1.

The child's will therefore must be guided, directed, and educated by the adults surrounding him. This is where there are many points of view,

Illustration 3

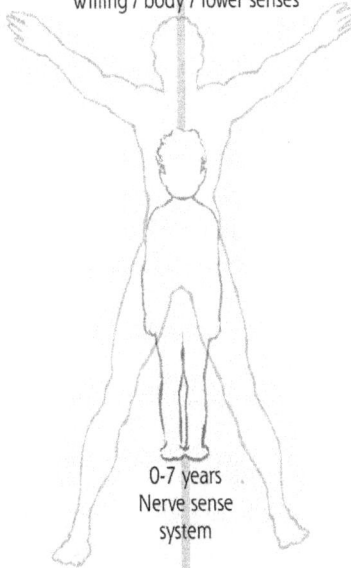

EMPHASIS OF DEVELOPMENT
OF WAKING-UP FORCES & THE 12 SENSES

Waking up

14-21 years
Thinking / spirit / higher senses

7-14 years
Feeling / soul / middle senses

0-7 years
Willing / body / lower senses

0-7 years
Nerve sense
system

7-14 years
Rhythmic system

14-21 years
Metabolic / limb
system

Growing down

EMPHASIS OF DEVELOPMENT OF GROWTH FORCES

spread out in a spectrum with many gradations in between. On one side of the scale is absolute freedom, and on the other, rigid restriction and discipline, to the point of psychological and corporal punishments. Each extreme viewpoint can have repercussions on the character and mental and emotional health of the child, which sooner or later affect the developing physical/life bodies. Very rigid parenting or education can lead to narrow-mindedness, inhibitions, and repressed emotional and will life. Parents who cannot control their anger may be inducing irregularity in the heart, or asthma. With too much freedom, the child can do anything he wants: eat any food he likes, sleep only when he is exhausted, watch television as long as he wants, play with anything, even if inappropriate, or behave without consideration of others. In other words, the child is becoming a slave of his mere likes and dislikes, and susceptible to the corresponding diseases (and consequences of inappropriate social behavior) that may be induced, as discussed earlier.

What then is the appropriate way to bring up children? One general principle is to provide them healthy boundaries that would ensure moderation in everything. These boundaries are determined by the properly informed and observant parents (and implemented ideally by all the adults surrounding the child). The goal is for the child to eventually learn how to control his own will, likes, and dislikes. Thus, inappropriate social behavior should immediately be corrected in a loving, firm manner. Children should engage in a variety of play modes and use diverse toys. They need to sleep early and for hours in the night. They should eat good nourishing food (as explained in Chapters 3 and 4 of Section 1) and not be limited only to what they want. Tantrums in children may indicate that the likes and dislikes are holding sway.

Another important principle is rhythm in the life of a child. One of its aspects is regularity of basic activities such as eating, sleeping, toilet time, bath, and the like. This rhythm provides the child with security. Once imbibed, it will become second nature and serve as the basis of discipline. Day to day challenges ("I don't want to eat, I am still playing") normally encountered by parents in bringing up children can be avoided. Parenting can be a more joyful experience rather than hard work, as many parents attest to nowadays. The second aspect is the alternating quality of activities—breathing in and out, expansion and contraction, sleeping and waking, concentrated forces and relaxation. To illustrate, indoor free play can be followed by a more structured activity like storytelling, then outdoor play, and so on.

b. Educating the Feeling Life[10]

From the ages 7 to 14 years, the child awakens more in his feelings and emotions, and is greatly swayed by likes or dislikes. Persuasion and sweet talk will hardly work. In learning new things, especially in school, the teacher must present the subject matter artistically and joyfully. In this period, the child thinks in pictures. Thus, whatever is beautiful and pleasing to the senses and imagination entices the child's interest, facilitating learning. This is the core methodology behind Steiner or Waldorf pedagogy. Mathematics, the sciences, history, or learning a new language must be fun rather than dry and boring, as is mostly the case today. Teachers of this age group should be loving authorities, earning the love and respect of the pupils. To know the biography of each child, his constitutional temperament, and likes or dislikes strengthens the connection between child and teacher, fostering the learning process. Everything the teachers say is true and right from the children's point of view.

The school life plays an important role in developing the capacity of children to manage their emotions, for better or for worse. Other than choosing a good school for the child, parents can further support the child's progress by minimizing stress and unnecessary expectations.[11] They should always make themselves available if and when the child needs them. If the will has been properly educated and an already established rhythm at home has led to self-discipline, the development of feeling life can proceed smoothly. Moreover, the child will have the strength to face the challenge of school work and possess the enthusiasm to learn.

Given that the first seven years of the child are the foundation years, most problems thereafter, which are related to learning, attitudes to life, and other human beings, can be traced back to certain aspects of the will; these may remain uneducated, hindered from being expressed freely, or misdirected (meaning the instinct, impulse, and desire of the body have not yet been taken hold of by the "I," and which can be transmuted later on more consciously by the "I" into motive[12]). These can still be redeemed and given form to some extent in this second stage of development, if the schooling system or the teacher understands the stages of development children undergo. If the school system cannot understand the child, then the part of the will that remains uneducated may eventually develop into more complicated, compounded, and complex expression, like burning out, anorexia, bulimia, schizophrenia, paranoia, bi-polar conditions, delusions of grandeur, prejudice, or racism, in varying degrees, sooner or later in life.

c. Educating the Life of Thinking

Roughly around the third 7-year period of life (ages 14 to 21 years), the child wakes up to his thinking—in concepts and ideas—and begins to form judgment. This is the time where the meaning of cause and effect becomes clearer in one's mind. The "I" asserts itself through the child's thinking. A child feels good if he defeats his father in a game of chess. He may often question the validity of what his parents say and what the teachers are teaching. This is the period of rebellion if not handled well by the adults. This is a heed to shift parenting style from being loving authorities to a facilitating companion/friend—that is, facilitating the process of decision making in sensitive areas of the adolescent life. Parents should learn how to be a big open *ear* to what the adolescent is narrating. Judgment must be founded on a considerable discussion of all angles of the matter.

Another new experience of the adolescent is attraction to the opposite gender. They will have crushes, idols, and may actually fall in "love." Parents and teachers should find ways to raise this developing capacity to love (a person) to the level of deep concern, love, and compassion for the world. This is the time to study biographies of people who, out of their love for others, engaged themselves in service for the good of the world— for example, scientists, who out of their altruism and using their talents, discovered new ways to heal people. The teaching of history and current events should make them comprehend the root causes of poverty and inequity in the world. Visiting victims of oppression and natural calamities and doing voluntary services every now and then should be part of the curriculum of upper grades. These are a few of the ways for the teenager's sense of love to encompass the whole of humanity and the world, and not to remain confined to personal love.

Another yearning and aspiration of the adolescent is self-discovery. The adolescent asks the questions (inwardly or outwardly) "Who am I?" "What am I here for?" "What are my capacities and talents?" "What then should I be doing with my life?" Parents and teachers must not only be aware of this, but also facilitate activities that may lead to potential answers to these questions. Camping in the forest as a class, where one's survival instinct is put to a test, is an example of a relevant activity. During a camp fire, the teacher could begin a conversation where each student mirrors his impressions about each of their companions, as a buddy, as someone who was tasked with a responsibility, as a classmate, as a friend, and so on. This way, the adolescent learns that his identity is also being molded by the impression he makes on others, and he can further refine his social relationships. It is hoped that eventually the adolescent will develop a sense that what he is, feels, and does positively or negatively affect others.

The normal adolescent today can easily lose interest in learning when these yearnings and aspirations are not being met. If and when he finds someone (or a peer group/gang) to direct his love and loyalty to, he may feel affirmed and fulfilled enough, and no longer aspire to complete his formal education. Others may remain in school simply to pass and earn a diploma. A worse scenario if these yearnings remain unfulfilled is to feel rejected both in school and at home, leading to suicide—and in even more severe cases, violence towards others.[13]

As was said earlier, the enthusiasm to learn and the love for life are cultivated in the child's first seven years through mindful parenting. A properly educated will brings about a healthy feeling life and eventually clarity in thinking. A will that is ill wakes up ill feelings and ill thoughts, and vice-versa.

3. Developing the Twelve Senses[14]—To Sense Oneself, the World, and Other Human Beings as Separate Entities, but also as a Unified Whole

One of the legacies of Rudolf Steiner in the understanding of the human being is the idea that we have twelve senses. These senses often work in synergy to give us a comprehensive picture of reality. For every perception (complete or incomplete), we have a corresponding comprehension (concept and idea) of the situation, then we respond and act out to make our permanent mark that will affect the environment and our fellow human beings, for better or for worse, and for all eternity. The ideal is for the twelve senses to fully develop and work harmoniously in every adult human being.

The twelve senses may be grouped into three: the willing/bodily/lower senses, the feeling/soul/middle senses, and the thinking/spiritual/higher senses. All of them are present and can be slowly awakened when the child is born. However, each group of senses has a particular period or emphasis of development, corresponding to the seven year phases of child development which we described above as Willing, Feeling, and Thinking. Thus it is best to nurture the senses at the appropriate time, so as not to divert the growth forces from their work in the body, and/or inhibit the effort of the "I" from mastering these senses, individually and later collectively, as will be explained towards the end of this discussion. (See again Illustration 3, p.143.) Our senses are used to perceive both what is outside us and what is within.[15]

a. The Will or Bodily or Lower Senses—
Touch, Life, Own Movement, and Balance

The *sense of touch* is found all over the free nerve endings of the skin and tactile corpuscles (concentrated in areas especially sensitive to light touch, such as the fingertips, palms, soles, lips, tongue, face, nipples, and the skin of the genitals). When one touches something or leans on a wall, it not only gives information about what is touched, but also informs the one touching that this (his skin) is the limit of "myself." At birth, the infant experiences the first touch while going through the birth canal. While being held by people who care, the child senses that "I am now in an enclosed space, bounded by what I feel around me as my skin." The loving touch is most especially important in the first few minutes, hours, and days of the child. The continuing experience of this loving touch confirms the child's existence on earth in a dense physical body, insures being welcomed, and gives the child trust in the environment and in other people.[16] Will/bodily development will then proceed as described above, without the initial possible aberration of the fight or flight (withdrawal) syndrome.

The *sense of life* is found in the vegetative nervous system. It is the part of the nervous system that regulates involuntary bodily functions, including the heart rate, activity of the intestines, and production of sweat. Experiences of comfort and harmony with his initial environment set the foundation for a good sense of life as the child gets older. Otherwise, the young child initially uses crying to convey any discomfort. The basic instinct of most parents is to find out what is wrong with the child, and through trial and error (or instinctively through the bond created between child and mother) they manage to ease the discomfort. In time, parents develop a sense of what each cry means and they respond appropriately. What nurtures a good sense of life? We already mentioned the loving and caring environment, the regular daily rhythm, and activities and other experiences appropriate to the age of the child. Thus, dissatisfaction, indulgence, stress, shock, lack of coherence, and consistent exposure to conflict, violence, and intimidation create insecurity and instigate the animal instinct of flight or fight. This insecurity develops anger, and sooner or later possibly hatred towards the world.

The bodily organ for the *sense of one's own movement* is found in the neuromuscular spindles within the fleshy portions of the muscles. Regular, repetitive, various gross and fine movements develop increasing perception and control of one's own movement. The ability to move brings about the experience of freedom, self-control, and further activity in life. The sensible sequence of movement, like in imaginative play, climbing trees to pick fruits, gardening, planting, and sweeping create harmonious interlinkages among the different cells of our four-fold brain system, enhancing intelligence in the child.[17] Thus it is important to arrange indoor (and outdoor) play to allow much freedom to explore anything and pursue free play. Children who are always followed around and forbidden to do certain things are inhibited in the full development of this sense. Activities that leave the child as a mere observer, such as the use of automated toys, television viewing, or merely sitting in a stroller or a moving vehicle, are not recommended. The growing child should be exposed to different terrains where he can perceive the uneven surfaces and adjust his movements accordingly. This sense is closely related to the sense of balance.

The *sense of balance* is centered in the semi-circular canals of the middle ear. Each child develops a relationship to the force of gravity and perceives himself in three-dimensional space: above and below, left and right, and front and back. It conveys in the child experiences of equilibrium and compensation, and a place of rest and self-confidence. To nurture this sense the child should engage in movement games, jumping, walking on a balance beam, seesaw, stilts, monocycles, and the like. In dealing with the child, the adult should have calmness and certainty. Moreover, the adult should be striving for balance within, and avoiding prolonged bouts of depression, resignation, restlessness, and the like.

New illnesses have emerged that are directly attributed to the mal-development of these four will/bodily/lower senses. For example, in an autistic child the sense of touch and of life are particularly oversensitive, such that if he is touched or looked at, he immediately withdraws and reacts as if he is in pain (then later on may develop hyposensitivity to touch). In the hyperactive and Attention Deficit Hyperactive Disorder, or ADHD child, the sense of touch may not be sensitive—to the point that when he bumps into things, he is barely hurt (until a bone is broken). For the ADHD child, the sense of own movement is not properly permeated or controlled by the "I." The muscles seem to move on their own and the child fails to learn how to control his movements at the appropriate moment, thus he bumps easily into things. For the autistic child, withdrawal from interaction with the world and with people would prevent him from properly developing his sense of own movement and balance, thus making his situation worse and more complicated. (Low muscle tone or floppiness, and movement stereotypes like rocking or hand-flapping, are some examples of autistic behavior and conditions.)

b. The Feeling/Soul/Middle Senses—Smell, Taste, Sight, and Warmth

The organ for the *sense of smell* is the olfactory mucosa at the root of the nose. It makes one feel connected with the aroma. Providing children with different smell experiences in plants, foods, and various situations in both city and countryside nurture this sense. A child who is continuously in stuffy rooms, surrounded by bad smells or disgusting impressions and behavior from adults, may be harmed in the development of this sense.

The taste buds are found in the mucus membranes of the tongue where the *sense of taste* is located. It works together with the sense of smell to give us different taste experiences such as sweetness, sourness, saltiness, bitterness, or pungency. Food prepared in such a way that its natural taste is released will positively affect this sense. Tasteful discerning of people and aesthetically designed environments will enhance this sense. Over-stimulation of the taste buds (especially between the ages 0 to 7 years), like excessive saltiness and sweetness, or frequent use of taste-enhancing substances like monosodium glutamate (MSG), will harm this sense. Tasteless comments, tactlessness, and inartistic environments will likewise damage its development.

In the eyes, the *sense of sight* gives us an experience of light and color. To nurture this sense and the experiences we get from it, we should draw attention to subtle color nuances in nature by showing interest in them. During the first seven years, the child's room should have predominantly pastel colors, and if possible no unnecessary images or prints that may tire the child's eyes. Reading, television viewing, loud colors—especially before 7 years old—may harm the development of the eyes and promote nearsightedness. Likewise, dark moods, lack of interest, or a colorless and dull environment can also be harmful influences.

All over the body, we have receptors of warmth and cold which convey such experiences to us. Thus quite early in the life of a child, we should provide adequate clothing to protect this *sense of warmth*. Likewise, providing the feeling of warmth in soul and spirit will enhance its development. Overheated or cold rooms, insufficient clothing, a cold and impersonal atmosphere, and an exaggerated, hypocritical "warm-heartedness" are some unfavorable influences.

As we stated earlier, adult actions and interactions with the child will either positively or negatively affect the development of the latter's feeling life and eventually sense of self. This set of senses invokes the feeling of sympathy or antipathy in the child. For example, strong-tasting food (sweets like cakes and candies, or salty food) becomes an automatic preference over more nutritious but less "tasty" ones. Thus the younger the child experiences these strong sympathies and antipathies in these four middle senses without regulation by the adults, the greater the possibility that the child's preferences will become fixated. Thus we frequently hear parents complaining, "but my child does not eat vegetables," because their taste buds have been corrupted prematurely. If the child starts being selective with regard to food, toys, scent, or activity, the parent should immediately break the habit. The key words are flexibility, diversity, and variety of activities within the day, the week, the month, and the year.

c. Senses that Relate Primarily to Thinking as Mental Capacity

Our ears and the *sense of hearing* give us experiences of sound/tone. In the early years, speaking softly, singing simple songs like pentatonic music, lullabies, hearing simple stories repeatedly, allowing time for inner pictures, tone, acoustic images to arise—these will nurture the development of this sense. As the child gets older, appropriate musical instruments can be played, like the recorder, violin or cello, flute, and percussion to refine this hearing sense. Classical pieces from Handel, Hayden, Bach, and Mozart will be most beneficial to play from nine years onwards. These will then form within the child a healthy inner soul realm. Thus, excessively loud music and other acoustics through the electronic media (lacking the personal human element), superficial or untruthful talk, and inhuman tone/voice may deter the development of this sense. The sense of hearing is directly related to—and a refinement of—the sense of balance.

The *sense of word* develops out of the child's perception of movement and language. It conveys the experience of form and physiognomy (sense of form), of grasping the meaning of body language, and the forming of sounds and words. The living tone/voice, the warmth of soul that accompanies the voice, awareness of body language, gestures and social cues, and ensuring inner experiences match outer expressions, cultivate this sense. Disparity between expressed intentions and deeds, cold neutral attitude, telling lies, and absentmindedness may be detrimental to the development of this sense.

The *sense of thought or meaning* develops as a result of the complex processes of perceiving outer events in life and discerning or having the feeling for what is "right" or "not right." This is seen in one's ability to immediately grasp a line of thought. To properly develop this sense, the child should be surrounded by what is true and right. Consistency and coherence of things and events in the life of a child, where the adult displays meaningful work, are most important. Thus meaningless actions, uncoordinated and erratic thinking, and distortion of facts are to be avoided in the presence of the child.

The *sense of the "I" of the other* develops out of and is a refinement of the sense of touch and contacts made at the periphery of one's own body. It conveys the experience of essential being, the immediate experience, cognition, and presence of the "I" of the other. Thus when the child experiences early in his life love between adults and towards himself, this sense is immediately affirmed. Continuous experience of people loving and caring for other people throughout childhood would further heighten the cultivation of this sense. As a family, a culture of visiting friends and other relatives and meeting new people where the genuine perception of the other is practiced by the adults, are other means to foster this sense. Lack of attention, disinterest, and other forms of lovelessness shown towards others would curtail the development of this sense. Early exposure to electronic media and virtual realities which do not let the child interact with real human beings are to be avoided, especially when the child is still younger than 12 years.

The harmonious development of these thinking senses would lead to a healthy life of thought and thinking. Willful thinking is a prerequisite for the "I" or the self to further develop and integrate all experiences in life into a coherent whole. This is the true meaning of freedom: ability to control, harmonize, and redirect the dictates of the lower passions, temperaments, and bodily predispositions in order to maintain mindfulness and equanimity of soul, as well as purposeful and meaningful deeds. This is the task of parenting and education.

Underdevelopment, miseducation, or incoherence of any sort in one's childhood, may be repaired through self-education after age 21 years (but at the expense of doing one's task in life). Some aimlessly drift here and there, unaware of what to do with life. Some can take on a criminal mind and pursue criminal activities. Others do find a job but bring their ill and incomplete thoughts, feelings, and deeds into their work. Thus, it is easy to resort to lies, cheating, or deception because the world is full of them anyway. A healthy, just, and equitable relationship may also be considered insignificant. Emphasis is given more on what can be taken from the world, and how cravings, power, and material gains can be satisfied. "This is the relationship I learned to live with, so what else is there to life?" Still, there could be others who will acknowledge and embrace their defects and inadequacies, so as to undergo conscious self-education. I hope that this book will also serve as a guide to this yearning in you.

Notes

1 See *www.actionbioscience.org* and *livescience.com* on this up-and-coming genetic determinism.

2 For example, it is common to hear of children born with hernia (failure of certain tissue to close at birth, usually around the abdomen), or a worse condition—one born with a "hole" in the heart or defective heart valves. All these and other examples may be caused by a weakening formative force body of the parents, due to toxins accumulated through the years or toxins from drugs, alcohol, and other exposure to environmental chemicals—as this appendix will continue to explain.

3 If you plan to get pregnant, then it is best to refrain from any chemical drugs, alcohol, and the like for at least three months. Try to live a balanced life as indicated in this book. This would facilitate detoxification of your body. You can also undergo certain simple detoxification procedures like fasting once a day, every week for a month. If you are above 35 years old, it is better to undergo a more thorough cleansing. See *mastercleanser.com* to get an idea of a safe way to fast.

4 The left brain is concerned with analytic functions, arithmetic, and processing language; while the right brain hemisphere is connected to simple spatial concepts, face recognition, some elements of music, and many aspects of emotions.

5 See Carpenter M. *The Core Text in Neuroanatomy*, Fourth Edition, Williams and Wilkins, Baltimore, 1991. "If fetal levels of testosterone are altered by maternal stress or other factors, the right hemisphere may become more developed and assume functions for language and handedness which the left hemisphere cannot support. The effects of testosterone on brain development are most pronounced in the male, which may account for higher incidence of left-handedness, dyslexia, and stuttering in the male." (p. 428). According to researchers from Cambridge University, UK, babies who produce high levels of testosterone while they are still in the womb have a higher chance of showing traits of autism later on. This could just be one possible after-effect of maternal distress. To read more about the link between autism and testosterone levels in the womb, see *www.medicalnewstoday.com/articles/7417.php*. There could be other effects not yet detected by research, thus the need to be more cautious when one is pregnant.

6 See Dunselman R. *In Place of Self: How Drugs Work*, Hawthorn Press, UK 1995. Drug and alcohol use is on the rise, undermining personal identity and maturity at a time when people are supposed to be open to spiritual experiences. Legalizing their use may only aggravate existing tendencies to addiction.

7 Early academic programs in the preschool were introduced only in the last 40 years or so. Before this, kindergarten was a play school—where play, singing, fantasy, imagination, the dreamy magical consciousness of the child, and interaction with nature are fostered—giving time for the body to be ready for academics in grade school. The word kindergarten (children's garden) reveals the original intention of preschool. Somehow materialistic educators and policy makers lost track of this original idea and became preoccupied with how to make children get ahead (in the rat race) at the expense of their proper and healthy development, as discussed in this appendix.

8 I have encountered in my practice young adults (below 30 years of age) with varying degrees of degenerative conditions like hypertension, diabetes, and even cancer. They belong to the generation who entered nursery schools and kindergartens with early academic programs. What Rudolf Steiner said 90 years ago about diverting the growth forces into early academics and thus depriving the bodily organs of full development, is becoming more evident now in the Philippines.

9 See Huseman/Wolff. *The Anthroposophic Approach to Medicine Vol. 1*, The Anthroposophic Press, Spring Valley NY, 1982, pp. 72-77 to know more about the significance of iron in the blood and why at puberty males and females diverge in their hemoglobin content.

10 The more common term for the education of feeling life is Emotional Intelligence. This is just the beginning of understanding this "new" intelligence. See Goleman D. *Emotional Intelligence: Why it Can Matter More Than IQ*, Bantam Books, New York, 1996. Another monumental work is on heart intelligence, as mentioned in note 12, Ch. 1, Section 2. See also Robert Sardello's *Love and the Soul: Creating a Future for Earth*.

11 For example, parents should not expect their children to pass examinations all the time, especially in the first four grade levels. Sometimes failing a test is a motivation to do better. If they continue to do so, then parents should look at as many angles as possible to find out what would motivate the child to learn, and not jump to nasty conclusions that would aggravate the matter, or resort to bribery (the way most parents do today).

12 Rudolf Steiner gives us a very comprehensive discussion on the subject of will. Will is first found in our instinct, and instinct is connected to our physical body. Instinct is taken hold of and made inward by our formative force body, and instinct is transformed into impulses. In the sensitivity body, the instinct and impulse are made more inward and both are lifted into consciousness, and in this way desire arises. When the human being takes up into his "I" the instinct, impulse, and desire of the body, then they are transmuted into motive. "It is only man who can raise the level of desire by bringing it into the soul world, hence comes the urge to conceive a true motive of will… in man,

instinct, impulse, and desire from the animal world still persist, but he raises them to motive." Steiner R. *The Study of Man*, Rudolf Steiner Press, London, 1966, pp. 60-62.

13 The recent killings in schools in the US and in Europe by "mentally deranged" pupils are truly a pathetic scenario. The increase in suicide rates of adolescents in most affluent urban centers of the world has not been taken as a distress signal by educators and policy makers. The killing of others is an aggravation of the situation, a much louder cry for help from the younger generation. Educators and parents from all over the world must begin to overhaul the whole system of modern child rearing and schooling soon, before another aggravated event happens.

14 See Aeppli W. *The Care and Development of the Human Senses*, Steiner Waldorf Schools Fellowship, Forest Row, UK, 1998, for a more thorough discussion of the twelve senses.

15 For the following discussion of the twelve senses I followed and elaborated the outline of Michaela Gloeckler in *"Education—A Pathway of 'Silent' Healing,"* found in Gloeckler, Langhammer, & Wiechert. *Health for Life: Education and Medicine Working Together for Healthy Development*, Medical and Pedagogical Section of the Goetheanum, 2006.

16 With our technological way of handling childbirth (drugged from painkillers and lack of blood, bright lights, mechanical suction, cold room, and no warm and familiar body in a nursery) the initial few minutes to affirm that the child is welcome can turn to distress and later withdrawal from the world. Could the hypersensitivity of the sense of touch in autistic children be due to the way they were handled in childbirth, or from overexposure to ultrasound and other electronic devices while still in the womb?

17 Yes, human beings have a four-fold brain system: the reptilian brain—the most ancient, corresponding to our will, our instinct to fight or flight: quick reflexive reaction; the old mammalian, limbic, or emotional-cognitive brain; the neocortex, or the new mammalian or verbal-intellectual brain, consisting of the left and right hemispheres; and the newest addition—our prefrontal lobes. The first three correspond to our faculty of willing, feeling, and thinking, while the fourth brain is more connected to our "I" and all its potential. The prefrontal lobes are being called by some neuroscientists "the "angel lobes," attributing to them our "higher human virtues" of love, compassion, empathy, and understanding, as well as our advanced intellectual skills. See Pearce J. *The Biology of Transcendence: A Blueprint of the Human Spirit*, Park Street Press, Rochester, Vermont, 2002. Like the previous discussion on the development of a child's faculty of willing, feeling, and thinking, the brain undergoes the same sequence of development. The full development of each part is very much determined by the environment/experience the child encounters in life, particularly the presence of a role model. A handicap in

the initial development can be magnified in the development of the other stages. "Miss one sequence and the entire structure is at risk" (Pearce, p. 47).

Appendix 2

Illustration 4: Schools of Thought in Medicine and Healing Arts
in a Four-fold Human Spectrum

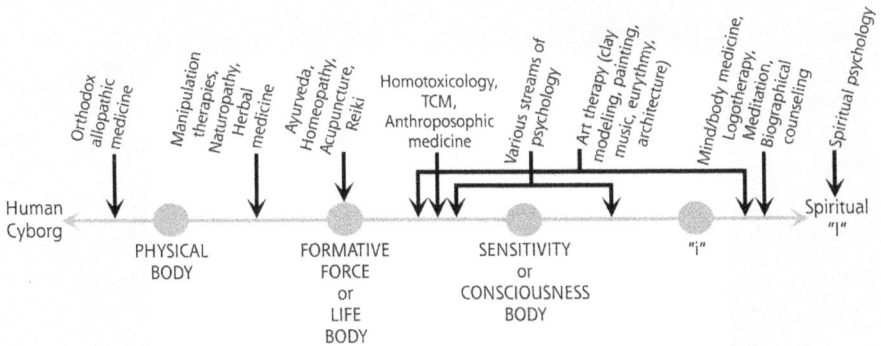

HUMANITY'S SEARCH FOR TRUE HEALING IN A
FOUR-FOLD HUMAN SPECTRUM

All healing arts and schools of thought in medicine can be put in a spectrum, addressing various aspects of the human being. Illustration 4 is my attempt to show how this is seen from the perspective of the four-fold human being. On one end of the scale is the physical body, while on the other is the "I" with the two other bodies (life and sensitivity bodies) in between. The scale is extended on each side to indicate possible tendencies of humanity as a whole, depending on the choices that will be made by the vast majority.

The basis of placing in this spectrum the various schools of thought in medicine, and the different old and new healing arts, is their professed theory of illness. For example, orthodox allopathic medicine is concerned more with the physical body. Its theory of disease involves germs and genes and a number of drugs which inhibit or replace the bio-chemical secretions of the body. Logotherapy (or meaning therapy) of Viktor Frankl, biographical counseling, and mind/body medicine are situated in the "I" pole because the meaning-giving principle in the human being is the "I." Spiritual psychology as expounded by Robert Sardello brings us to a level of consciousness of the spiritual "I" and the process of rediscovering our relationship with "I" and Soul of the World.[1]

Energy medicine, as it is called by the National Center for Complementary and Alternative Medicine, stimulates particularly the formative force/life body. Different healing arts and alternative medical systems such as homeopathy, ayurveda, traditional Chinese medicine, and anthroposophic medicine do not just address the energy body, but harmonize the sensitivity body and "I" with the life and physical bodies to a certain extent by the nature of their remedies. Furthermore, the emotional, relational, and lifestyle factors in the illness may have been brought to light of consciousness *depending on the practitioner.*[2] Thus, the consultation with the practitioner alone may have also stimulated some participation of the "I" in the processing and adjustment of lifestyle and habits.[3]

I am unable to put all the healing arts in the spectrum due to space limitation. I leave it to you to find out where the rest (as you encounter them) can be placed in the said spectrum. The most popular ones are there, along with the new and emerging ones. As it is, it can give the reader a sense of how to make use of the different schools of thought in medicine and healing arts in one's path to healing.

The illustration also suggests the evolution of human consciousness. Traditional schools of thought in medicine, like traditional Chinese medicine, ayurveda, and Greek medicine had an image of the human being beyond the physical (as discussed in Chapter 2 of Section 1). In its original form, they would allude to or perhaps publicly speak of the human spirit that needs to gain full control of human life.

Original Greek medicine as articulated by Hippocrates was inspired by the lofty philosophies of Socrates, Plato, Aristotle, and many others. Through the centuries, Greek medicine contracted into orthodox medicine (as explained in Chapter 3 of Section 1), where the only reality is the physical body—a biochemical machine (a fall into materialism and reductionism). Chiropractic and various manipulation techniques, naturopathy, herbal folk medicine, gymnastics (in its original design as purposeful movement, but now only a sport)—these are actually remnants of Greek medicine, while homeopathy is a rediscovered remnant (as discussed in Chapter 1 of Section 1). They retained the idea of a life/vital body as the higher principle in homeostasis, but have lost a clear understanding of the other members of the human being (or, the higher members are taken together as soul or mind).

Chinese medicine, inspired mainly by Taoist thought, is in the process of splintering into independent healing arts. Thus, there are specific therapies for purposeful movement, like taichi and chigong. Acupuncture uses the allopathic principle (reducing or tonifying the "chi"); herbal medicine often uses the homeopathic principle of like cures like, but with no dilution (the new facet of homeopathy). Their manipulation therapies are tuina, shiatsu, and various methods of massage connected to stimulating the energy meridians. Relaxation, contemplation, and meditation techniques are plentiful (because of their Buddhist/Taoist history). Culinary arts to support healing exist as well. Chinese medicine is also undergoing a "fall" into materialistic explanation and understanding, as I mentioned in the beginning of Chapter 3 of Section 1.

On the one hand, trends in orthodox scientific research coming from biotechnology (stem cells, cloning, etc.), nanotechnology (electronic limbs, eyes, and other body parts), artificial intelligence, and cognitive technology (voice, DNA, ECG recognition) are bringing into medicine a narrower and extremely deterministic image of the human being—a mineral, biochemical, biomechanical, cybernetic body.[4] Thus, I have to extend the spectrum further to the left and to the right to show the trends in human evolution.

The emerging new therapies, on the other hand, are mind-body medicine, logotherapy, meditation, biographical counseling, spiritual psychology, anthroposophic medicine, art therapy (painting, music, clay work), and eurythmy (a new form of movement). They address more consciously the "higher" bodies or principles, as well as the ethical-moral aspect of the human being. These therapies summon the spiritual "I" to be in charge of daily life—developing, engaging, and enhancing cognitive feeling, positive and constructive thoughts, purposeful and meaningful deeds. These therapies are articulating and working with a clearer understanding of the whole human being and pointing to a different direction of human evolution. In this different direction, human beings are evolving toward a more mindful, conscious "I," fully living and engaged in social transformation towards the development of new hygienic communities and a new earth.[5]

Notes

1   See Sardello R. *Love and the Soul: Creating a Future for Earth*, new and expanded edition, North Atlantic Books Berkeley, CA, Goldenstone Press, Benson, NC, & Heaven & Earth Publishing, East Montpelier, Vermont, 2008, and his other work, *The Power of Soul: Living the Twelve Virtues*, Hampton Roads Publishing Co. Inc., Charlottesville, VA,

2002. This second book shows us how we can "educate the emotions, refine the soul, and develop character." This is a stage one should undergo before engaging in serious meditation.

2 A more recent work is by Cowan T., et.al, *The Fourfold Path to Healing: Working with the Laws of Nutrition, Therapeutics, Movement and Meditation in the Art of Healing,* New Trends Publishing, Inc. Washington DC, 2004. "The goal of medicine should be healing on all levels and all of us are moving towards that goal."

3 It could also be that practitioners of the alternative medical system work like a prescription dispenser and do not elicit the active participation of the patient, therefore the patient will not have a clue as to what else he needs to do to achieve complete healing (and the illness may just recur or a new illness can emerge). The practitioner is still crucial even in an alternative medical system. This is the main reason why this book advocates developing a participative relationship with your doctor. In cases where this is not possible, take charge!

4 Behind these four technologies, the implementation of the idea of the human cyborg is slowly being realized. As of this time, human cyborgs are people who use cybernetic technology to repair, replace, or overcome the physical and mental constraints of their physical bodies. Science fiction has prepared the modern human being for this eventuality. Its full blown application and realization, however, may still be in the far future (or perhaps sooner, depending on our choices today). See Wikipedia and *www. techradar.com* for the latest in the development of the human cyborg, or type *human cyborg* in your internet search engine.

   If one has a debility of the body, the human cyborg is a very enticing idea. The wealth of modern civilization is being used in all this research in the guise of solving the problems of the world (human weaknesses: diseases, wars, strife, addiction, selfishness). But as this book tries to explain, a technological solution is only a palliative. The real solution is consciousness development (the process of realizing and engaging your true spiritual "I"). A technical solution with a reduced image of the human being can only bring the whole of humanity further down into materialism.

5 It is thus important to see how through the centuries exceptional human beings (Hippocrates and the Greek philosophers, the avatars of India, Lao Tze, Buddha, Rudolf Steiner) perceive and articulate trends in the evolution of human beings and the reorganization and development of society. They and their followers then develop the schools of medicine and healing arts that address, cultivate, and nurture these emerging aspects in the hope that the best human quality and virtue will be expressed—not only for oneself, but for the improvement of everyone in society and the world.

Section Two

Make Your Own
Homeopathic Remedies

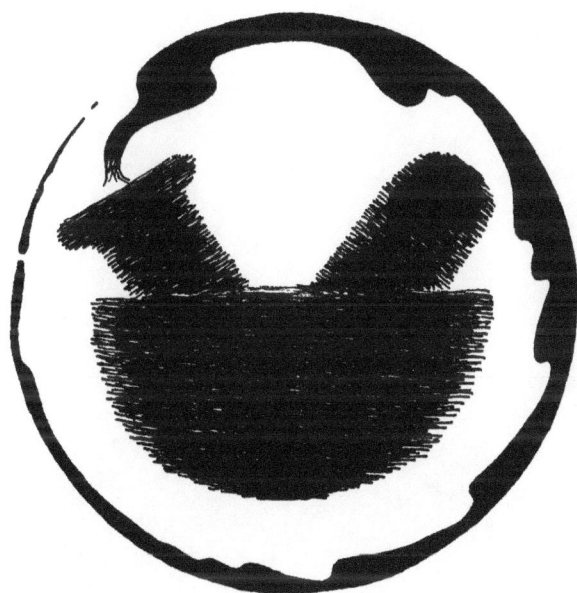

Chapter One

❧

The Preparation of Mother Tinctures and the Process of Potentizing the Remedies

There are various ways of making the mother tincture or mother substance. We advocate the process termed *maceration.*[1] It is quite simple. (Another method called *tituration* is described separately for raw materials that cannot be dissolved in water or alcohol, like most mineral preparations.)

The following are the materials needed to make the tinctures for home use. For community-scale production, simply increase the volume of raw materials and use larger bottles for processing.

For liquid tinctures:

- Mortar and pestle
- Wide-mouth brown or clear bottles for processing tinctures
- Narrow-mouth brown bottles for storing tinctures
- 40% to 95% ethyl alcohol (vodka, gin, and other clear alcohol are acceptable for home use. They contain 40% to 45% ethyl alcohol, good for making most of the tinctures)
- Cheesecloth, around 6 x 6 inches
- Funnel or bowl

Three types of alcohol are described in this book:

- Strong alcohol is from 75% to 95% ethyl alcohol
- Medium-strong is from 35% to 70% ethyl alcohol
- Weak alcohol is from 10% to 15% ethyl alcohol

There are two main uses of alcohol in preparing the tincture: as solvent, and as preservative.[2] The homeopathic procedure strictly follows the required percentage of alcohol for particular plants, which mostly fall under the 75% to 95% range. Homeopaths instituted this as a standard among manufacturers. In our case, we can only approximate this standard. We will make mother tinctures with the concentration ranging from 40% to 60% alcohol. For the dilution medium, an alcohol concentration of 10% to 12% is suggested here.

The wide range of alcohol concentration is acceptable and will in no way lessen the efficacy of the remedies. Most of the extracted tinctures will be used in a diluted or potentized form. Their power to stimulate the higher members of the human being will essentially be the same. Very precise concentration demands high-quality precision instruments and research work which are not readily accessible to ordinary households. For practical purposes, what is available in one's kitchen should suffice to get started. The main consideration in the making of mother substances is to extract the plant essence in a convenient manner and preserve it in its potent form for as long as possible.

In each description of the remedies in this section under the subtitle PARTS UTILIZED, the suggested concentration of alcohol is indicated. Medium-strong alcohol is recommended for most remedies, but occasionally strong alcohol is called for (but for home use medium-strong alcohol is acceptable, as stated earlier).

A. MAKING THE MOTHER TINCTURE

Mother tinctures are usually about 10% to 20% mineral, plant, or animal essence, 40% to 50% alcohol, and 30% to 50% water. Under the sub-heading PARTS UTILIZED, the material to be used for the tinctures is described. Some plants can be harvested only at certain times of the year, for example during the flowering stage or only in the cold season. Please take note of this detail if it is indicated.

The first step is to know the amount of mother tincture you want to make. Reading this entire section will help you make this decision. For home use, you may need only about 20 to 30 milliliters of plant substance, which means for example, pounding a matchbox-size ginger to make a tincture.

Gathering plants as raw materials must be done within two hours before and two hours after sunrise. Inspect the materials and remove blemishes and foreign matter, such as insects. Wash the materials thoroughly with fresh tap water. The final rinsing should be in distilled water, conveniently available as bottled water in supermarkets. Cut the plant parts into smaller pieces using a knife, or shred them with your hands. With a

Steiner, she performed a series of plant experiments using wheat seeds. She studied the effects of solutions of substances subjected to varying degrees of rhythmical dilutions or potentized solutions. In the 1950s, Theodore Schwenk, another anthroposophical scientist, verified her work.[7]

Kolisko and Schwenk have improved upon five aspects of the potentizing process since Hahnemann.

The first aspect is the length of time necessary to reach the optimum dynamization or potentization of remedies. Samuel Hahnemann developed the procedure called *succussion*, i.e., holding the phial of liquid mixture in the right hand and striking it forcefully against a felt pad 100 times. Today, in special homeopathic laboratories, the same procedure is accurately reproduced by sophisticated electronic machines. Dr. Kolisko, however, tried different durations: one half minute, one minute, one and a half minutes and so on, until fifteen minutes. She used the various potentized solutions to germinate the wheat seeds, measured their growth, and plotted them in graphs. She concluded that two and a half minutes and five minutes are the optimum length of time to achieve the harmonious potentization of remedies.

Secondly, because "rhythm is life," the rhythmical movement of the solution in a vessel is equally important for anthroposophic pharmaceuticals. Life as manifested in the rhythms of the earth, nature, and human beings is applied to the process of potentization.

The anthroposophic pharmaceutical firm WALA Heilmittel GMBH makes use of the *vortex* in the potentizing process. The vortex imitates the way the life force precipitates into matter. Galaxies and typhoons are spiral shaped. Water, as it flows down, goes into a vortex[8]. Theodore Schwenk in his pioneering work *Sensitive Chaos* throws much light on the water's forming forces. WALA's potentizing process was inspired by Schwenk's work.

The third aspect or contribution by Kolisko and Schwenk is the determination of the effective potencies, which are under the subtitle "Basic Procedure in the Process of Dilution." Kolisko pinpointed the minimum and maximum points along the 1 to 30 range of potencies. This later became the basis for determining the relationship and application of the various potencies to the three living systems in the human being, namely, the nerve sense and the rhythmic and metabolic systems.

The fourth contribution concerns the best time to potentize. The sun is the source of all life and the origin of the formative force principle. Therefore, potentization should be done when there is sunlight. However, anthroposophic pharmaceuticals do not potentize between 10

a.m. and 2 p.m. Rudolf Steiner indicated that during this time the kind of
cosmic forces at work in the atmosphere may have adverse effects on the
potentization process.

The time one hour before sunrise till 10 a.m., and from 2 p.m. till an
hour after sunset, is the best time to potentize. Dr. Guenther Wachsmuth's
pioneering work, *The Etheric Formative Forces in Cosmos, Earth and Man:
A Path of Investigation into the World of the Living*, gave clear experimental
evidence to this.[9] The regular double daily wave phenomenon (still
inadequately explained by orthodox science) in barometric pressure
reading is particularly involved here. This double daily wave occurs during
and after sunrise and before and during sunset. During these times there
is maximum vertical current, maximum potential gradient, and maximum
barometric pressure in the lower atmosphere. At midday and at midnight
the reverse is true. These measurements indicate the movement of the
formative forces which help release and strengthen the dynamic forces still
attached to the mother substance during potentization.

However, potentization should be avoided during solar and lunar
eclipses. Kolisko made many experiments before, during, and after eclipses
and found that eclipses distort the formative force coming from the
sun.[10] Maria Thun, another anthroposophical scientist, provided further
understanding of this phenomenon. She was asked by a Swiss company
which manufactures ball bearings to investigate the reason why twice in
a month their machines produced slightly oblongated ball bearings. Ms.
Thun took note of the dates when these occurred and found that all of
them happened during the astronomical period called "moon's node."
(This is when the path of the moon crosses that of the sun. At certain
times this crossing of paths leads to eclipses.) The ball bearings were noted
to be most deformed during eclipses. Ms. Thun then made a calendar of
all future moon's nodes and told the company not to produce on those
dates. They never had the same problem again.[11] For our purposes, we
should avoid potentizing during eclipses.

The fifth and final contribution is about the whole mood of soul that
accompanies the process of making remedies. Reverence, humility, and
full knowledge of the deed should inspire workers in anthroposophical
pharmaceuticals. They should avoid using machines for processes that can
be enhanced by human hands and heart.[12]

The reader is encouraged to adopt this said mood while preparing
mother tinctures and potentizing remedies. This is one way of realizing the
interconnectedness of things around us, i.e., how one kingdom of nature
sacrifices itself for the human kingdom to be healed and enabled to move

forward in its evolution. This mood will also give us the feeling that what one is doing is an act of spiritualizing nature, a task which humanity needs to do from here on.

2. Materials Needed

In potentizing the remedies we need the following materials:

- Preferably distilled water, but fresh spring water is acceptable
- One measuring device, preferably a graduated cylinder (a teaspoon, a dropper, a jigger, or small bottles may also be used if a graduated cylinder is not available)
- One 25 ml test tube with rubber stopper or one clear gin bottle with rubber stopper
- Any alcoholic drink of 40% to 50% alcohol
- Small brown bottle for storing the remedies

3. Making the Diluting Medium

The diluting medium should be about 10% to 12% alcohol. Take one part of gin, vodka, or other alcoholic drink and add another 2 to 3 parts of distilled water. If you have a stronger alcohol of known percentage, use the table on the next page to get about a 10% alcohol concentration.[13]

4. Basic Steps in the Process of Dilution and Dynamization

- Take 1 ml or one part (jigger, teaspoon) mother tincture. Add to it 9 ml or nine parts (jigger, teaspoon) 30% ethyl alcohol. Shake rhythmically for two and a half minutes to get the second decimal potency, D2 or 2X.
- Take 1 ml or one part D2. Add to it 9 ml or nine parts 10% ethyl alcohol. Shake rhythmically for two and a half minutes to get the third decimal potency, D3 or 3X.
- Repeat the steps to get the succeeding higher potencies.

This process is very easy to do, but it requires time, care, and concentration. To make potencies 2 to 30 for one remedy, we will need twenty-nine more small bottles. For ten types of remedies to be readily available, there must be 290 bottles. These occupy much space for storage. However, the saving grace is that not all remedies are used in high potencies. Under the subtitle DOSE where each of the remedies is described, the recommended potencies are specified. The discussion below is a guide to the use of the various potencies.

DILUTION TABLE FOR ETHYL ALCOHOL Amount of water needed (in ml) to dilute 1000 ml of ethyl alcohol (20°C)													
Original alcohol concentration (%)	Adjusted Alcohol Concentration (%)												
	30	35	40	45	50	55	60	65	70	75	80	85	90
35	167												
40	335	114											
45	505	290	127										
50	674	436	255	114									
55	845	583	384	229	103								
60	1017	730	514	344	207	95							
65	1189	878	644	460	311	190	88						
70	1360	1027	774	577	417	285	175	81					
75	1535	1177	906	694	523	382	261	163	79				
80	1709	1327	1039	812	630	480	353	246	153	70			
85	1884	1478	1172	932	738	578	443	329	231	144	68		
90	2061	1630	1306	1052	847	677	535	414	310	218	138	65	
95	2239	1785	1443	1174	957	779	629	501	391	295	209	133	64

Specific potencies address the three living systems of the human being. They are as follows:

D1 to D6 ———Illnesses of the Metabolic system and any degenerative condition

D8 to D15 ———Illnesses of the Rhythmic system and chronic inflammatory or sub-acute conditions

D20 to D30———Illnesses of the Nerve Sense system and acute inflammatory conditions

The effective potencies are 1, 2, 3, 4, 6, 8, 10, 12, 15, 20, 25, 30. Once potentized, remedies can have a shelf life of five years.

C. SUGGESTIONS FOR GETTING STARTED

To get started in making remedies for home use, I suggest the ten most familiar ones—red onion, garlic, ginger, corn silk, table salt, radish, dandelion, beet, tomato, and cayenne pepper. They should be all organically grown.

Make mother tinctures of these plants, perhaps one a day, depending upon your time availability. Read through the descriptions of the remedies. Try to visualize and memorize what they are for.

If the remedy is recommended in a potentized form, potentize it to the first effective potency indicated. Leave it on the shelf until you encounter a situation where it can be used. In deciding which remedy is appropriate, make sure that the ill person exhibits as many of the symptoms described in the *materia medica* (begins p. 181) as possible. Remember, the principle of medicine applied here is to utilize the inherent processes and forces of the remedy to stimulate the higher members of the human being to make use of such forces. This is still within the principle of "like cures like." Thus if the plant produces rashes, in a potentized form or with a minimum dose, our immune system and our higher members will be stimulated to use the (rash-producing) force imprinted in the liquid and effect a cure, for example, in an allergy. In other words, we are strengthening our higher members by the force inherent in the remedy.

If there is no time to potentize the remedy, give one-half teaspoon of the mother tincture (please note that this is possible only for the non-toxic tinctures) mixed with one-half cup of water.[14] This mixture should be stirred for two and a half minutes and taken internally under the tongue, one-half teaspoon every half hour in acute cases, or every four hours in chronic cases.

The most important consideration in using this form of medicine is the close correspondence between symptoms exhibited by the patient and those associated with the remedy (as described in this book). The potentization process is resorted to only to avoid the aggravation of symptoms and help our three systems absorb the healing force more readily. If the remedy is given at the tincture level or in a low potency despite the recommended high potency, then a cure can still be expected. Our three systems will potentize it themselves.

D. FREQUENCY OF DOSE

One-half teaspoon of a potentized remedy is given as often as every thirty minutes for acute symptoms. This frequency is tapered off to every three hours after a positive response occurs. What counts is the frequency of stimulation, not the quantity. In other words, drinking a whole bottle will bring about the same amount of stimulation desired as half a teaspoon.

When the remedy is almost consumed, potentize the remaining amount to the next effective potency level. This can be continuously given to the sick person until a cure is achieved.

If there is no positive response within a day or two, choose the next available remedy that approximates the range of symptoms and wait for results. Do not rely solely on the oral remedy. Complement it with naturopathy. For example, in a fever give plenty of liquids. Do not suppress the fever. If the fever rises to about 40.5 to 41 degrees centigrade for children and 39 to 39.5 for adults, apply tap water on the extremities to maintain the temperature.[15] Let the fever run its own course. Remove animal flesh from the diet and give fresh vegetable soup and rice.[16] In an inflammation, provide more warmth (as hot as the body can tolerate) over the inflamed area four times a day for twenty to thirty minutes each time.

Starting out is really the most difficult phase. But once you have focused your attention on it, it will not be long before you can master many of the remedies listed here. One only needs determination and brief moments of concentrated study to achieve mastery over time.

E. A BRIEF DESCRIPTION OF THE PROCESS OF TITURATION

Tituration is resorted to whenever the material is not soluble in water or alcohol, such as most mineral preparations. Lactose or milk sugar (available commercially) is used as the diluting medium. The raw material is ground into a fine powder. Preferably the powder should be passed through a 60X mesh.

To make the first decimal potency, take 10 grams of the powdered raw material. Mix it in a mortar and pestle (or glass bowl) with 90 grams milk sugar by stirring it for one hour in a counterclockwise direction, creating a spiral, i.e., from the circumference to the center. (See figure below.)

Repeat the procedure to make the succeeding potencies.

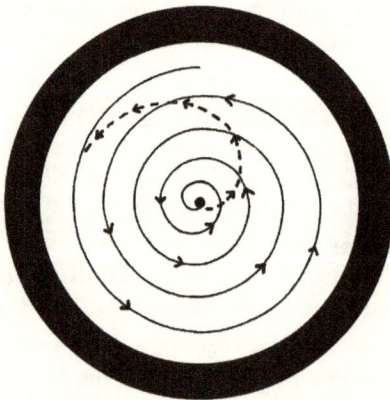

F. MAKING COMBINATIONS OF REMEDIES

One can also combine the remedies to make new remedies. There are two ways to make a combination. The first is to combine the various potencies of a single remedy. The final product can have the following dilutions: 2, 12, and 30. To do this, take one part each of dilution 1, 11, and 29 and take seven parts of the diluting medium. Potentize them together for two and a half minutes, and then you have a single remedy combination. This combination can address the three living systems.

The second way is to take various remedies that are similar in action, such as remedies that would address the specific weakness of the metabolic system. One could take several tinctures at their lower potency and dynamize them together to their effective potencies. One should first have studied the action of the substances before resorting to this. If you are doing your concentrated studies well on the various remedies described in this section, your spiritual "I" will guide you in your choices and decisions.

I hope that with these relatively simple procedures, you will be encouraged to look after your health and become your own doctor. As we gain mastery of the use of these remedies, we should pass on what we have learned to others. As discussed in Section 1, each one now has the capacity to be one's own authority, a capacity which was formerly relegated only to priests and specialized healers such as doctors. Trust your creativity and insights but learn also from your errors. This is healthy common sense, which is one of the talents we have lost because of our present predicament. By learning to heal yourself, you are likewise redeeming this lost capacity.

Notes

1 Anthroposophical pharmaceuticals use various degrees of warmth to produce different mother tinctures from plants. Maceration is considered a cold extract. Fermentation and digestion use temperatures ranging from 25 to 37 degrees centigrade. Infusion, decoction, and distillation are in a temperature range of 90 to 150 degrees centigrade, while toasting, carbonating, and incinerating require a temperature of 170 to 700 degrees centigrade. As a general rule, the higher the temperature used, the more the remedy is directed to the metabolic system. The medium temperature gives remedies for the middle system, while maceration is for the nerve sense system. See Ullrich C. The pharmaceutical process: from natural substance to remedy. In *Man and Remedy*.

WELEDA Newsletters for Physicians, 1986.

2 Dr. Rudolf Hauschka pioneered the use of water to extract the plant essence. He perfected the method after more than 20 years of research. This is now the main feature of the products of WALA Heilmittel GMBH, an anthroposophical pharmaceutical firm in Ekwaelden, Germany. The plants are carefully selected, washed in distilled water, pounded in mortar and pestle, and immersed in distilled water for seven days. This is all done by hand. During the seven days, the plant solution is kept in a special box lined with peat moss to protect it from cosmic influences. A temperature of 37 degrees centigrade is likewise maintained. One hour before and after sunrise and sunset, the solution is brought out of the box, exposed to the rising and setting sun, and immersed in ice water to bring down the temperature to 4 degrees centigrade. This rhythm of alternating warmth and cold and the effects of the forces of sunrise and sunset assist in preserving the formative force of the plant solution. The solution undergoes fermentation with the previously insoluble parts of the plant getting dissolved in water. Alcohol then need not be used either as solvent or as preservative. Afterwards, the solution is filtered using cheesecloth. It is squeezed out by hand. The extracted liquid is stored in brown bottles and made to rest for one year in a cool dark place prior to use. During my training at WALA, mother substances made more than twenty years ago were still "alive" and being used to prepare potentized remedies.

WELEDA, the original anthroposophic pharmaceutical firm, also came out with its own water-based extraction process called RH. It follows the same rhythms described above, but not necessarily the same procedure. Rudolf Steiner once said, "Rhythm is life." This statement has been made practical and useful in developing a genuinely living medicine.

Recently, a pharmacist from Sonnen Apotheke in Waiblingen, Germany taught me another water extraction method he is using. One must have plain distilled water, and added to it are 10 drops of Easter water (water taken from a clean spring before 6 a.m. on Easter Sunday), after which one can put in any part of the plant (even minerals), whole (no need to crush it). One must only wait for 49 days (shaking the solution twice a day like above) before the tincture is ready for extraction (using a specialized membrane filter). If you wish to try this method, please do so.

3 The explanation regarding the action of the plant is not found in Hahnemann's writings. Hahnemann claimed that the production of a second but temporary disease triggers the vital body to react to the toxins and stimulates it to get rid of them. Once stimulated, the vital body can eventually work on the original toxins. Now this explanation may be true for remedies that contain toxins. But for those medicinal plants and animals that do not, this does not hold. Anthroposophical understanding of plants includes the logic of toxicity, but goes beyond it. It sees mineral, plant, and animal kingdoms as extrusions of forces and substances which were formerly part of

humanity. The human spirit extruded them in the course of evolution. The forces in these substances can be absorbed and utilized by humans for healing purposes. For example, a plant rich in iron and possessing the forces to process and incorporate this mineral into its being, would give someone who cannot properly absorb or incorporate iron into oneself, the capacity to do so. Thus, knowledge of the processes inherent in plants, animals, and the mineral kingdom is important in determining their true healing value, i.e., making a human being (and eventually the entire humanity) whole again. To make whole, not only to balance, is the core principle of every healing process.

4   A related new discovery on how water is able to be imprinted with these spirit-like qualities comes from the works of Masaru Emoto. See Emoto M. *The True Power of Water: Healing and Discovering Ourselves.* Hosoyamada N, trans. New York: Atria Books; 2005. "My fascination led me to study water deeply... I became convinced that water took in information... I'm referring to external factors that affect mind and body." To prove that this is so he froze water and found a way to take pictures of frozen ice crystals. He compared different kinds of water (from various taps: filthy, bottled, etc.) and found out that the quality of the water crystals can be changed by one's consciousness. "When you send your gratitude to water, its quality improves. When you call water by names or ignore it, it deteriorates [p xii]." For updates on the work of Masaru Emoto just type *emoto water* in your internet search engine.

5   Moreover, homeopaths do not clearly distinguish their idea of the different higher members of the human being. They tend to mix up the symptoms associated with the sensitivity body, the ego, and that of the vital body. We do not yet aim to be as precise as the anthroposphic doctors. It is enough to know at this juncture that we can still go into a finer distinction in our diagnosis in order to be able to give a more specific remedy. This is something to aspire for.

6   Kolisko L. *Physiologischer and Physikalischer Nachweis der Wirksamkeit Kleinster Entitaten: Herausgegeben durch die Arbeitsgemeinschaft anthroposophischer Arzte.* Stuttgart, 1921.

7   Schwenk T. *The Basis of Potentization Research.* Spring Valley, New York: Mercury Press; 1988.

8   In the northern hemisphere, the formative force goes in a counterclockwise direction, while in the southern, it goes in a clockwise direction. You can try this out yourself by watching how the water drains in your bath tub. Or, if there is a typhoon, a tornado, or some other weather disturbance, try looking at the weather satellite on the internet, which would show the form of the weather disturbance as I stated above. Observe also the indigenous plants in your garden; they would normally follow this pattern as they emerge and grow.

9   Wachsmuth G. The ethereric formative forces in cosmos. In *Earth and Man*, pp 48-56.

10 Kolisko L. *Spirit in Matter*. Bournemouth: Kolisko Archive Publication.

11 This story was narrated to the author by a colleague while training at the WALA Heilmittel GMBH, April to November 1992.

12 Current research by scientists of the HeartMath Institute shows that the heart emits an electromagnetic field called a *torus* about 12 to 15 feet away in all directions. This is what we feel/perceive when someone is approaching us or when we are intensely listening to someone. Thus, love for the deed, like making mother tinctures or potentizing them, would enhance the medicinal effects of the remedies. See the Institute of HeartMath at *www.heartmath.org*. These scientists have rediscovered with scientific precision (and proof) that the heart *thinks*, and that one can again learn to develop the intelligence of the heart. The Institute of HeartMath is dedicated to conducting research and providing programs for schools and families to facilitate heart-based living. This is the kind of science we need to bring humanity closer to one of its goals in evolution: spiritualization (developing conscious wisdom) of every aspect of the human being and of nature and the accompanying possibility to change the world through change of our lifestyle.

13 Taken from *Common Medicinal Plants of the Cordillera*, with the permission of the author, Leonard Co.

14 To distinguish the toxic plants from the non-toxic ones, study carefully the recommended dosage. Most non-toxic remedies are given at low potencies, i.e., tincture to dilution 5 (D5), while toxic ones are usually prescribed beyond dilution 10 (D10).

15 See note 55 in Chapter 2, Section 1 for a review of the role of fever in healing.

16 If the high fever persists after three days, then giving an antipyretic and going to the hospital for laboratory tests (to find out other possible causes of the fever) is justified.

Chapter Two

🌿

Seventy-Nine Remedies
One Can Make Locally

The remedies described in this book are classified into mineral, plant, and animal.[1] The descriptions have been abridged from several homeopathic *materia medica*, and medical terminologies are defined in parentheses to enable ordinary folks to fully learn from them.[2] I did not generalize the content but retained much of the detailed symptoms because I wanted the reader to appreciate them. By having access to these details, one is able to see coherence or a "drug picture."[3] Moreover, these details help us understand how a weakened vitality is expressed in the different parts of the body, in various forms and degrees.

Whenever possible, I first indicated briefly the properties of the substances and their action on the particular part of the body.[4] A description of their common uses follows. This gives one a quick reference or key words as to what illnesses are addressed by the remedies.

Under "Other Conditions and/or Collaborating Symptoms," the reader is given a more specific characterization of a variety of symptoms that may be experienced in the different parts of the body (in bold letters), including, in a number of cases, emotional signals, sleeping behavior, or the quality of the fever. For example, is the rheumatism right-sided only? Is it accompanied by a severe headache? Tonsillitis? Or rashes? The remedy may still be given for any one of the cited cases—rheumatism, headache, tonsillitis, skin rashes—but will be most appropriate if all symptoms are present. In other words, the more symptoms you find matching the descriptions of a remedy, the surer you can be that this single remedy alone can address all the symptoms.

Another reason why I included details of symptoms that may appear in the different parts of the body is to show that even if only one symptom appears or is obvious, you may try the remedy. This will train you to be more perceptive or observant of the various feelings in the body, and the quality of each feeling. For example, a sense of dryness in the mouth may indicate an excessive salt intake in the diet. Before it gets worse, one should stop taking salty foods and begin taking one of the remedies described in this section, potentized table salt (at 30x), to help overcome the excess salt. In other words, one should not ignore seemingly harmless symptoms. They may indicate an imbalance or the beginning of a weakness in the vitality.

In a number of cases, there are a variety of descriptions of symptoms in particular body parts. For example, in the first mineral remedy (calcium carbonate), the symptoms that may be found in the "Head" section are described as follows:

> Head feels hot and heavy, with pale face. Headache with cold hands and feet. Vertigo or dizziness on ascending, and when turning the head. Headache from overlifting, from mental exertion, with nausea. Icy coldness in, and on the head, especially the right side. Head is enlarged with much perspiration, wetting the pillows. Itching of the scalp.

These are the different descriptions of a weakened vitality expressed in the head region that calcium carbonate can address. It also means that different individuals may express the same weakened vitality in one or several of the described symptoms. If any of the symptoms appear and are collaborated by signals from other parts of the body, then you can try this remedy.

I also categorized the descriptions according to our three living systems, namely: nerve sense, middle/rhythmic, and metabolic/limb systems, in order for you to begin learning to think in the three-fold way. Knowing the kinds of symptoms that appear in the three living systems, you can already discern where you are out of balance.[5] (This also reveals the underlying affinity of the remedy to our three living systems.) You can resort to other forms of therapy to counteract them. For example, if symptoms related to the nerve sense system predominate, like numbing, hardening, or tendency to atrophy, then relaxation, meditation, and eating more living foods are the complementary therapies. If symptoms come more from the middle/rhythmic system, then engaging in artistic therapy like playing a musical instrument or painting may be necessary, and/ or equanimity and positivity exercises should be heightened. Dominant symptoms from the metabolic/limb system require such therapy as gardening, physical activity, or engaging in a new socially or ecologically relevant initiative for long-term cure.

It may take some time for you to get into the inner logic of all these other therapies and see how they work. You can do it if you have the will to learn. The first step is to do it yourself. Once you have done it, it will be easier to accumulate learning and insights from the experience. Soon you will know how it can help others also.

With regard to some technical terms still found in the description of the remedies, I purposely retained them and put in parentheses a layman's description in order for you to start learning some medical terminology. This will bridge the gap between physicians who use specialized language and the general public. If you find yourself conversing with medical professionals or reading medical journals, you will not be lost in their jargon. If there are still some terms not simple enough, please consult a medical dictionary.

For those plant remedies you cannot identify despite the illustration, please consult local herbalists or go to a herbarium to learn how to identify them.

Notes

1 On the internet, one can now easily access any homeopathic remedy. Just type the name in your internet search engine and you can have immediate access to the full description of the remedy. Thus, most of the minerals, plants, and animals presented here are only sample remedies one can make. I took care to include very common ones, or those that are edible and available in the supermarket, or can be planted in your garden or in pots.

2 Most of the descriptions of the remedies came from the *Homeopathic Materia Medica* of Boericke. I inserted some of the descriptions from Clark and Reckeweg whenever necessary. Please see the bibliography for their publication details.

3 The "drug picture" is the overall picture one can discern or see as the true essence of the remedy. For example, the drug picture of table salt, or natrum muriaticum, has the tendency to watery secretions or retentions. They weep easily, or have watery nasal secretions. The water drops and drips from them, or, in the opposite pole, water is unnecessarily retained in the form of various edemas. The picture that is created in our mind is that of our interweaving bodies' ability to manage water. With this in mind, we can then figure out (by more study) what particular organ this remedy is invigorating or stimulating. It is particularly addressing the relationship between the liver and the kidney through the supra-renal glands. I cannot go into a detailed discussion here. But those who are ready to go further may consult the various books on anthroposophic medicine listed in the bibliography. The author is willing to conduct seminars for those

interested in learning more about anthroposophic medicine and other complementary healing arts.

4   The generic and specific properties and actions of the mineral remedies were enhanced from the descriptions given by Huseman and Wolff. *The Anthroposophical Approach to Medicine: An Outline of a Spiritually Oriented Medicine.* Anthroposophical Press Inc. 1985; vol 2:117-182.

5   Knowing the various plants and their affinity to our three living systems, one can then use them as ingredients to make combination remedies as described in the preceding chapter.

Chapter Three

🌿

Minerals

1. ARGENTUM METALLICUM

Other Name: *Silver*

Generic Properties and Action:

Silver, in general, rules all constructive processes that create living substances. Thus the processes of vitalization, regeneration, and reproduction are particularly referred to. This includes the functions of the reproductive organs and the formation of new tissues. It is important to note that the formation and growth of living substances are bound to (inner and outer) light (that is found, for example, in food, the refinement of feelings, or the realization of eternal truths). The life body of the human being has also the light processes within it. Thus in using potentized argentum, the silver process takes up light and leads it over into life.

Conditions Most Used For:

In general, argentum works by enhancing the connection of the life body with the physical body, and in particular, with the anabolic side of metabolism. Thus argentum is best for watery diarrhea, various gastric disturbances, dry mucous membranes of the mouth, neck and larynx, and the appearance of dry skin. Growing children who are pale, dreamy, often underweight, and look older than their age indicate that their life building processes are too weak. Argentum could also be used in sleep-walking and bed wetting.

Other Conditions and/or Collaborating Symptoms:

a. Nerve Sense System

Head - Neuralgia or headaches of the left side, gradually increasing and ceasing suddenly. Scalp very tender to touch. Vertigo on looking at running

water. Head feels empty and hollow. Eyelids are thick and red. Pain between left eye and forehead or in the facial bones.

b. Middle/Rhythmic System

Throat - Raw, hawking, gray, jelly-like mucous, and throat is sore on coughing. Morning expectoration profuse but easy, with phlegm looking like boiled starch. **Respiratory System** - Hoarseness with loss of voice. Raw, sore feeling when coughing. There is great weakness of the chest, but worse on the left side, especially the left lower ribs.

c. Metabolic/Limb System

Back - Severe backache to the point that one must walk bent with pain in the chest. **Urine** - Urine is profuse but turbid. It may have a sweet odor. Polyuria (frequent urination). **Extremities** - Rheumatic pains of the joints, especially the elbow and the knee. Swelling of ankles. Legs are weak and trembling, becoming worse when descending stairs. Involuntary contractions of fingers, partial paralysis of forearm; writer's tendency to cramps. **Male** - Crushing pain in the testicles. Seminal emissions without sexual excitement. Frequent urination with burning sensation. **Female** - Ovaries feel too large, sore or painful. Pain only in the left ovary. Sore feeling throughout the abdomen, becoming worse by jarring. Prolapse of the womb. Eroded spongy cervix. Vaginal discharge, foul and excoriating. Menopausal hemorrhage. **Fever** - Hectic fever at noon.

DOSE - Sixth potency and higher. Stop when result is achieved. Do not use too often.

2. ARGENTUM NITRICUM

Other Name: *Silver Nitrate*

Specific Properties and Action:

Allopathic orthodox medicine primarily uses this substance as an astringent, a disinfectant, and a caustic (a substance that destroys living tissues). It is an irritant of the mucous membranes, producing violent inflammation of the throat, and a marked gastroenteritis. In homeopathic potency, argentum nitricum has obvious effects on the autonomic nervous system, and on vagotonous conditions (an abnormal increase in the activity of the vagus nerves, especially abnormal slowness of the heartbeat, causing faintness and sudden loss of strength) in particular.

Conditions Most Used For:

Argentum nitricum is best used for distention in the upper abdomen, gastro-cardiac symptom-complex, amelioration from belching, and most gastric crises including bleeding ulcers; when diarrhea is caused by stage fright, excitement vertigo, or when stool is flecked, green, mucoid—like chopped spinach. It can also be used in catarrh and hoarseness of voice after over-exertion, catarrh of the pharynx, ears and conjunctiva; in epilepsy, when the pupils are enlarged for hours or days before the attack; in states of weakness and exhaustion, primarily of the calves and lower arms; finally, in emotional states such as agoraphobia, neurasthenia, restlessness, and worry.

Other Conditions and/or Collaborating Symptoms:

a. Nerve Sense System

Head - Headache, ameliorated by tight binding of the head. Headache with coldness and trembling, or from mental exertion. Emotional disturbances cause the appearance of hemi-cranial attacks. Brain fag, with general debility and trembling. Vertigo, with buzzing in the ears and with nervous affections or with tinnitus. **Eyes** - Inner canthi are swollen and red. One sees spots before the vision. Great swelling of the conjunctiva (as an eye drop); discharge abundant and purulent. Acute granular conjunctivitis. Chronic ulceration of the margin of the lids. Unable to keep eyes fixed steadily. Eye-strain from sewing becoming better in warm room. Useful in restoring power to the weakened ciliary muscles. Cornea opaque. Ulcer in the cornea. **Nose** - Loss of smell. Ulcers in septum (wall dividing the nostrils). Nasal congestion with chilliness, lacrimation (secretion of tears), and headache. **Face** - Old man's look: sunken, pale, and bluish; tight drawing of the skin over the bones. **Mouth** - Gums are tender and bleed easily. Tongue has pimple, tip is red and painful. Canker sore or stomatitis. **Back/Spine** - Much pain. Spine is sensitive and painful at night. Paraplegia; posterior spinal sclerosis. **Skin** - Brown, tense, and hard. Drawing in skin, as from a spider-web, or dried albuminous substance, withered and dried up. Irregular blotches.

b. Middle/Rhythmic System

Emotional State - Great craving for sweets. One thinks his understanding will and must fail. Fearful and nervous; there is impulse to jump out of the window. Melancholic; apprehensive of serious disease. Memory is weak, there is error in perception. Time passes slowly. Impulsive; wants to do things in a hurry. **Throat** - Thick mucous in the throat and mouth causing much hawking cough. Throat is raw, rough, and sore or dark red. There is sensation of a splinter upon swallowing. Strangulated feeling. Catarrh of smokers as if there is hair in throat. **Respiratory System** - High notes cause cough. Chronic hoarseness. Difficulty in breathing: chest as if a bar were around it. **Heart/Circulatory** - Palpitation, pulse is irregular and intermittent, becoming worse while lying on the right side. Angina pectoris with nightly aggravation. Painful spots in chest.

c. Metabolic/Limb System

Stomach - Belching accompanies most gastric complaints. Flatulence with painful swelling of the pit. Pain radiates to all parts of the abdomen from the stomach. Trembling and throbbing in the stomach. Enormous distention. Ulcerative pain in the left side of the ribs. **Abdomen** - Colic, with much flatulence. Ulcerative pain on the left side of the stomach, below the short ribs. **Bowel Movement** - Watery, noisy, flatulent, offensive; green, like chopped spinach, with mucous and enormous distention of the abdomen. Diarrhea immediately after eating or drinking. Fluids go right through after sweats. Flatulence after feeling any emotion. Itching of the anus. **Urinary System** - Urine passes unconsciously, day and night. Urine scanty and dark. Emission of a few drops after having finished. Urine goes out in divided streams. Urethra inflamed, with pain, burning, itching. Early stage of gonorrhea; profuse discharge and terrible cutting pains. Bloody urine. **Male** - Impotence. Erection fails when intercourse is attempted. Cancer-like ulcers on the genitals. Genital shrivels. Desire wanting. Intercourse painful. **Female** - Gastralgia at the beginning of menses. Uterine hemorrhages, two weeks after menstruation. Painful affection of the left ovary. Profuse vaginal discharge, with erosion of the cervix, bleeding easily. **Extremities** - Trembling, with general debility. Paralysis, with mental and abdominal symptoms. Rigidity or debility of the calf muscles. Numbness of the arms. Post-diphtheritic paralysis. **Sleep** - Sleepless, from fanciful imagination; horrible dreams of snakes, and of sexual gratification. Drowsy stupor or dullness. **Fever** - Chills with nausea. Chilly when uncovered, yet feels suffocated if wrapped up.

DOSE - Third to thirtieth potency of aqueous solution.

3. ARGENTUM SULFURATUM

Other Names: *Natural Silver Sulfide, Argentite*

Specific Properties and Action:

Argentite brings the metabolism into movement through the sulfur component in it. It can cause the excretory processes in the kidneys and digestive area to flow again when blocked, and at the same time stimulates the anabolism of protein.

Conditions Most Used For:

Argentite is best applied in persons with weak anabolism or building-up processes, general ill-health, and faulty diet usually linked to wasting diseases such as tuberculosis and cancer, and in genital hypoplasia (underdeveloped genitals). In children who are small-headed, and are excessively exposed to early intellectualization, argentite will be most appropriate. Those who have arteriosclerosis, inclination to spasm and stone formation, rheumatoid arthritis, and anorexia, will also be helped by this remedy.

DOSE - Four to the thirtieth potency.

Other Salts of Argentum

Other salts of argentum can be of use to address specific ailments. Pyargerite (natural antimony silver sulfide)—through its silver content, the structuring component of antimony and the vitalizing action of sulphur—is indicated in chronic inflammation of the genital region in lower potencies (4 to 8x). Dyscrasite (natural antimony silver) is used for somnambulism or similar states, i.e., when a person overflows physically or psychologically, and in blurring of memory. In these situations, the higher potencies (above 12x) may be required.

4. AURUM METALLICUM

Other Name: *Gold*

Generic Properties and Action:

The metal gold attacks the blood, glands, and bone, producing deteriorations of the bodily fluids and alterations in the tissues, very similar to syphilitic infections and mercury poisoning. It can produce the deepest depression, suicidal tendency, and disgust for life coupled with heart complaints, missed heart beats, pressure and constriction of the chest. Palpitations are usually hard and pumping with visible beating of the arteries in the temples and neck.

On another level, gold summons and strengthens the creative soul forces of every human being. The heart as the central organ binds body, soul, and spirit harmoniously and intensively. The "I" then through gold gives one the possibility to harmonize and balance the polarities of life on many levels such as earth and cosmos, incarnation and excarnation, gravity and levity, mania and depression, pain and sorrow. The therapy for these various levels are, however, strongly dependent on the potency.

Conditions Most Used For:

In lower potencies, gold mediates the necessary heaviness, e.g., in mania and the tendency to rages. In higher potencies, aurum can lift one from the earth environment. It is thus indicated in depressions, especially connected with fear of death, and self-reproach. Low potencies can be used in the disturbance of the formation of the bones, especially in youth, or in threatened miscarriage to firm up the connection with the body, while a premature tendency to excarnate during menopause points to the use of higher potencies. Older persons who cannot let go and are unable to find access to the spirit are also helped by higher potencies of gold. Aurum 30x works right into the thinking, giving it quality and direction.

Other Conditions and/or Collaborating Symptoms:

a. Nerve Sense System

Head - Violent pain becoming worse at night or with outward pressure. Vertigo. Pain in the bones extending to the face. Boils on the scalp. **Eyes** - Extreme photophobia. Great soreness all around the eyes and into the eyeballs. Interstitial keratitis (inflammation of the cornea). Trachoma with pannus (cornea is filled with blood vessels and grainy tissue just under the surface). Double vision with upper half of the objects invisible. **Ears** - Chronic nerve deafness. External meatus (the tunnel from the external ear to the ear drum) bathed in pus. Caries of the ossicula and of the mastoid bones. **Nose** - Ulcerated, painful, swollen, obstructed. Inflammation of the nose with fetid, purulent, or bloody discharge. Horrible smell from the nose and mouth. **Mouth** - Foul breath in girls during puberty. Ulceration of the gums. Putrid and bitter taste of the mouth. **Throat** - Stitches when swallowing; pain in the glands. Caries of the palate. **Scalp/Bones** - Pain in the bones of the head, lumps under the scalp, exostosis (abnormal bony growth on the surface of bones) with nightly pains.

b. Middle/Rhythmic System

Emotional State - Feeling of self-condemnation and utter worthlessness. Profound despondency with increased blood pressure, disgust of life and suicidal tendency. Great fear of death. Peevish and vehement at the least contradiction. Anthropophobia. Mental derangements. Constant rapid questioning without waiting for a reply. Oversensitivity to noise, excitement, and confusion. **Respiratory System** - Difficulty in breathing, especially at night. Frequent deep breathing; stitches in the sternum. **Heart** - Sensation as if the heart stopped beating for two or three seconds, immediately followed by a tumultuous rebound, with sinking in the epigastrium. Palpitation. Pulse is rapid, feeble, and irregular. Enlarged heart. **High Blood Pressure** - Valvular lesions of arteriosclerotic nature. (30x).

c. Metabolic/Limb System

Stomach - Appetite and thirst increased, with feeling of uneasiness, doubt or misgivings. Swelling of the epigastrium. Burning and hot belching. **Abdomen** - Right hypochondrium (soft part of the body below the cartilage of the breastbone) hot and painful. Swelling and suppuration of the inguinal (near the groin) glands. **Urinary System** - Urine is turbid, like buttermilk with thick sediment. Painful retention of urine. Uterine fibroids and other hardened tissues. **Bowel Movement** - Constipation with stools hard and knotty. Diarrhea at night with burning in the rectum. **Female** - Great sensitivity of the vagina. Uterus is enlarged and prolapsed. Sterility; vaginismus (fear of painful entry before intercourse or pelvic examination). **Male** - Pain and swelling of the testicles. Chronic induration (hardening) of the testicles. Atrophy of the testicles in boys. Hydrocele (watery fluids in the scrotum or spermatic cord). Prostatorrhea. **Bones** - Destruction of bones like secondary syphilis. Soreness of the affected bones becoming better in the open air but becoming worse at night. **Extremities** - All the blood seems to rush from the head to the lower limbs. Edema of the lower limbs. Paralytic, tearing pains in the joints. Knees weak. **Sleep** - Sleepless. Sobs aloud in sleep. Frightful dreams.

DOSE - Third to thirtieth potency.

Other Salts of Aurum

Gold generally resists oxidation and chemical transformation. Thus, there are very few naturally occurring compounds of aurum. One such salt is aurum sulfuratum (gold monosulphide), a useful remedy to strengthen metabolism. The vitalizing component of gold is guided by sulphur into the metabolism. Thus at potencies 6 to 12x, it can address, among other symptoms, indigestion, liver dysfunction, depression, and menopausal syndrome. Aurum muriaticum natronatum (sodium chloroaurate) has the most pronounced effect on the female organs. Thus they are used in inflammatory and degenerative illness such as uterine tumors, ulceration of the neck of the womb and vagina, ovarian edema, ossified uterus, at potencies 2 to 3x.

5. CALCAREA CARBONICA

Other Names: *Calcium Carbonate, Carbonate of Lime*

Specific Properties and Action:

Calcium is an important mineral needed by the body for the development of various tissues. In the skeletal system, calcium is required and stored in large quantities. Calcium is also closely related to the functioning of the glands, especially the thyroid glands where calcium metabolism is regulated.

Its chief action then is centered in the metabolic/limb system, and is especially effective in treating impaired nutrition. Changes that are brought about in the glands, skin, and bones such as in the pituitary, thyroid, tonsils, hilius (a notch where nerves and vessels enter an organ) and mesenteric glands should be carefully observed. Any perceived imbalance of functions in these glands should be treated with this remedy.

Conditions Most Used For:

Calcium carbonate is used in the treatment of gall and kidney stones, in umbilical colic, growth of polypi, especially in the nose, ear, and uterus, or catarrhs (inflammation) of the mucosa. It can treat tickling cough, fleeting chest pains, nausea, and acidity of the stomach. The patient who would need calcium carbonate on a regular basis belongs to the phlegmatic temperament, a temperament which tends towards constitutional obesity.

In children, the development of a large head, delayed closing of the fontanelles, hydrocephalus, delayed dentition and walking, may also be treated by this remedy.

Other overall symptoms associated with calcium carbonate include a great sensitivity to cold, chilliness, and to fresh air with partial sweating. The hands and feet feel cold as if wrapped in wet socks.

Other Conditions and/or Collaborating Symptoms:

a. Nerve Sense System

Head - Head feels hot and heavy, with a pale face. Headache, with cold hands and feet. Vertigo or dizziness on ascending, and when turning the head. Headache from over-lifting, from mental exertion, with nausea. Icy coldness in and on the head, especially the right side. Head is enlarged with much perspiration, wetting the pillows. Itching of the scalp. **Eyes** - Eyes are easily fatigued, sensitive to light, far-sighted. Vision is dimmed, as if looking through a mist. Spots and ulcers in the cornea. Lachrymal (tear) ducts are closed from exposure to the cold. Opthalmia (inflammation of the eye). Itching eyelids, swollen, scurfy. Chronic dilation of the pupils. Cataract. **Ears** - Throbbing; stitches; pulsating pain as if something would press out. Deafness from working in the water. Polypi (projecting growths of a membrane) which bleed easily. Perversions of hearing; hardness of hearing. Eruption on and behind the ear. Cracking noises in the ear. Sensitive to cold about the ears and neck. **Nose** - Dry, sore, ulcerated nostrils. Blocked air passages with fetid, yellow discharge. Offensive odor in the nose. Polypi that swell at the root of the nose, but not bleeding. Epitaxis or nose bleeding. Developing cold at every change of the weather. Nasal congestion alternates with colic. **Face** - Swelling of the upper lip. Face is pale, with deep-seated eyes, surrounded by dark rings. Itching of pimples in the whiskers. Pain from the right mental foramen (opening) along the lower jaw to the ear. **Mouth** - Persistent sour taste. Offensive smell from the mouth. Dryness of the tongue at night. Burning pain at the tip of the tongue, becoming worse from anything warm taken into the stomach. Bleeding of the gums. Difficult and delayed dentition. Toothache, excited by a current of air, anything cold or hot. **Throat** - Swelling of the tonsils and sub-maxillary glands; stitches on swallowing. Goiter. **Skin** - Chilblains, boils, or carbuncle. Warts on the face and hands. Skin is unhealthy; readily ulcerating; flaccid. Small wounds do not heal readily. Glands are swollen. Nettle rash, becoming better in the cold air. **Back** - Nape of the neck is stiff and rigid. Back pain as if sprained; can scarcely rise; from over-lifting. Scoliosis, curvature of the dorsal vertebrae. Pain between the shoulder blades, impeding breathing. Rheumatism in the lumbar region; weakness in the small of the back.

b. Middle/Rhythmic System

Emotional State - Apprehensive, forgetful, confused, low-spirited, becoming worse towards the evening. Fear of the loss of reason, misfortune, contagious diseases, going crazy. Anxiety is accompanied by the palpitation of the heart. Obstinacy (resistant to treatment); slight mental effort produces a hot head. Averse to work and exertion. **Respiratory System** - Tickling cough is troublesome, especially at night, but is dry and free from expectoration in the morning. Expectoration only during the day; thick, yellow, sour mucus. Scanty and salty expectoration. Bloody expectoration, with sour sensation in the chest. Difficult or painful breathing. Suffocating spells; tightness, burning, and soreness in the chest, becoming worse on going up stairs; on the slightest ascent, one must sit down. Sharp pains in the chest going to the back. Chest is very sensitive to touch, or to pressure. Longing for fresh air. Painless hoarseness of the voice becoming worse in the morning. **Heart** - Palpitation at night and after eating. Palpitation with feeling of coldness, with restless oppression of the chest, or after suppressed eruption.

c. Metabolic/Limb System

Stomach - Aversion to meat, boiled things; craving for indigestible things—chalk, coal, pencils; also for eggs, salt, and sweets. Milk disagrees. Frequent sour burping; sour vomiting. Loss of appetite when overworked. Heartburn and loud belching. Cramps in the stomach, becoming worse with pressure, or cold water. Voracious appetite. Swelling over the pit of the stomach. Repugnance to hot food and to fats. Painful to touch in the epigastric region. Thirst; longing for cold drinks, aggravated by eating. **Abdomen** - Swollen and sensitive to the slightest pressure. Cutting sensation in the abdomen. Liver region is painful when stooping. Incarcerated flatulence. Inguinal and mesenteric glands are swollen and painful. One cannot bear tight clothing around the waist. Gall stone colic. Umbilical hernia. Trembling; weakness, as if sprained. **Bowel Movement** - Constipation; stool at first hard, then pasty, then liquid. Crawling and constriction in the rectum. Stool large and hard; whitish, watery, sour. Hemorrhoids, burning, and stinging. Diarrhea of undigested food, fetid, with ravenous appetite. Children's diarrhea. **Urinary** - Urine is dark, brown, sour, fetid, abundant, with white sediment, bloody. Irritable urinary bladder. Bed wetting. Renal colic. **Male** - Coition (sexual intercourse) is followed by weakness and irritability. Frequent seminal emissions. Increased sexual desire. Premature ejaculation. **Female** - Premenstrual syndrome:

headache, colic, chilliness, and leucorrhea (whitish discharge from the womb). Dysmenorrhea: cutting pains in the uterus during menstruation. Menses too early, too profuse, too long, with vertigo, toothache, and cold, damp feet; the least excitement causes their return. Sterility with copious menses. Uterus is easily displaced. Polyp growth in the uterus. Much sweat about the external genitals. Burning and itching of the vaginal area before and after menstruation, especially in little girls. Increased sexual desire. Hot swelling breast. Breast tender and swollen before menses. In lactating mothers, milk is too abundant or disagreeable to the child. Deficient lactation, with distended breasts in lymphatic women. **Extremities** - Rheumatoid pains. Sharp sticking pain, as if parts were wrenched or sprained. Cold knees, cramps in the calves. Weakness of the extremities. Swelling of the joints, especially the knees. Tearing in the muscles. Burning of the soles of the feet. Sweaty hands. Arthritis. Cold, damp feet; feeling as if damp stockings were worn. Soles of the feet are raw. Feet feel cold and dead at night. Sour foot-sweat. Old sprains. **Fever** - Hectic fever. Chill at 2 p.m.; begins internally at the stomach region. Fever with sweat. Pulse full and frequent. Chilliness and heat together; heat at night during menstruation, with restless sleep. Partial sweats. Night sweats, especially on the head, neck, and chest. Sweat over the head in children, so that pillow becomes wet. **Sleep** - Sleepy in the early part of the evening. Ideas crowding in the mind preventing sleep. Some disagreeable idea always arouses one from light slumber. Horrid vision when opening the eyes. Night terrors. Dreams of the dead. Starting at every noise; frequent waking at night.

DOSE - First to the thirtieth potency. This remedy should not be repeated too frequently in elderly people.

PARTS UTILIZED - Grind the white portion of oyster shells into a fine powder. Potentize only in lactose.

6. CALCAREA FLUORICA

Other Names: *Calcium Fluoride, Fluorite*

Specific Properties and Action:

Within a healthy human organism one can find numerous processes necessary to make life on earth possible. One of these processes is fluorine. It acts to demit life and the connection with the earth. It is the plastic artist in everyone, restraining the radiating magnesium forces and delimiting them, for example, in the formation of teeth. In the formation of dentine the magnesium process can be discerned, while the formation of enamel belongs to the fluorine process. Magnesium works from within outwards, while fluorine delimits and mineralizes from without. A balance of these two polar forces is essential to a healthy life.

Conditions Most Used For:

Fluorite is a powerful tissue remedy for hard, stony glands, varicose and enlarged veins, arteriosclerosis, and the malnutrition of the bones. Fibrocystic breast diseases, mammary tumors, Meibomian cysts and styes, and many cases of cataract are characteristic of this remedy. Fluorite can also be considered for the treatment of enamel defects and caries, and generally to firm up the connective tissues, e.g., ligaments of the joints and osteoporosis.

Other Conditions and/or Collaborating Symptoms:

a. Nerve Sense System

Head - Creaking noise in the head. Ulcers on the scalp with callous, hard edges. Blood tumors of newborn infants. **Eyes** - Flickering and sparks before the eyes, spots on the cornea; conjunctivitis; cataract. Subcutaneous cysts of the eyelids. **Ears** - Calcium deposits on the tympanum; sclerosis of ossicula and petrous portion of the temporal bone, with accompanying deafness, ringing, and roaring of the ear. Chronic pus formation of the middle ear. **Nose** - Cold in the head; stuffy cold, dry coryza; ozaena (decrease in the bony ridges and mucus membranes inside the nose). Copious, offensive, thick, greenish, lumpy, yellow nasal catarrh. Atrophic rhinitis, especially if crusts are prominent. **Face** - Hard swelling of the cheek, with pain or toothache. Hard swelling of the jaw bone. **Mouth** - Gum boil, with hard swelling on the jaw. Cracked appearance of the tongue, with or without pain. Unnatural looseness of the teeth with or without pain. Toothache, with pain if any food touches the tooth. **Throat** - Follicular sore throat; plugs of mucus are continually forming in the crypts of the tonsils. **Skin** - Marked whiteness of skin. Scar tissue with a tendency to adhesion after operation. Chaps and cracks in the palms and hands, or hardened skin. Fissures of the anus. Pus formation with callous, hard edges. Indolent, fistulous ulcers, secreting thick, yellow pus. Knots, kernels, hardened glands in the female breast.

a. Middle/Rhythmic System

Emotional State - Great depression; groundless fears of financial ruin. **Respiratory System** - Hoarseness. Croup. Cough with expectoration of tiny lumps of yellow mucus, with tickling sensation becoming worse on lying down. Spasmodic cough. Fibroid deposits about the endocardium. **Circulatory System** - Vascular tumors with dilated blood vessels, and for varicose and enlarged veins. Arteriosclerosis. Aneurism. Valvular disease, when tuberculous toxins attack the heart and blood vessels.

b. Metabolic/Limb System

Stomach - Vomiting of infants. Hiccough. Flatulence. Weakness and daintiness of appetite; nausea and distress after eating in young children who are overburdened with their studies. Acute indigestion from fatigue, and brain-fag with much flatulence. **Bowel Movement** - Diarrhea in gouty subjects. Itching of the anus. Fissures of the anus, and intensely sore crack near the lower end of the bowel. Bleeding hemorrhoids. **Male** - Hydrocele (watery fluid in the scrotum or sperm duct). Indurations of the testicles. **Extremities** - Ganglia and encysted tumors at the back of the wrist. Gouty enlargements of the joints of the fingers. Bony growth on the fingers. Chronic synovitis of the knee-joint. **Back** - Chronic lumbago becoming aggravated at the beginning of movement, becoming better on continued motion. Osseous tumors. Rachitic (rickets) enlargement of the femur in infants.

Raw material comes from the naturally occurring mineral fluospar, which consist principally of calcium fluoride, $CaF2$.

DOSE - Third to the thirtieth potency.

7. CALCAREA PHOSPHORICA

Other Names: *Calcium Phosphate, Phosphate of Lime, Apatite*

Specific Properties and Action:

Calcium phosphate unites with the organic substance albumin, giving solidity to the bones, building up the teeth, and playing an important part in assimilation and digestion. In the latter, it is needed in all-important secretions of the body, such as the blood, gastric juice, and efficient glandular function, among others.

Conditions Most Used For:

Apatite is most useful particularly when the life processes in the metabolic/ limb system predominate, producing a watery constitution as expressed in exudative diathesis, lymphoid hypertrophy, tendency to perspiration, and glandular swelling. It is also indicated in late dentition, mending of fractured bones, and in school children's headache. In the latter case, the catabolism becomes stronger than anabolism because of an overburdened nerve sense system, giving rise to the headache. Apatite in the blood diverts the activity of the "I" to the metabolism, restores the balance, and unburdens the head. All symptoms become worse from any change of weather.

Other Conditions and/or Collaborating Symptoms:

a. Nerve Sense System

Head - Headache becoming worse near the region of the sutures. Headache with abdominal flatulence. Head hot, with smarting of the roots of the hair. Headache of school children about puberty. Fontanelles remain open too long. Cranial bones soft and thin. **Eyes** - Diffused opacity in the cornea following an abscess. **Mouth** - Swollen tonsils. Complaints during teething such as slow teeth development or rapid decay of teeth. Adenoid growths. **Neck and Back** - Rheumatic pain from draught of air with stiffness and dullness of the head. Soreness in sacroiliac symphysis, as if broken.

b. Middle/Rhythmic System

Emotional State - Peevish, forgetful, after grief and vexation. Always want to go somewhere. **Respiratory System** - Involuntary sighing. Hoarseness. Chest sore. Cough tends to be suffocating, becoming better while lying down. Pain through the lower left lung.

c. Metabolic/Limb System

Stomach - Infant wants to nurse all the time and vomits easily. Much flatulence. Great hunger with thirst, flatulence temporarily relieved by sour belching. Heartburn. Easy vomiting in children. **Abdomen** - At every attempt to eat, produces colicky pain in the abdomen. Colic, soreness, and burning around the navel. Abdomen sunken and flabby. **Urinary System** - Increased flow of urine with sensation of weakness. Pain in the region of the kidneys, especially when lifting or blowing the nose. **Extremities** -

Stiffness and pain, with cold, numb feeling becoming worse from any change of weather. Crawling and coldness. Buttocks, back, and limbs asleep. Pain in the joints and bones. Weary when going upstairs. **Bowel Movement** - Bleeding after excretion of hard stool. Diarrhea from juicy fruits or cider, or during dentition. Stool is green, slimy, hot, sputtering, undigested, with foul flatus. **Female** - Menses too early, excessive, and bright in girls. If late, blood is dark; sometimes, first bright, then dark, with violent backache. Nymphomania with aching, pressing, or weakness in the uterine region. Sexual excitement during lactation. Child refuses breast; milk tastes salty. Vaginal discharge like egg white.

The attenuations are prepared from natural occurring mineral apatite, found in most volcanic rock.

DOSE - Third to the thirtieth potency.

8. CUPRUM METALLICUM

Other Name: *Copper*

Generic Properties and Action:

The copper process enables our interweaving bodies to transform living substances that are capable of sensation. Here, the living substance is not utilized for continuous growth, reproduction, repair, or revitalization of tissues, but is so transformed that our life of sensation (and later the "I" activity of thinking and willing) is made possible. One of the many activities of copper is the conversion of living substances into blood. This occurs particularly in the lymphatic/glandular systems, and the organ where it happens is the liver. The liver is most rich in copper. It is the organ that takes up the venous portal blood. The copper content in the liver makes it able to transform living substances in order that our physical/life body is able to take up soul/spiritual impulses.

Conditions Most Used For:

Hypochromic anemia is one expression of a disturbed copper process, or an inadequate penetration of our sensitivity body in our physical/life bodies. Another is various cramping states. Here the sensitivity body is primarily unable to work in the metabolism, but instead finds its way into the nerve-sense system and thus cramps are produced. Copper is indicated in most abdominal spasms, leg cramps, pertussis, asthma, epilepsy, spastic constipation, and many more. With copper's connection with the venous system, it can be used in venous thromboses, crural ulcers, hemorrhoids, in circulatory diseases, and edematous swellings. To a large degree, copper maintains blood in a living flow.

A sensitivity body that is working excessively strongly may result in hyperthyroidism or Graves' disease. Copper is able to detoxify thyroxin and help control excessively strong astrality and other fundamental disturbances.

The anthroposophical understanding of the kidney system is similar to the copper process. One of the tasks of the kidney system is to break down the impulses of the nervous system into a guided anabolic stream equivalent to the ensoulment of living substances, as described earlier. It is the organ that mediates the proper incorporation of the sensitivity body with the life body. Copper, then, is one of the important remedies in any kidney therapy.

Other Conditions and/or Collaborating Symptoms:

a. Nerve Sense System

Head - Purple, red swelling of the head, with convulsions. Meningitis. Giddiness accompanies many ailments, head falls forward on the chest. **Eyes** - Aching over eyes. Fixed, starry, sunken, glistening, turned upward. Cross-eyed. Quick rolling of eyeballs, with closed eyes. **Face** - Distorted, pale bluish, with blue lips. Contraction of jaws with foam at the mouth. **Nose** - Sensation of violent congestion of blood to the nose. **Mouth** - Strong metallic, slimy state, with flow of saliva. Constant protrusion and retraction of the tongue, like a snake. Paralysis of the tongue. Stammering. **Skin** - Bluish, marbled skin. Ulcers, itching spots, and pimples at the creases of the joints. Chronic psoriasis.

b. Middle/Rhythmic System

Emotional State - Fixed ideas, malicious and morose. Fearful. Feeling of emptiness. Craves cool drinks. **Respiratory** - Cough has a gurgling sound, becoming better by drinking cold water. Suffocative attacks becoming worse by 3 a.m. Spasm and constriction of the chest; spasmodic asthma, alternating with spasmodic vomiting. Whooping cough with vomiting, spasms, and purple face. Spasm of the glottis. Angina with asthmatic symptoms and cramps. Tuberculosis of the larynx. **Heart** - Angina pectoris. Slow pulse, or hard, full, and quick. Palpitation, precordial anxiety, and pain. Fatty degeneration. Arteriosclerosis.

c. Metabolic/Limb System

Stomach - Hiccough preceding the spasms. Nausea. Vomiting, relieved by drinking cold water; with colic, diarrhea, spasms. **Abdomen** - Tense, hot, and tender to touch; contracted. Neuralgia of the abdominal viscera. Intestinal spasm. Intussusception (intestinal blockage where one part of the intestine sink into the other like a telescope). **Bowel Movement** - Black stool, painful, bloody, with tenesmus (ineffective urging) and weakness. Cholera, with cramps in the abdomen and calves. Ulcerative colitis. **Kidney System** - Nephrosis and kidney diseases which proceed with hypotension. Left-sided renal colics. **Female** - Menses too late, protracted. Cramps, extending into the chest, before, during, or after suppression of menses, or from suppressed foot sweats. Bubbling up of blood; palpitation. Dysmenorrhea. **Extremities** - Jerking, twitching of the muscles. Coldness of hands. Cramps in the palms. Great weariness of the limbs. Cramps in the calves and the sole of the feet. Clenched thumbs. Clonic spasms, beginning in the fingers and toes. Epilepsy; auro begins in the knees and ascends to the hypogastrium; then one becomes unconscious, mouth foams, and one falls to the ground. Sydenham's chorea (St. Vitus' dance). **Sleep** - During sleep there is constant rumbling in the abdomen. Sleep is deep but with shocks in the body.

Pains are ameliorated by cold drinks and pressure, but aggravated by hot water at night and before menses.

Raw materials come from powdered metallic copper.

DOSE - Third to the thirtieth potency.

Other Salts of Copper

The copper process can be guided to the specific region of the organism by using various compounds. Copper sulfate (3 - 10x) is active in the intestines in spastic constipation and lymphatic and venous congestion, and can enhance the constructive processes there. Cuprum aceticum (3 - 12x) is best for asthma, pertussis, or whooping cough. Malachite (3 - 10x), a naturally occurring copper carbonate, harmonizes the functions of the stomach and the intestines and is used to treat gastritis, gastroptosis, and cramps in the intestines. The crystal chalkosin (2 - 15x) or chalcocite (copper sulphide) is best in thyrotoxemia and Grave's disease. The combination of arsenic and copper in olivenite (4 - 30x) works into the venous circulation and kidney system. It is particularly indicated in varicoses, hypogenitalism, cryptorchidism (undescended testes), and leg cramps. Natural copper silicate or dioptase (6 - 10x) works on the skin, sense organs, and the nervous system. Cuprite (natural copper oxide at 3 to 8x) works more in the metabolism and is also good for hyperthyroidism, various forms of anemia, motility disorders of the digestive tract, recurrent and highly febrile infections, and malaria.

Generally, these copper compounds can also be used for conditions indicated in the mother substance, i.e., metallic copper.

9. FERRUM METALLICUM

Other Name: *Iron*

Generic Properties and Action:

Iron is primarily the metal of incarnation—it makes it possible for the "I" to work with his soul and spirit, right into the bodily substances, to take hold of it and actively shape it. Iron is therefore found in the hemoglobin of the blood, serum of tissues, cytochrome enzymes (important in cell respiration), and the nervous system. Iron has a different task in each of these bodily substances and system.

After the sixth fetal month, the iron levels reach a little over 23 gms per 100 ml in the blood until birth, and goes down to about 12 to 13 gms by the second week of life. Then the iron level rises again right before and during puberty. The amount of iron rises in boys (16 gms), while it reaches a plateau for girls (14 gms). This indicates that men incarnate more deeply into the physical/life bodies than women, bringing about the fundamental difference between the sexes. Thus regular experiences of weaknesses, fatigue, circulatory disturbances, and other scattered symptoms observed between 10 to 12 years of age may indicate an inadequate iron process. Moreover at puberty, the developing child must also come to terms with protein formation—another process ruled by iron. Therefore, two typical diseases occur frequently at this time—acne as a symptom of a disturbed protein metabolism, and anemia. The human being's relationship to iron throughout one's life then is a direct index of his/her incarnation process. The knowledge of the use of iron with all its compounds becomes very useful to manage this process.

Another property of iron is its strong affinity to light. In porphyria, the increase of a body substance called porphyrin (a protein, and therefore considered as a problem of protein metabolism) is the reason for the heightened sensitivity to light. Here, iron therapy makes possible the correct assimilation and utilization of light. On another level, light is the element that forms the substance of thought. With clear thinking (an activity of the "I"), one sees light, an inner light.

In the metabolism, iron stimulates the flow of bile. Bile acid not only helps in the digestion, but stimulates one to activity and eventually affects consciousness. In the heart, the energy of iron is metamorphosed into courage, and therefore affects our feeling life. In the nerve sense system, iron is found in the nucleus ruber and substantia nigra and therefore has a significant function in the brain. Lastly, iron is essential against infection and any life foreign to one's own life. Iron enters the organ of defense called the reticular endothelial system, and maintains the self against foreign invasion.

Conditions Most Used For:

Ferrum metallicum harmonizes the form and function of the whole organism. It is best used in illnesses of the nerve sense system such as in cerebral sclerosis, migraine, Parkinsonism, and degenerative and chronic infection of the nerves, air passages, and constitutional anemia. It is also for young weakly persons with pseudo-plethora (too red color of skin) who flush easily; oversensitive; worse after any active effort.

Other Conditions and/or Collaborating Symptoms:

a. Nerve Sense System

Head - Vertigo upon seeing flowing water. Stinging headache with pain extending to the teeth and with cold extremities. Pain in the back of the head with roaring in the neck. Scalp painful. **Eyes** - Watery, dull red; photophobia; letters run together. **Face** - Fiery red and flushed from the least pain, emotion, or exertion. Red parts become white, bloodless, and puffy. **Nose** - Mucous membrane relaxed, boggy, anemic, pale. **Mouth** - Pain in the teeth but relieved by icy-cold water. Earthy, pasty taste like rotten eggs. **Skin** - Pale; flushes readily; pits remain on pressure.

b. Middle/Rhythmic System

Emotional State - Irritable with the slightest noise becoming unbearable. Excited from the slightest opposition. Sanguine temperament. **Respiratory**

System - Chest oppressed; breathing difficult. Surging of blood to the chest. Hoarseness. Cough dry and spasmodic. Hemoptysis. Risk of tuberculosis. **Heart** - Palpitation becoming worse during movement. Pulse full, but soft and yielding; also small and weak. Heart suddenly bleeds into the blood vessels, and as suddenly draws a reflex, leaving pallor of surface. Anemic murmur.

c. Metabolic/Limb System

Stomach - Voracious appetite, or absolute loss of appetite. Loathing of sour things. Attempts to eat bring on diarrhea. Eructation of food after eating without nausea. Nausea and vomiting after eating. Vomiting after midnight. Intolerance of eggs. Heat and burning in the stomach. Soreness of the abdominal walls. Flatulent dyspepsia. **Bowel Movement** - Stool at night with undigested food, but painless. Ineffectual urging; stool hard, followed by backache or cramping pain in the rectum. Prolapse recti; itching of the anus, especially in young children. **Urinary System** - Involuntary urine becoming worse during daytime. Tickling in the urethra extending to the bladder. Cystitis, enuresis, nephritis. **Female** - Menses remit a day or two and then return. Discharge of long pieces from the uterus. Women who are weak, delicate, chlorotic, yet have a fiery-red face. Menses too early, too profuse, last too long; pale, watery. Sensitive vagina. Tendency to abortion. Prolapse of the vagina. Amenorrhea or heavy menstruation with long intervals. Sterility. Indifferent to sexual intercourse. **Extremities** - Rheumatism of the left shoulder. Dropsy (edema) after the loss of vital fluids. Lumbago becoming better by slow walking. Pain in the hip joint, tibia, sole, and heel. **Fever** - General coldness of extremities; head and face hot. Chill at 4 a.m. Heat in palms and soles. Profuse debilitating sweat. Fever with thirst during chill.

Potentized remedies are prepared from the metallic iron.

DOSE - Third to the thirtieth potency.

10. FERRUM PHOSPHORICUM

Other Names: *Ferrum Phosphate, Phosphate of Iron*

Specific Properties and Action:

As already indicated in the description of iron, it is the metal with a strong affinity to light, including the ability to see inner light, an activity performed by the spirit or the spiritual "I." The phosphorus in this iron compound gives special emphasis to the "I" and light character of iron. In acute infection such as pneumonia or any fever, ferrum phosphoricum stimulates the ego in the metabolism, making fever unnecessary. In this case, its seemingly anti-pyretic quality is totally different from the allopathic concept of antipyresis.

Ferrum phosphoricum as a tissue salt is found in the blood as an essential constituent of hemoglobin—which carries oxygen to all parts of the body. It gives strength to the circular walls of the blood vessels, especially the arteries.

Conditions Most Used For:

Ferrum phosphoricum is the remedy for all kinds of fever and inflammation. It is indicated in the relaxed condition of the muscular tissue and in abnormal conditions of the corpuscles of the blood. A little powder, externally applied, will promote clean and rapid healing of the injured tissue and hemorrhage, relieve pain, and resolve inflammation.

Other Conditions and/or Collaborating Symptoms:

a. Nerve Sense System

Head - Sore to touch, cold, noise, or jar. Rush of blood to the head. Ill effects of sun heat. Throbbing sensation. Vertigo. **Eyes** - Red, inflamed, with burning sensation. Feeling of sand under the lids. Hyperamia of optic disc and retina, with blurred vision. **Ears** - Noises, throbbing. First stage of otitis. Membrana thympani red and bulging. **Nose** - First stage of colds in the head. Predisposition to colds. Epitaxis; bright red blood. **Face** - Flushed; cheeks sore and hot. Florid complexion. Facial neuralgia becoming worse when shaking the head and when stooping.

b. Middle/Rhythmic System

Respiratory System - First stage of all inflammatory affections. Congestion of the lungs. Hemoptysis; short, painful tickling cough; croup. Hard, dry cough, with sore chest. Hoarseness. Expectoration of pure blood in pneumonia. Pneumonia. Cough that becomes better at night. Bronchitis in young children. Acute exacerbation of tuberculosis. **Throat** - Mouth hot; throat red, inflamed. Ulcerated sore throat. Tonsils red and swollen. Eustachian tubes inflamed. Sub-acute laryngitis with fauces inflamed and red. First stage of diptheria. Ranula (large sac-like swelling in the floor of the mouth, mostly caused by a blockage of the ducts of the salivary gland) in vascular, sanguine constitutions. **Heart** - Palpitation with rapid pulse. First stage of cardiac disease. Short, quick, soft pulse.

c. Metabolic/Limb System

Stomach - Aversion to meat and milk. Desire for stimulants. Vomiting of undigested food. Vomiting of bright red blood. Sour eructations. **Abdomen** - First stage of peritonitis. First stage of dysentery, with much blood in the stool. **Urinary System** - Urine spurts with every cough. Nocturnal enuresis and diurnal incontinence of urine. Irritation of the neck of the bladder. Polyuria. **Extremities** - Articular rheumatism. Rheumatism of the right shoulder with pain extending to the chest and wrist. Palms hot. Hands swollen and painful. **Female** - Menses every three weeks, with bearing down sensation and pain on top of the head. Vaginismus. Vagina dry and hot. **Sleep** - Restless and sleepless. Anxious dreams. Night sweats of anemia. **Fever** - Chill daily at 1 p.m. All catarrhal and inflammatory fevers; first stage.

Potentized remedies are prepared from ferric phosphate, $FePO_4$, or from the mineral vivianite (ferrous phosphate). Vivianite is formed through the weathering of iron minerals in the region of phosphoric acid containing minerals. It may also be formed through the decomposition of plant or animal substances which contains phosphoric acid. Though it is white and cheese-like when newly exposed, it turns blue upon contact with air. In some lead mines, it is found as indigo blue transparent crystals.

DOSE - Third to the thirtieth potency.

Other Salts of Iron

By knowing the proper salt or iron compound, the iron impulse can be guided therapeutically. Siderite (natural iron carbonate) at potency 3x to 6x works best in the metabolic region for problems such as pancreatopathy, fermentation, and indigestion, especially during puberty. Pyrite (iron sulphide) brings harmony between breathing and circulation and is indicated in the upper respiratory tract illnesses such as bronchitis, tracheitis, pharyngitis, and laryngitis. Skorodite (iron arsenate) brings together iron (for the "I") and arsenic (for the sensitivity body) to properly incarnate during times of fatigue and hypotonia, hypotension, and the difficulty to become awake (and incarnated) in the morning (6 to 10x potencies). Ferrum sidereum (meteoric iron) works in a balancing, vitalizing, and healing way on the nervous system such as in nephrosis, hypotension, and depression (esp. in erroneous attitude towards life, better taken together with aurum). In medium potencies (8 - 15x) can work against fear, compulsive, and anxious conditions, and in higher potencies (20x) for states of nervous fatigue and lack of will.

11. KALIUM

Other Name: *Potassium*

Generic Properties and Action:

Any living fluid found in plants or animals has potassium in it. The life body is able to enliven living fluids by making use of potassium dissolved in the water. Potassium is thus found in all living cells and tissues and is particularly important for the liver and the heart. With little potassium, fluids will stagnate and lead to certain forms of edema, poor circulation, or cramps and pains.

Conditions Most Used For:

Each compound of potassium has a distinctive use as a remedy. Like the compounds of other minerals and metals, they are able to address particular tissues or organs of the organism. The general symptomatology of all potassium salts is usually expressed in soft pulse, coldness, general depression, and very characteristic stitches, i.e., sharp and cutting, which are felt in any part of the body. All pains nearly become better by motion. This is indicated in fleshy, aged people with a tendency to edema and paralysis.

12. KALIUM BICHROMICUM

Other Name: *Potassium Bi-chromate*

Specific Properties and Action:

Potassium bi-chromate specifically addresses the mucous membrane of the stomach, gastro-intestinal tract, the female genitalia, and air passages. It also affects the kidneys, heart, and liver.

Conditions Most Used For:

The potentized form of potassium bi-chromate may be used in catarrh of the pharynx, bronchi, and nose that produces tough, stringy, viscous secretion. It is of service in balanitis (inflammation of the penis), prostatitis (with pain on movement), in incipient urinary obstruction with copious deposits, and in purulent vaginal discharge. It is indicated in nephritis, cirrhosis of the liver, and in general weakness that is bordering on paralysis. It is especially indicated for fleshy, fat, light-complexioned persons with a history of the above ailments. Symptoms usually are worse in the morning; pains migrate quickly while rheumatic and gastric symptoms alternate. This remedy is more adapted to sub-acute rather than the violent acute stages of a disease.

Other Conditions and/or Collaborating Symptoms:

a. Nerve Sense System

Head - Vertigo with nausea when rising from the seat. Headache over the eyebrows, preceded by blurred vision. Aching and fullness in the glabella (a flat triangular area of bone of the forehead). Semi-lateral headaches in small spots, and from suppressed catarrh. Frontal pain; usually over one eye. Bones and scalp feel sore. **Eyes** - Supra-orbital neuralgia, right side. Eyelids burn, swollen, edematous. Discharge ropy and yellow. Ulcers on the cornea; no pain or photophobia. Croupous conjunctivitis; glanular lids, with pannus (eye filled with blood vessels and grainy tissue). Iritis, with punctate (marked with dots and tiny spots) deposits on the inner surface of the cornea. Slight pain with severe ulceration or inflammation. **Ears** - Swollen with tearing pains. Thick, yellow, stringy, fetid discharge. Sharp stitches in the left ear. **Nose** - Snuffles of children, especially fat, chubby babies. Pressure and pain at the root of the nose, and sticking pain in the nose. Septum (wall dividing the nostrils) ulcerated; round ulcer. Fetid smell. Discharge thick, ropy, greenish-yellow. Tough, elastic plugs from the nose; leave a raw surface. Inflammation extends to the frontal sinuses, with distress and fullness at the root of the nose. Dropping from posterior nares. Loss of smell. Much hawking. Inability to breathe through the nose. Dryness. Violent sneezing. Profuse, watery discharge. Chronic inflammation of the frontal sinus with stopped-up sensation. **Face** - Florid complexion. Blotchy, red appearance. Acne. Bones sensitive, especially beneath the orbits. **Mouth** - Dry, viscous saliva. Tongue mapped, red, shining, smooth, and dry, with dysentery; broad, flat, indented, thickly coated. Feeling of a hair on the tongue. **Throat** - Fauces red and inflamed. Dry and rough. Parotid glands swollen. Uvula relaxed, edematous, bladder-like. Pseudo-membranous deposit on the tonsils and soft palate. Burning extended to the stomach. Aphthae (small white spot caused by a fungus). Diphtheria, with profound prostration and soft pulse. Discharge from the mouth and throat, tough and stringy. **Skin** - Acne. Papular eruptions. Ulcer with punched-out edges, with tendency to penetrate and tenacious exudation. Pustular eruption, resembling small-pox, with burning pains. Itching with vesicular eruption.

b. Middle/Rhythmic System

Respiratory System - Voice hoarse, becoming worse in the evening. Metallic, hacking cough. Profuse, yellow expectoration, very glutinous and sticky, coming out in long stringy, and very tenacious mass. Tickling in the larynx. Catarrh laryngitis cough has a brassy sound. True membranous croup, extending to the larynx and nares. Cough, with pain in the sternum, extending to the shoulders, becoming worse when undressing. Pain at bifurcation of trachea on coughing; from mid-sternum to the back. **Heart** - Dilatation, especially from coexisting kidney lesion. Cold feeling around the heart.

c. Metabolic/Limb System

Stomach - Nausea and vomiting after taking beer. Load immediately after eating. Feels as if digestion stopped. Dilation of the stomach. Gastritis. Round ulcer of the stomach. Stitches in the region of the liver and spleen through to the spine. Dislikes water. Cannot digest meat. Desire for beer and acids. Gastric symptoms are relieved after eating, and the rheumatic symptoms appear. Vomiting of bright yellow water. **Abdomen** - Cutting pain in the abdomen, soon after eating. Chronic intestinal ulceration. Soreness in the right hypochondrium. Fatty infiltration of the liver and increase in soft fibrous tissue. Painful retraction, soreness, and burning. **Bowel Movement** - Jelly-like, gelatinous stools becoming worse in the mornings. Dysentery; tenesmus, stools brown, frothy. Sensation of plug in the anus. Periodic constipation, with pain across the loins, and brown urine. **Urinary System** - Burning in the urethra. After urinating, a drop seems to remain which cannot be expelled. Ropy mucus in the urine. Urethra becomes clogged up. Congestion of the kidneys; nephritis, with scanty, albuminous urine and casts. Pyelitis; urine mixed with epithelial cells, mucus, pus, or blood. **Male** - Itching and pain of the penis, with pustules. Ulcers, with paroxysmal stitches aggravated at night. Constriction at the root of the penis, at night on awakening. Syphilitic ulcers, with cheesy, tenacious exudation. **Female** - Yellow, tenacious leucorrhea (vaginal discharge). Pruritus of the vulva, with great burning and excitement. Prolapsus of the uterus becoming worse in hot weather. **Back** - Cutting pain through the loins; cannot walk; extends to the groins. Pain in the coccyx and sacrum extending up and down. **Extremities** - Pains fly rapidly from one place to another. Wandering pains along the bones, aggravated by cold. Left-sided sciatica becoming better by moving. Bones feel sore and bruised. Very weak. Tearing pains in the tibia; syphilitic rheumatism. Pain, swelling, and stiffness and crackling of all joints. Soreness of the heels when walking. Tendon Achilles swollen and painful. Pains in small spots.

Potentized remedies are made from potassium bi-chromate, $K_2Cr_2O_7$.

DOSE - From the third to the thirtieth potency.

13. KALIUM CARBONICUM

Other Name: *Potassium Carbonate*

Specific Properties and Action:

This compound is closest to the description given earlier of potassium. That is, it gives the life body the possibility to permeate water that remains excessively stagnant or physical. This means that "cold" water can be revitalized, making it accessible for excretion. It acts also on the mucosa and the heart.

Conditions Most Used For:

Kalium carbonate is of particular use to persons who catch cold easily or develop scurvy-like symptoms like stomatitis, periodontitis, or acne. In catarrhal conditions of various kinds (nose, bronchi, chronic intestinal catarrh, hemorrhoids), this remedy can be the first choice. It is used in pleurisy, especially on the right side, and stabbing pains also on the right side and unrelated to respiration. It may be given in great weakness and unsteadiness, such as muscular weakness and rheumatism, or in weakness of the bladder. It has been found useful in helping repair damaged heart muscle with arrhythmia due to an infectious disease.

Other Conditions and/or Collaborating Symptoms:

a. Nerve Sense System

Head - Vertigo on turning. Headache from riding in the cold wind.

Headache comes on with yawning. Great dryness of the hair; falls out. **Eyes** - Stitches in the eyes. Spots, gauze, and black points before the eyes. Lids stick together in the morning. Swelling over the upper lid, like little bags. Swelling of the glabella between the brows. Asthenopia. Weak sight from excessive sexual indulgence. On closing the eyes, painful sensation of light penetrating the brain. **Ears** - Stitches in the ears. Itching, cracking, ringing and roaring. **Nose** - Thick, fluent, yellow discharge. Post-nasal dropping. Sore, scurfy nostrils; bloody nasal mucus or nosebleed on washing the face in the morning. Crusty nasal openings or ulcerated nostrils. **Mouth** - Gums separate from teeth; pus oozes out. Pyorrhea. Tongue white. Much saliva constantly in the mouth. Bad slimy taste. **Throat** - Dry, parched, rough. Sticking pain, as from a fish-bone. Swallowing difficult; food goes down the esophagus slowly. Mucous accumulation in the morning. **Skin** - Burning as from a mustard plaster.

b. Middle/Rhythmic System

Emotional State - Despondent. Alternating moods. Very irritable. Full of fear and imaginations. Anxiety felt in the stomach. Sensation as if bed were sinking. Never wants to be left alone. Never quiet or contented. Obstinate and hypersensitive to pain, noise, or touch. Desire for sweets. **Respiratory System** - Cutting pain in the chest becoming worse on lying on the right side. Hoarseness and loss of voice. Dry, hard cough about 3 a.m., with stitching pains and dryness of pharynx. Bronchitis, whole chest is very sensitive. Expectoration scanty and tenacious, but increasing in the morning and after eating. Hydrothorax (build up of chest fluids). Expectoration must be swallowed; cheesy taste; copious, offensive lump. Coldness of the chest. Wheezing. Tendency to tuberculosis becoming better in warm climate. **Heart** - Sensation as if heart were suspended. Palpitation and burning in the heart region. Weak, rapid pulse; intermits, due to digestive disturbance. Threatened heart failure.

c. Metabolic/Limb System

Stomach - Flatulence. Feeling of a lump in the pit of the stomach. Dyspepsia of old people; burning acidity, bloating. Gastric disorder from ice-water. Nausea becoming better lying down. Constant feeling as if stomach were full of water. Anxiety felt in the stomach. Epigastric pain to the back. **Abdomen** - Stitches in the region of the liver. Old chronic liver troubles, with soreness. Jaundice and edema. Distention and coldness of the abdomen. Pain from left hypochondrium through the abdomen; must turn on the right side before he can rise. **Bowel Movement** -

Large, difficult stools, with stitching pain an hour before. Hemorrhoids, large, swollen, painful. Itching, ulcerated pimples around the anus. Large discharge of blood with normal stool. Pain in the hemorrhoids when coughing. Burning or itching in the rectum and anus. **Urinary System** - Obliged to rise several times at night to urinate. Pressure on the bladder long before urine comes. Involuntary urination when coughing, sneezing, etc. **Male** - Deficient sexual instinct. Excessive emissions followed by weakness. Complaints from coition. **Female** - Menses early, profuse or too late, pale and scanty, with soreness about the genitals; pains from the back passing down through the gluteal muscles, with cutting in the abdomen to the chest. Delayed menses in young girls, with chest symptoms or ascites. Difficult first menses. Complaints after giving birth. Uterine hemorrhage; constant oozing after copious flow, with violent backache, relieved by sitting and pressure. **Back** - Great exhaustion. Stitches in the region of the kidneys and right scapula. Small of the back feels weak. Stiffness and paralytic feeling in the back. Burning in the spine. Severe backache during pregnancy, and after a miscarriage. Hip disease. Lumbago with sudden, sharp pains extending up and down the back and to the thighs. **Extremities** - Backs and legs give way. Uneasiness, heaviness, and tearing in the limbs, and jerking. Tearing pain in the limbs, with swelling. Tearing in arms from shoulder to wrist. Lacerating in wrist-joint. Limbs go to sleep easily. Tips of toes and fingers painful. Sole very sensitive. Pain from hip to knee. **Sleep** - Drowsy after eating. Wakes up about two in the morning and cannot sleep again.

Potentized remedies are made from potassium carbonate, K_2CO_3.

DOSE - From the third to the thirtieth potencies.

14. KALIUM MURIATICUM

Other Names: *Chloride of Potassium, Potassium Chloride, Kali Mur.*

Specific Properties and Action:

Kalium muriaticum unites with albumin, forming the stringy protein fibrin, which gives semi-solid character to a blood clot. Fibrin is found in every tissue of the body except the bones. A deficiency of this compound in the tissues brings about the release of albumin that can cause phlegm formation that is thick, white, sticky in character. The tongue coating becomes white or grey and the blood thickens and tends to form clots.

Conditions Most Used For:

This remedy is indicated in naso-pharyngeal and the eustachian tube catarrh with mucous, as described above. It is the best for spasmodic croup, diarrhea, and bronchitis to control the exudation. It may be given also in ulcerative keratitis or inflammation of the cornea of the eye.

Other Conditions and/or Collaborating Symptoms:

a. Nerve Sense System

Head - Headache with vomiting. Crusta lactea. Dandruff. Imagines he must starve. **Eyes** - White mucous, purulent scabs. Superficial ulcer. Trachoma. Corneal opacities. **Ears** - Chronic, catarrhal conditions of the middle ear. Glands about the ear swollen. Snapping and noise in the ear. Threatened mastoid. Great effusion about the auricle. **Nose** - Catarrh; phlegm white, thick. Vault of pharynx covered with adherent crust. Stuffy cold. Nosebleed. **Face** - swollen, painful cheeks. **Mouth** - Aphtha; thrush; white ulcers in mouth. Swollen glands about the jaw and neck. Coating of the tongue grayish-white, or slimy. **Throat** - Follicular tonsillitis. Tonsil enlarged so much that one can hardly breathe. Grayish patches or spots in the throat and tonsils. Adherent crust in vault of pharynx. Eustachian catarrh. **Skin** - Acne, erythema, and eczema, with vesicle containing thick, white contents. Dry, flour-like scales on the skin. Bursitis.

b. Middle/Rhythmic System

Respiratory System - Loss of voice; hoarseness. Asthma, with gastric derangements; mucous white and hard to cough up. Loud, noisy stomach cough, cough short, acute, and spasmodic, like whooping cough; expectoration thick and white.

c. Metabolic/Limb System

Stomach - Fatty and rich food causes indigestion. Vomiting of white, opaque mucus; water gathers in the mouth. Pain in the stomach with constipation. Bulimia; hunger disappears by drinking water. **Abdomen** - Abdominal tenderness and swelling. Flatulence. Thread worms, causing itching at the anus. **Bowel Movement** - Constipation; light colored stools. Diarrhea, after fatty food; clay-colored, white, or slimy stools. Dysentery; purging, with slimy stools. Hemorrhoids; bleeding; blood dark and thick, fibrinous, clotted. **Female** - Menstruation too late or suppressed, checked, or too early; excessive discharge; dark-clotted, or tough, black blood, like tar. Leucorrhea; discharge of milky-white mucus, thick, non-irritating, bland. Morning sickness with vomiting of white phlegm. Bunches in breast feel quite soft and are tender. **Extremities** - Rheumatic fever; exudation and swelling around the joints. Rheumatic pains felt only during motion, or increased by it. Nightly rheumatic pains becoming worse from warmth of the bed. Lightning-like pains from the small of the back to the feet; one must get out of bed and sit up. Hands get stiff while writing.

Potentized remedies are made from potassium chloride, KCl.

DOSE - Third to the twelfth potency.

15. KALIUM PHOSPHORICUM

Other Names: *Potassium Phosphate, Phosphate of Potassium, Kali Phos.*

Specific Properties and Action:

In situation of nervous exhaustion and neurasthenia, the sensitivity body is activated too strongly by the nervous system. Here, the phosphorus (the vehicle of the "I") in kalium phosphoricum can lead the "I" into the stream of watery metabolism and bring relief and proper nourishment to the nervous system. Moreover, it is a constituent of all tissues and fluids of the body, notably of the brain and nerve cells. It is in this sense that kalium phosphoricum is a great nerve nutrient.

Conditions Most Used For:

Kalium phosphoricum is given to those who experience exhausted mental states or sluggish conditions of the mind following continued exertion or great emotional strain. A deficiency of this compound produces brain-fag, melancholia, irritability, fearfulness, timidity, or lack of nerve power. It can restore debilitated muscles and impaired nerve function brought about by an acute infectious disease. The above symptoms are aggravated by noise, physical or mental exertion, or motion after a rest or cold air. Symptoms become better by gentle motion, eating, rest, excitement, or by anything which diverts the mind.

Other Conditions and/or Collaborating Symptoms:

a. Nerve Sense System

Head - Occipital headache becoming better after rising. Vertigo from lying down, on standing up, from sitting, and when looking upward. Cerebral anemia. Headache of students and those worn out by fatigue. **Eyes** - Weakness of sight; loss of perceptive power; after diphtheria or from exhaustion. Drooping of the eyelids. **Ears** - Humming and buzzing in the ears. **Nose** - Nasal disease, with offensive odor; fetid discharge. **Face** - Livid and sunken, with hollow eyes. Right-sided neuralgia, relieved by cold applications. **Mouth** - Breath offensive, fetid. Tongue coated brownish, like mustard. Excessively dry in the morning. Toothache with easily bleeding gums; they have a bright red seam on them. Gums spongy and receding. **Throat** - Gangrenous sore throat. Paralysis of the vocal cords.

b. Middle/Rhythmic System

Emotional State - Anxiety, nervous dread, lethargy. Indisposition to meet people. Extreme lassitude and depression. Very nervous, starts easily, irritable. Brain-fag; hysteria; night terrors. Somnambulance. Loss of memory. Slightest labor seems a heavy task. Great despondency about business. Shyness; disinclined to converse. **Respiratory System** - Asthma; least food aggravates it. Shortness of breath on going upstairs. Cough with yellow expectoration.

c. Metabolic/Limb System

Stomach - A nervous "gone" sensation at the pit of the stomach. Feels seasick without nausea. **Abdomen** - Diarrhea; foul, putrid odor; occasioned by fright, with depression and exhaustion. Diarrhea while eating. Dysentery; stools consist of pure blood; patient becomes delirious; abdomen swells. Cholera; stools have the appearance of rice water. Prolapse of the rectum. **Female** - Menstruation too late or too scanty in pale, irritable, sensitive, lachrymose females. Too profuse discharge, deep-red or blackish-red, thin and not coagulating; sometimes with offensive odor. Feeble and ineffectual labor pains. **Male** - Nocturnal emissions; sexual power diminished; utter prostration after sexual intercourse. **Urinary System** - Enuresis. Incontinence of urine. Bleeding from the urethra. Very yellow urine. **Extremities** - Paralytic lameness in the back and the extremities. Pains, with depression, and subsequent exhaustion. **Fever** - Sub-normal temperature.

Potentized remedies are made from potassium dihydrogen phosphate, KH_2PO_4.

DOSE - From the third to the twelfth potency.

16. KALIUM SULPHURICUM

Other Name: *Potassium Sulfate*

Specific Properties and Action:

Kalium sulphuricum works together with the iron in the blood to carry oxygen to every cell in the organism, especially the skin. In bringing the blood to the surface, it promotes perspiration and opens the pores of the skin.

Conditions Most Used For:

Kalium sulphuricum can address many skin ailments. A deficiency of it gives rise to symptoms of chilliness, shifting inflammatory pain and a desire for fresh, cool air. This substance has an affinity for oil, hence in inflammatory conditions the secretion is light yellow, slimy, sticky, watery, or greenish matter. It is also useful in stimulating the full shedding of eruptions of measles, chicken pox, and other ailments that uses the skin to eliminate toxins.

Other Conditions and/or Collaborating Symptoms:

a. Nerve Sense System

Head - Rheumatic headache beginning in the evening. Bald spots. Dandruff and scaldhead. **Ears** - Eustachian deafness. Discharge of yellow matter. Chronic otitis media with yellow discharge. **Nose** - Colds, with yellow, slimy expectoration. Nose obstructed. Smell lost. Engorgement of the nasal pharyngeal mucous membrane, mouth breathing, snoring, etc., remaining after the removal of the adenoids. **Face** - Aches in heated room. **Mouth** - Tongue coated yellow and slimy. Insipid, pappy taste. Gums painful. **Skin** - Psoriasis. Ezcema; burning, itching, papular eruption. Nettle-rash. Polypi. Seborrhea. Favus. Ring-worm of scalp or beard with abundant scales.

b. Middle/Rhythmic System

Respiratory System - Coarse rales. Rattling of mucus in the chest. Post-grippal cough, especially in children. Bronchial asthma, with yellow expectoration. Cough, worse in the evening and in hot atmosphere. Croupy hoarseness.

c. Metabolic/Limb System

Stomach - Burning thirst, nausea, and vomiting. Load feeling. Dread of hot drinks. **Abdomen** - Colicky pains; abdomen feels cold to touch; tense. Yellow, slimy diarrhea. Constipation with hemorrhoids. **Extremities** - Pain in the nape, back, and limb becoming worse in a warm room. Shifting, wandering pains. **Male** - Gonorrhea; discharge slimy, yellowish-green. Orchitis. (inflammation of the testicles). **Female** - Menses too late, scanty, with feeling of weight in the abdomen. Metrorrhagia.

Potentized remedies are made from potassium sulphate, K_2SO_4.

DOSE - From the third to the thirtieth potency.

Other Salts of Potassium

Other compounds of potassium are still used today to address specific ailments. Potassium arsenite ($KAsO_2$) or kalium arsenicosum (4 - 12x) is usually given to those with nephrotic syndrome, chronic eczemas, dry, slack skin, itching psoriasis, lichen ruber, or numerous papules with white scales and fissures in the crease of the elbows and knees. The symptoms are accompanied by a quarrelsome, peevish, discontented mood, or apathy. Potassium acetate, CH_3COOK, or kalium aceticum is given in diabetes, diarrhea, and edema.

17. MAGNESIUM

Generic Properties and Action:

To understand the action of magnesium, one must see it in the light of its polarity, calcium. In the human body, magnesium is found intracellularly while calcium is primarily found extracellularly. In nature, magnesium is more related to the plant kingdom because it is an important ingredient in chlorophyll, while calcium is connected more to the animal kingdom through the bone formation. Magnesium, then, has a deep relationship to light and the forces of the sun. For example, when magnesium is burned, it emits a radiant light. Iron (as mentioned in ferrum phosphoricum) has a similar relation to light. Magnesium and iron is another polarity which manifests in nature as chlorophyll and hemoglobin, green and red, vegetative and animal life. Magnesium therapy then may be necessary when iron cannot be properly assimilated by the organism.

Half of the magnesium in a human body is found in the bones. This indicates that magnesium provides an inner light structure for the bones that is adequate for the penetration of the "I." The other half is found partly bound to protein, in the liver, striated muscles, kidneys, and brain. Here, magnesium is living and active. For example, it activates the bile production and the intracellular enzymes, which catalyzes the metabolism of glucose, known as phosphorylisation of carbohydrates.

Magnesium blocks the liberation of acetylcholine, a substance that allows messages to travel from one nerve to another. It is thus applied as a remedy for pain and cramps brought about by the excessive penetration of the sensitivity body into the nerves and muscles.

Conditions Most Used For:

The guiding idea behind the use of magnesium is that of an exhausted, overstressed life body, particularly in excessively nervous, thin people. It cushions the effects of shock, blows, and mental distress. In illnesses where there is a decreased magnesium level, such as in cirrhosis of the liver or hyperthyroidism, magnesium will be helpful together with other remedies. In these two illnesses, cirrhosis is an indication of a weakened life body through time or indulgence, while hyperthyroidism is an expression of an excessively strong sensitivity body. The latter also leads to a weakened life body and therefore needs magnesium.

Magnesium is particularly needed in the first seven years of life to actively bring about the structuring and formative processes that stream from within to the periphery. (See the description of fluorine in calcium fluoride to better understand this idea.) This activity of magnesium should be discerned from the radiating faces of growing children.

18. MAGNESIUM CARBONICUM

Other Names: *Carbonate of Magnesia, Magnesite, Magnesium Carbonate*

Other Conditions and/or Collaborating Symptoms:

a. Nerve Sense System

Head - Sticking pain in the side of the head on which he lies, as if the hair was pulled; becoming worse on mental exertion. Itching of the scalp becoming worse in damp weather. Pain above margin of the right orbit. Black motes before the eyes. Dryness of the mucosa (eyes, nose, pharynx). **Ears** - Diminished hearing. Deafness; comes suddenly and in varying degrees. Numbness of the outer ear. Feeling of distention of the middle ear. Subdued tinnitus. **Face** - Tearing pain in one side becoming worse when quiet; one must move about. Toothache, especially during pregnancy, becoming worse at night, when cold and quiet. Teeth feel too long. Ailments from cutting wisdom teeth. Pain in malar bone becoming worse during rest, at night, or exposure to cold wind. **Mouth** - Dry at night, sour taste. Vesicular eruption; bloody saliva. Sticking pain in the throat; hawking up fetid, pea-colored particles. **Skin** - Earthy, sallow, and parchment like; emaciation. Itching vesicles on the hands and fingers. Dry, itching skin. Nodosities under the skin. Sore; sensitive to cold.

b. Middle/Rhythmic System

Respiratory System - Tickling cough with salty, bloody expectoration. Constrictive chest pains, difficult breathing. Sore chest during motion.

c. Metabolic/Limb System

Stomach - Desire for fruit, acids, and vegetables. Sour belching, and vomiting of bitter water. Craving for meat. **Abdomen** - Gastro-intestinal catarrh with marked acidity. Very heavy feeling; contractive, pinching pain in the right iliac region. **Bowel Movement** - Preceded by griping, colicky pain. Green, watery, frothy stool like a frog's pond's scum. Bloody mucous stools. Milk passes undigested in nursing children. **Extremities** - Tearing in shoulders as if dislocated. Right shoulder painful, unable to raise it. Arthritis of the shoulder joints. Whole body feels tired and painful, especially the legs and feet. Swelling in the folds of the knee. **Children's Symptom** - Whole child smells sour and disposed to boils. **Female** - Sore throat, or coryza and nasal catarrh before the menses appear. Menses too late and scanty, thick, dark, like pitch; mucous leucorrhea. Menses flow only in sleep; more profuse at night or when lying down, but ceases when walking. Broken-down, "worn out" women, with uterine and climatic disorders or numbness and distention in various parts, and nerve prostration.

Potentized remedies are made from the mineral magnesite.

DOSE - Third to the thirtieth potency.

19. MAGNESIUM PHOSPHORICUM

Other Name: *Magnesium Phosphate*

Specific Properties and Action:

With the combination of phosphorus in this form of magnesium, we now have two light elements. Through this substance, the "I" is directed into the light aspect of the life body. Its overall effect is relaxing, and it builds up and gives direction to the life body. Magnesium phosphate then is the great anti-spasmodic remedy. It soothes the cramping of muscles and neuralgic pains that are relieved by warmth. It is especially suited to tired, languid, exhausted individuals.

Other Conditions and/or Collaborating Symptoms:

a. Nerve Sense System

Head - Vertigo on moving, falls forward upon closing the eyes, becoming better on walking in the open air. Headache after mental exertion, with chilliness. Sensation of fluid in the head as if parts of the brain were changing places. **Eyes** - Supra-orbital pains. Increased lachrymation. Twitching of the eyelids. Eyes hot, tired, vision blurred, colored lights before the eyes. **Ears** - Severe neuralgic pain; worse behind the right ear becoming worse by going into cold area or by washing the face and neck with cold water. **Mouth** - Toothache becoming better by heat or hot drinks. Ulceration of the teeth, with swelling of glands of the face, throat, and neck, and swelling of the tongue. Complaints of teething children. Spasms without fever.

b. Middle/Rhythmic System

Emotional State - Laments all the time about the pain. Inability to think clearly. Sleepless because of indigestion. **Throat** - Soreness and stiffness especially the right side; parts seem puffy, with chilliness, and aching all over. **Respiratory System** - Asthmatic oppression of the chest. Dry, tickling cough. Spasmodic cough and whooping cough especially at night and while lying down. Voice hoarse, larynx sore and raw. Intercostal neuralgia. **Heart** - Angina pectoris. Nervous spasmodic palpitation. Constricting pains around the heart.

c. Metabolic/Limb System

Abdomen - Intestinal pain, relieved by pressure. Flatulent colic, forcing one to bend; relieved by rubbing, warmth, or pressure; accompanied by belching of gas but with no relief. Bloated, full sensation in the abdomen. Gall stone colic. Renal colic. **Extremities** - Involuntary shaking of the hands. Paralysis agitans. Cramps in the calves. Sciatica with boring shooting pains, changing location and aggravated by light touch. Sydenham's Chorea with contortion of the limbs. Rheumatism of the joints. Weakness in the arms and hands, fingertips stiff and numb. General muscular weakness. Twitching. **Female** - Menstrual colic and dysmenorrhea with neuralgic complaints, relieved by the onset of the flow. Menses too early, dark, stringy. Swelling of external parts. Ovarian neuralgia. Vaginismus. **Fever** - Chilliness after dinner, in the evening. Chills run up and down the back, with shivering, followed by a suffocating sensation.

Potentized remedies are taken from magnesium hydrogen phosphate, Mg2PO4. Another form comes from magnesium phosphoricum acidum, MgHPO4.

DOSE - Third to twelfth potency.

20. MAGNESIUM SULFURICUM

Other Names: *Natural Magnesium Sulfate, Kieserit, Epsom Salt, Magnesia Sulphurica*

Specific Properties and Action:

Magnesium sulfate has a purgative action. Its purgative quality, however, is not due to increased intestinal peristalsis, but it causes a rush of fluid into the intestine producing a distention of the bowels thus inducing evacuation. The pure salt is then best employed to purge mercurial and other cases of poisoning, including parasitic worms. It acts within one to two hours, more quickly if taken in hot water and in the morning before breakfast. Homeopaths apply it locally to illnesses of the skin, and in potentized form in urinary problems, especially among women.

Other Conditions and/or Collaborating Symptoms:

a. Nerve Sense System

Head - Vertigo, head heavy during menses. Eyes burn, noises in the ears. Toothache. **Skin** - Small pimples over the whole body that itch violently. Suppressed itch. Crawling in the tips of the fingers of the left hand, becoming better by rubbing. Warts. Erysipelas, poison ivy itches, cellulitis and other local skin inflammations (applied locally as a saturated solution). **Neck and Back** - Bruised ulcerative pain between the shoulders, with a feeling as of a lump as large as the fist, and therefore cannot lie on the back or side, but relieved by rubbing. Violent pain in the small of the back, as if bruised, and before menstruation.

b. Metabolic/Limb System

Stomach - Frequent belching, tasting like bad eggs. Rising of water in the mouth. Sore pain in the sacrum. **Abdomen** - Gallstone colic (take 2 - 4 teaspoonfuls in a glass of hot water. Improve the taste by adding sugar or lemon juice). **Bowel Movement** - Dysentery. Diarrhea of children. **Urinary System** - Stitches and burning in the orifice of the urethra after urinating. Stream intermits and dribbles. The urine passed in the morning copious, bright yellow, soon becomes turbid, and deposits a copious red sediment. The urine is greenish as passed; is of a clear color, and in a large quantity. Diabetes. **Female** - Thick leucorrhea, as profuse as the menses, with weary pain in the small of the back and thighs, on moving about. Some blood from the vagina between menses. Menstruation returned after fourteen days with the discharge thick, black, and profuse. Menses too early, intermit. **Fever** - Chill from 9 to 10 a.m. Shuddering in the back; heat in one part and chill in another.

Raw materials are taken from the mineral kieserit or epsom salt.

DOSE - The pure salt (dissolved in water) and up to the thirtieth potency in titurated or liquid form.

21. MERCURIUS VIVUS

Other Names: *Quicksilver, Mercury*

Generic Properties and Action:

Mercury contains mediating and combing forces. Living substances vitalized by the life body and the silver process are led over into the soul and spiritual members of the human being. Mercury mediates and combines the vitalized substances in order that they will be under the control of the organism's higher members. In ancient times, the original meaning of illnesses had something to do with excess or deficiency in the organism.

We can still see a glimpse of this in the theory of traditional Chinese medicine. The original meaning of healing then lies in the adjustment of this syndrome, i.e., true healing is to strive to remove an excess (causing congestion) and put it in its rightful place. In many illnesses, there is an inadequate mediation that underlies them. The mercury process then can bring movement in stagnation and dissolves congestion. (This is especially true for congestion that is of the excessive type. For congestion caused by a deficiency, the silver or copper process is indicated to stimulate vitality).

Water is the carrier of life. Mercury shows its relationship to water (and therefore life) by its current liquid state and its tendency to form drops. This intensive connection of mercury to life is also responsible for its great toxicity. When ingested at a certain concentration, mercury is able to permeate the whole organism. It can pass from the mother to the suckling infant, destroying life. The nervous system is particularly affected in chronic mercury poisoning. It begins with tremors, then later polyneuritis and pseudotabes develop leading to paralysis. Stannum, the polar metal of mercury, at potency 6 to 10x can arrest the adverse effects of mercury.

All glands can be affected by mercury especially those glandular functions that are connected with the watery, mucoid processes, including partly the nutritional. When nutritional substances enter the lympathic system by way of the portal vein to the liver, this process of mediation (from the intestine into the blood, through which the venous system is involved, and where actual formation of human substances takes place) is ruled by the mercury process.

Conditions Most Used For:

Malignant tumors and catarrhs are examples of life processes that have become separated from the overall function of the organism. Mercury therapy in tumors guides the life processes back into the control of the organism's higher members while in catarrhs, the excretions are dissolved and can again be integrated and reabsorbed.

Other Conditions and/or Collaborating Symptoms:

a. Nerve Sense System

Mind - Thinks he/she is losing his/her head. Slow in answering questions. Memory weakened and loss of will-power. **Head** - Vertigo, when lying on back. Band feeling about the head. One-sided, tearing pains. Tension about the scalp, as if bandaged, or oily sweat on head. Catarrhal headaches; much heat in the head. Stinging, burning, fetid eruptions on scalp. Loss of hair. Exostosis, with feeling of soreness. **Eyes** - Lids red, thick, swollen. Profuse, burning, acrid discharge. Floating black spots. Parenchymatous keratis of syphilitic origin with burning pain. Iritis, with hypopyon (pus in front chamber of eye between cornea and iris). **Ears** - Thick, yellow discharge; fetid and bloody. Otalgia (ear ache) becoming worse in warmth of bed; at night, sticking pains. Boils in external canal. **Nose** - Much sneezing. Sneezing in sunshine. Nostrils raw, ulcerated; nasal bones swollen. Yellow-green, fetid, pus-like discharge. Coryza (acute nasal congestion), acrid discharge, but too thick to run down the lip, becoming worse in a warm room. Pain and swelling of the nasal bones, and caries, with greenish fetid ulceration. Nose-bleeding at night. Copious discharge of corroding mucus. Coryza, with sneezing; sore, raw, smarting sensation, becoming worse in damp weather; profuse, fluent. **Face** - Pale, earthy, dirty-looking, puffy. Aching in the facial bones. Syphilitic pustules on the face. **Mouth** - Sweetish metallic taste. Saliva greatly increased; bloody, cohesive, and sticky. Saliva fetid and coppery. Speech difficult because of trembling tongue. Gums spongy, receding, bleed easily. Sore pain on touch, and from chewing. Whole mouth moist. Crowns of teeth decay. Teeth loose, feel tender and elongated. Furrow in the upper surface of the tongue lengthwise. Tongue heavy, thick; moist coating; yellow, flabby, teeth-indented; feels as if burnt, with ulcers. Fetid order from the mouth; can smell it all over the room. Alveolar abscesses becoming worse at night. Great thirst, with moist mouth. **Throat** - Bluish-red swelling. Constant desire to swallow. Putrid sore throat; worse at the right side. Ulcers and inflammation appearing at every change in weather. Stitches into the ear on swallowing; fluids return through the nose. Tonsillitis, with difficulty in swallowing, after pus has formed. Complete loss of voice. **Skin** - Almost constantly moist. Persistent dryness of the skin contraindicates the use of mercurius. Excessive odorous sticky perspiration becoming worse at night. General tendency to free perspiration, but the patient is not relieved. Vesicular and pustular eruptions. Ulcers, irregular in shape, edges undefined. Pimples around the main eruption. Itching becoming worse from warmth of bed. Crusta lactea; yellowish-brown crusts, considerable suppuration. Glands swell every time the patient takes cold. Buboes (swollen lymph nodes).

b. Middle/Rhythmic System

Emotional State - Mistrustful. Weary of life. **Respiratory System** - Soreness from fauces to sternum. Cannot lie on the right side. Cough, with yellow muco-purulent expectoration. Paroxysms of two becoming worse at night, and from warmth of bed. Catarrh, with chilliness; dread of air. Stitches from the lower lobe of the right lung to the back. Whooping-cough with nosebleed.

c. Metabolic/Limb System

Stomach - Putrid eructations. Intense thirst for cold drinks. Weak digestion, with continuous hunger. Stomach sensitive to touch. Hiccough and regurgitation (return of swallowed food). Feels replete and constricted. **Abdomen** - Stabbing pain with chilliness. Boring pain in the right groin. Flatulent distention, with pain. Liver enlarged; sore to touch, indurated. Jaundice. Bile secreted deficiently. **Bowel Movement** - Greenish, bloody, and slimy stool, with pain and tenesmus. Never-get-done feeling. Discharge accompanied by chilliness, sick stomach, cutting colic, and tenesmus. Whitish-gray stools. **Urinary System** - Frequent urging. Greenish discharge from the urethra; burning in the urethra on beginning to urinate. Urine dark, scanty, bloody, albuminous. **Male** - Vesicles and ulcers; soft chancre (skin sore usually from syphilis) Cold genitals. Prepuce irritated; itches. Nocturnal emissions, stained with blood. Orchitis (inflamed testicles). **Female** - Menses profuse, with abdominal pains. Leucorrhea (vaginal discharge) excoriating, greenish and bloody. Sensation of rawness in parts. Stinging pain in ovaries. Itching and burning, becoming worse after urinating, but better after washing with cold water. Morning sickness with profuse salivation. Breast painful and full of milk at menses. **Extremities** - Weakness of the limbs. Bone-pains and in the limbs becoming worse at night. Patient very sensitive to cold. Oily perspiration. Trembling extremities, especially the hands; paralysis agitans. Lacerating pain in joints. Cold, clammy sweat on the legs at night. Edema of the feet and legs. **Back** - Bruised pain in the small of the back, especially when sitting. Tearing pain in the coccyx becoming better by pressing on the abdomen. **Fever** - Generally gastric or bilious, with profuse nightly perspiration; debility, slow and lingering. Heat and shuddering alternately. Yellow perspiration. Profuse perspiration without relief. Creeping chilliness becoming worse in the evening and into the night. Alternate flashes of heat in the single parts.

Potentized remedies are made from the metallic mercury, Hg.

DOSE - Sixth to thirtieth potency.

Other Salts of Mercury

There are a number of salts or compounds of mercury which can bring the mercury process to the particular area of the organism. Cinnabar, natural mercurius sulphide, is particularly useful in chronic catarrhal states of the neck and sinus areas (Pharyngitis, tonsillitis, Eustachian tube congestion, etc.). Mercury cyanide, $Hg(CN)_2$, 4x to 15x, is best for diphtheria, angina tonsillitis, dark hemorrhages from the nose, syphilitic ulceration of the cornea with danger of perforation and dysentery. Mercurius aurantus (gold amalgam), prepared from 2 parts by weight of mercury with 1 part weight of gold, is good for indurated glandular tumors and tertiary syphilis with granuloma; if given in low potencies and at middle potency (15x) is especially indicated in psychological imbalance, enhanced sensitivity, and rigidified depressive states. Mercurius dulcis (calomel), 4 to 6x, prepared from mercurius chloride, Hg_2Cl_2, is indicated for kidney dysfunction (at 4x), diabetes mellitus, enteritis with green stools, corneal ulcers, and Eustachian catarrhs. Red oxide of mercury, HgO, or mercurius praecipitatus ruber is best for periostitis (inflammation of fiber-like covering of bones) and nocturnal pains in the bones, fistulae in bones, and cerebral abscess. One can try it also in pemphigus (disease of skin and mucus membranes) neonatorum, night attacks of asthma and suffocation occurring during sleep, and pustular acne.

22. NATRUM

Other Name: *Sodium*

Generic Properties and Action:

Potassium and sodium are chemically similar to each other. Both have an intense relation to water. These substances, however, have a polar relationship to each other. Potassium pervades the plant world, while sodium is almost poisonous to it. In the animal and human organisms, potassium is found intracellularly, while sodium is found in extracellular fluids. Our life body is able to enliven fluids through the potassium in it, while our sensitivity body (astral body) takes hold of the same water organism by way of sodium. Thus the presence of sodium in plasma, urine, the cerebrospinal fluid, and in the fluid in the anterior chamber of the eye are indications where the sensitivity body is more dominant. All sodium compounds stimulate cellular activity and increase oxidation and metabolism.

Conditions Most Used For:

Various salts of sodium would be directed to particular processes of the body depending on the compound. Generally, sodium compounds are used to harmonize the excessive or inadequate engagement or activity of the sensitivity body, such as the formation of acids, blood pressure, poliomyelitis, encephalitis, and other illnesses of the nerves.

23. NATRUM CARBONICUM

Other Names: *Carbonate of Sodium, Soda, Sodium Carbonate*

Other Conditions and/or Collaborating Symptoms:

a. Nerve Sense System

Mind - Unable to think; difficult, slow comprehension. Mental weakness and depression. **Head** - Aches from the slightest mental exertion. Headaches with the return of hot weather. Vertigo from exposure to the sun, or after school. **Nose** - All troubles of the external nose which may attain a morbid size—pimples and puffiness. Constant coryza; obstruction of the nose. Bad smell of nasal secretion. Hawking much mucus from the throat, becoming worse from the slightest draught. **Face** - Freckles, yellow spots, pimples. Swelling of the upper lip. Pale, with blue rings around the eyes and swollen lids. **Skin** - Tendency to perspire easily, or dry, rough, cracked skin. Eruption on finger-tips, knuckles, and toes. Vesicular eruption in patches and circles. Veins full. Soles of feet raw and sore.

b. Middle/Rhythmic System

Emotional State - Worries; very sensitive to noise, colds, or change of weather. Anxious and restless during thunderstorm, becoming worse from music. Marked gaiety. Sensitive to the presence of certain individuals. **Respiratory System** - Dry cough, when coming into a warm room from outdoors. Cough with coldness of the left side of the breast.

c. Metabolic/Limb System

Stomach - Feels swollen and sensitive. Hungry at 5 a.m. Very weak digestion, caused by the slightest error of diet. Milk causes diarrhea. Depressed after eating. Bitter taste. Dyspepsia, relieved by soda biscuits. **Bowel Movement** - Sudden call to defecate. Escapes with haste and noise.

Yellow substance like pulp of orange in the stool. **Female** - Induration of the cervix. Pudenda sore. Heaviness, becoming worse by sitting, becoming better by moving. Menses late, scanty, like meat-washings. Vaginal discharge offensive, irritating, preceded by colic. **Extremities** - Old sprains. Great weakness of the limbs, especially in the morning. Easy dislocation and spraining of ankles. Foot bends under. Soreness between toes and fingers. Heel and tendo-achilles affected. Ulcers on the heel. Chapped hands. The hollow of the knee is painful on motion. Icy cold up to knees. **Sleep** - Wakes too early in the morning. Amorous dreams. Drowsy during the day.

Potentized remedies are prepared from the mineral trona, or desiccated sodium carbonate, Na_2CO_3.

DOSE - Third to the sixth potency. Sodium carbonate or soda can be externally applied in poliomyelitis and other illnesses of the nerves such as encephalitis (as a follow-up treatment). Take 20 - 30 grams of soda mixed in a bath tub of water. Here Rudolf Steiner indicates that the sensitivity body is diverted to the skin and is released from imprisonment in the illness. This can also be used as prophylaxis against flu.

24. NATRUM MURIATICUM

Other Names: *Sodium Chloride, Common Table Salt*

Specific Properties and Action:

The prolonged intake of too much salt can lead to the excessive retention of fluids in the tissues, including the blood. This situation may then produce disorders in nutrition, alteration of the blood's chemistry, and other symptoms.

Conditions Most Used For:

Ordinary salt in its potentized form can address the following ailments: Edema, dropsy, chlorosis and gout (the excessive fluids in the body or a part of the body), goiter and hyperthyroidism, hypertension or high blood pressure, anemia (the lack of red blood cells), menstrual disorders, diabetes (inability of the body to handle sugar), Addison's disease (underactivity of the adrenal glands), complaints of alimentary tract or digestion, intermittent fever and malaria, rheumatism, and neuralgias.

Other Conditions:

a. Nerve Sense System

Head - Frontal headache, especially in the temples, becoming worse towards noon. Headache is throbbing, blinding, and may be chronic, congestive, and semi-lateral. This may happen in the morning, after menstruation, or from sunrise to sunset. The face is pale. Patient feels like vomiting or may actually vomit. Frontal sinuses are inflamed. **Eyes** - Eyelids feel heavy, bruised, or swollen. Letters are seen running together. Fiery zigzag appearance around all the objects. A burning sensation in the eyes, which may appear wet. The lachrymal duct is inflamed or infected. Asthenopia: strained eyes with headache and dizziness. Cataract begins to form. Intra-orbital neuralgias. **Ears** - One hears noises such as roaring and ringing in the ears. **Nose** - Violent, fluent nasal congestion or coryza, lasting from one to three days, then stopping but making breathing difficult. Discharge from the nose is thin and watery. Sense of smell and taste is lost. Inside of the nose may be sore and dry. **Face** - Face has an earthy complexion. Face is oily and shiny. **Mouth** - Tongue has a frothy coating with bubbles on the sides. There is dryness, numbness, or tingling of the tongue, lips, and nose. Lips and the corners of the mouth are dry, ulcerated, and cracked. A deep crack in the middle of the lower lip is present. **Skin** - Oily or greasy, especially on the hairy parts. Dry eruptions, especially on the margin of the hairy scalp and bends of the joints. Warm blisters. Eczema; raw, red, and inflamed; becoming worse on eating salty food, and at the seashore. Blisters affect hair follicles, making the hair fall. Urticaria and hives: itching and burning after exertion. Crusty eruptions in the bends of the limbs, margin of the scalp, or behind the ears. Warts on the palms of the hands.

b. Middle/Rhythmic System

Emotional State - The person is pale, looking relaxed, easily irritated, despondent, pessimistic, emotional and tends to cry, but aggravated by consolation. He gives reproachable answers when asked. When grief, anger, fright, and other strong emotions are experienced, this remedy can caution their ill effects. **Respiratory System** - Cough coming from a tickling in the pit of stomach, accompanied by stitches in the liver and spurting of urine. Stitches all over the chest. Cough, with bursting pain in the head. Shortness of breath, especially on going up stairs. Whooping cough with flow of tears. **Heart** - Tachycardia (rapid beating of the heart) coming on in sudden attacks. Sensation of coldness in the heart. Heart and chest feel constricted. Palpitation with arrhythmias, especially at rest.

c. Metabolic/Limb System

Stomach - There is unquenchable thirst. Sweating while eating. There is craving for salt and highly seasoned foods, throbbing in the pit, and/or sticking sensation in the cardiac orifice. **Abdomen** - Experience of a cutting pain in the abdomen, especially when coughing. **Bowel Movement** - Burning pains and stitching after defecation. Anus is contracted, torn, bleeding. Constipation with hard, dry, crumbling stools. Painless and copious diarrhea, preceded by a pinching pain in the abdomen. **Male** - Impotence with retarded seminal emission. **Female** - Menses are irregular but usually profuse. Vagina is dry. Acrid and watery vaginal discharge. Prolapse of the uterus. Ineffectual labor pains. Menses suppressed. Hot sensation during menses. **Extremities** - Pain in the back, with a desire for some firm support. Arms and legs, especially knees, feel weak. Ankles turn easily. Cracking in the joints on motion. Rheumatism, neuralgias, and coldness of the legs with congestion reaching the head, chest, and stomach. Palms hot and perspiring. Hangnails. Dryness, cracking, and fissures in the nails. Numbness and tingling in the fingers and lower extremities. **Sleep** - Sleepy towards forenoon. Nervous jerking during sleep. Dreams of robbers. Sleepless from grief. **Fever** - Chill between 9 and 11 am: violent thirst that increases with fever. Coldness of the body, and a continued chilliness is very marked. Chronic malarial states with weakness, thirst, violent headaches, constipation, and loss of appetite. Fever and all other symptoms are ameliorated by sweating.

DOSE - One can start taking the sixth potency. The very highest potencies (30 and above) often yields most brilliant results and may be taken for only a few times.

PREPARATION: Dissolve 10 grams of sodium chloride in 90 milliliters of water to make the mother tincture. Or 10 grams of coarsely powdered sodium chloride titurated in 90 grams of lactose.

25. NATRUM PHOSPHORICUM

Other Names: *Phosphate of Sodium, Sodium Phosphate*

Specific Properties and Action:

Through the combination of sodium and phosphorus, the ego is able to intervene in the realm of sodium and therefore check the excessive activity of the sensitivity body. For example, all excess acidity mainly resulting from over-indulging in sugar and fats can be addressed by this compound of sodium.

Other Conditions and/or Collaborating Symptoms:

a. Nerve Sense System

Head - Feels dull in the morning, full feeling and throbbing. **Eyes** - Discharge of golden yellow, creamy matter from the eyes. Dilation of one pupil. Whites of eyes dirty yellow. **Ears** - One ear red, hot, frequently itchy, accompanied by gastric derangement and acidity. **Nose** - Offensive odor. Itching of the nose. Naso-pharyngeal catarrh, with thick, yellow, offensive mucus. **Face** - Paleness of bluish, florid appearance of the face. **Mouth** - Canker sores of the lips and cheeks. Blisters on the tip of the tongue, with stinging in the evening. Thin, moist coating on the tongue. Yellow, creamy coating at the back part of the roof of the mouth. Dysphagia (difficulty in swallowing). Thick, creamy membrane over the tonsils and soft palate. Inflammation of any part of the throat, with sensation of a lump in the throat. **Skin** - Yellow. Itching in various parts, especially the ankles. Hives. Smooth, red, shining. Erysipelas. Feet icy cold in the daytime, burn at night. Swelling of the lymphatic glands.

b. Metabolic/Limb System

Stomach - Sour eructation, sour vomiting, greenish diarrhea. Spits mouthful of food. Dyspepsia. **Extremities** - Rheumatism of the knee-joint. **Back** - Weariness; aching in the wrist and finger-joints. Hamstrings sore. Synovial crepitation. Rheumatic arthritis. Crackling of joints. **Female** - Menses too early; pale, thin, watery. Sterility, with acid secretion from the vagina. Leucorrhea; discharge creamy, honey-colored, or acid and watery. Sour smelling discharge from the uterus. Morning sickness with sour vomiting. **Male** - Emissions without dreams, with weakness in the back and trembling in the limbs. Desire without erection. Gonorrhea.

Potentized remedies are made from sodium monohydrogen phosphate, Na_2HPO.

DOSE - Third to the twelfth potency. In jaundice use the first potency or 10%. For Graves disease, thyroidism, and constitutional iodism (excess use of iodine) take 75 grams of phosphate soda daily.

26. NATRUM SUPHURICUM

Other Names: *Glauber's Salt, Sulphate of Sodium, Sodium Sulphate*

Specific Properties and Action:

Sodium sulphate is found only in the intercellular fluids, primarily serving to regulate the quantity of water in the tissues, blood, and other fluids of the body. It works with the bile and maintains it in normal consistency. It also stimulates the secretions of the intestines, liver, and pancreas, and helps in treating simple functional disturbances of these organs.

Conditions Most Used For:

Sodium sulphate is a liver remedy, especially when there is dark green stool from excess of bile; jaundice; and/or bitter taste. It may be given in intermittent fever with vomiting of bile; in vomiting during pregnancy, with bitter taste, watery secretions on the skin; in erysipelas, with smooth, red, shiny, or swollen skin. Symptoms become worse by using water in any form, by living in low, marshy places, damp buildings, basements, or from eating water plants, fish, or others, while one feels best in warm, dry air.

Other Conditions and/or Collaborating Symptoms:

a. Nerve Sense System

Head - Occipital pain. Piercing stitches in the ears. Vertigo, relieved by sweat on the head. Bursting feeling on coughing. Boring in the right temple, preceded by burning in the stomach. Ill effects of fall and injuries to the head, and mental troubles arising therefrom. **Eyes** - Conjunctiva yellow. Granular lids. Photophobia. **Nose** - Nasal catarrh, with thick, yellow discharge and salty mucus. Epistaxis (nosebleed). Ethmoiditis (spongy bone forming walls of upper nasal cavity). **Ears** - Sticking pain, earaches, lightning-like stitches in damp weather. **Mouth** - Slimy, thick, tenacious, white mucus. Bitter taste, blisters on the palate. **Tongue** - Bitter, brown coating. **Spine** - Spinal meningitis; opisthotonos (continuous muscle spasm). Violent pains in the back of the neck and at the base of the brain. **Skin** - Itching while undressing. Jaundice, watery blisters. Sycotic excrescences; wart-like red lumps all over the body.

b. Middle/Rhythmic System

Emotional State - Lively music saddens. Melancholy, with periodic attack of mania. Suicidal tendency; must exercise restraint. Inability to think. Dislikes to speak, or to be spoken to. **Throat** - Thick, yellow mucus, drops from posterior nares. **Respiratory System** - Difficulty in breathing during damp weather. Humid asthma; rattling in the chest, at 4 and 5 a.m. Cough, with thick, ropy, greenish expectoration. Asthma in children as a constitutional remedy. Delayed resolution in pneumonia. Pain through the lower left chest. Every fresh cold brings on the attack of asthma.

c. Metabolic/Limb System

Stomach - Vomit sour. Thirst for something cold. Bilious vomiting, acid dyspepsia, with heartburn and flatulence. **Abdomen** - Duodenal catarrh; hepatitis; icterus and vomiting of bile; liver sore to touch, with sharp, stitching pains; cannot bear tight clothing around the waist, becoming worse on lying on the left side. Flatulence; wind colic in ascending colon becoming worse before breakfast. Burning in the abdomen and the anus. Bruised pain and urging to stool. Stools involuntary when passing flatus. Great size of fecal mass. **Urinary System** - Urine loaded with bile. Brick-dust sediment. Excessive secretion. Diabetes. **Female** - Nosebleed during menses, which are acrid and profuse. Burning in pharynx during menstruation. Herpetic vulvitis. Leucorrhea yellowish green, following gonorrhea in female. **Male** - Condylomata (venereal wart); soft, fleshy excrescenses; greenish discharges. Gonorrhea; discharge thick, greenish with little pain. **Extremities** - swelling of axillary glands. Inflammation around the root of nails. Burning in soles; edema of the feet; itching between the toes. Gout. Pain in the limbs, compels frequent change of position. Pain in hip-points. Stiffness of the knees, crackling of joints. Rheumatism becoming worse in damp cold weather.

Potentized remedies are made from dehydrated sodium sulphate or Glauber's salt, Na_2SO_4.

DOSE - First to the twelfth trituration.

27. PLUMBIUM METALLICUM

Other Name: *Lead*

Generic Properties and Action:

To properly understand the action of lead in the human organism, one must understand first the relationship of life, death, and how consciousness emerges from the interaction of the two. Life has the tendency to expand and grow. Part of this process is the transformation of living substances into the minerally dead. In the human organism we see this as the process of bone and tooth formation, the most dense and mineralized part of the physical body. This polarity of the dynamics of life and death forces within the human organism results in the formation of the human form. For without the limiting (and forming) action of the death forces, human beings would not be able to attain their present form, but would look like something else. Because life is limited and held in check by death, consciousness arises, and with this the possibility for "I" consciousness. Lead delimits and promotes formation and hence promotes the death process in the human organism.

We all know the possibility of the lead poisoning. Patients suffering from it exhibit anorexic, anemic, and finally cachectic (wasting) conditions. The toxic effects appear later in the nervous system. But one could start experiencing anesthenias (lack of normal sensation, esp. to pain), parasthesias (the skin becoming sensitive to pressure and cold air), neuralgias and cramps in various places, and visual disturbances which could lead to complete blindness. Lead poisoning also affects strongly the cerebral cortex, while the spinal ganglia a little less. Of the cranial nerves, the larynx, tongue, eyes, and optic nerves are more affected by this poison. These are the nerves that are more involved in thinking and speaking, the main function of the "I" in each one of us.

Conditions Most Used For:

Now that we know the properties and action of lead, in a potentized form we can safely use it for various conditions. It should, however, not be used continuously. Lead therapy is indicated for many forms of sclerosis and degenerative diseases (where a particular organ prematurely degenerates (dies) more than the rest of the organism). In arteriosclerosis, for example, vital substances undergo a hardening and deposition process instead of being broken down and excreted (e.g. cholesterol into bile acids and excreted), typical of the conditions of very old people. High potencies (20 - 30x) of lead are used here.

For symptoms where the life processes are too strong and consciousness is inadequately experienced, the lower potencies (6 - 10x) are used. (At this potency, it should only be given for a few weeks, one in the morning and another at noon. Then the positive effect of lead is stabilized by copper. In cases when symptoms of lead poisoning are observed, one can counteract the adverse effect by giving argentum 6x.) In children with deficient bone formation, as in rickets or cranial tabes, whenever there is an imbalance of vitality and dullness and consciousness is inadequate, or when there is inadequate delimitation against the environment, as in most cases of allergies and hay fever, one can resort to lead therapy.

Alcoholism is another condition indicated for lead therapy. Alcohol paralyzes the "I" functions as expressed in the slurred speech, incoherent thinking, and the difficulty to maintain uprightness. Loss of inhibitions, drives, and cravings are not anymore under the control of the "I," and the sensitivity body becomes expressed in its animal nature. Alcoholics have a relative soul-spiritual weakness of the "I," for whatever reason. Lead therapy can provide the possibility to help the addiction but cannot, however, cure it. The person's individuality or "I" must still be consciously activated and is the true healer if and when one succeeds in consciously willing the addiction out.

Other Conditions and/or Collaborating Symptoms:

a. Nerve Sense System

Head - Delirium alternating with colic. Pain as if a ball rose from the throat to the brain. Hair very dry. Tinnitus. **Eyes** - Pupils contracted. Yellow. Optic nerve inflamed. Intraocular, suppurative inflammation. Glaucoma, especially if secondary to spinal leson. Optic neuritis, central scotoma (dark area in the visual field). Sudden loss of sight after fainting. **Face** - Pale and cachetic. Yellow, corpse-like; cheeks sunken. Skin of the face greasy, shiny. Tremor of the naso-labial muscles. **Mouth** - Gums swollen, pale; distinct blue lines along the margins of the gums. Tongue tremulous, red on the margin. Cannot put out the tongue, as if paralyzed. **Back** - Spinal cord sclerosed. Lightning-like pains; temporarily better by pressure. Paralysis of the lower extremities. **Skin** - Yellow, dark-brown liver spots. Jaundice. Dry. Dilated veins of the forearms and legs.

b. Middle/Rhythmic System

Emotional State - Mental depression. Fear of being assassinated. Quiet melancholy. Slow perception; loss of memory; amnesic aphasia. Hallucinations and delusions. Intellectual apathy. Memory impaired. Paretic dementia. **Heart** - Cardiac weakness, pulse soft and small, dichrotic. Wiry pulse, cramp-like constriction of the peripheral arteries. Arteriosclerosis with fatty heart and ventricular hypertrophy.

c. Metabolic/Limb System

Stomach - Contraction in esophagus and stomach; pressure and tightness. Gastralgia. Constant vomiting. Solid cannot be swallowed. **Abdomen** - Excessive colic, radiating to all parts of the body. Abdominal wall feels drawn by a string to the spine. Pain causes desire to stretch. Intussusception; strangulated hernia. Abdomen retracted. Obstructed flatus, with intense colic. Colic alternates with delirium and pain in atrophied limbs. **Bowel Movement** - Constipation; stools hard, lumpy, black, with urging and spasm of the anus. Obstructed evacuation from impaction of the feces. Neuralgia of the rectum. Anus drawn up with constriction. **Urinary System** - Frequent ineffectual tenesmus. Albuminous; low specific gravity. Chronic interstitial nephritis, with great pain in the abdomen. Urine scanty. Tenesmus of the bladder. Emission drop by drop. **Extremities** - Paralysis of single muscles. Cannot raise or lift anything with the hand. Extension is difficult. Paralysis from overexertion of the extensor muscles in piano players. Pains in muscles of the thighs; come in paroxysms. Wrist drop. Cramps in calves. Stinging and tearing in limbs, also twitching and tingling, numbness, pain or tremor. Paralysis. Feet swollen. Pain in the atrophied limbs alternates colic. Loss of patellar reflex. Hands and feet cold. Pain in the right big toe at night, very sensitive to touch.

Potentized remedies are taken from the metal lead.

DOSE - Sixth to the thirtieth potency.

Other Salts of Lead

Plumbium aceticum (lead acetate) is used preferably in chronic diseases characterized by violent pains, spasms, and paralysis, which are aggravated at night. It is also indicated in trembling and weakness of the limbs, accompanied by optic and auditory nerve symptoms and esophageal and stomach cramps. Colicky and flatulent complaints with constipation resulting from a depressed intestinal activity; pain and inflammation of the testes (for males), mastitis, spasm of the uterus (for females), uterine pain; and pulmonary congestion with hemoptysis can be addressed by this remedy. Use the fourth to the twentieth potency.

Minium (natural lead oxide, 3 to 6x) is the mineral used mainly for the possibility to overcome addiction.

Plumbium iodatum (lead iodide) is indicated for arteriosclerosis, progressive muscular atrophy, one-sided facial atrophy, and placid paresis of all kinds. It has been historically used by homeopaths in various forms of paralysis, sclerotic degenerations (especially of the spinal cord), pellagra (lack of B-vitamins); indurations (hardening of tissues) of the mammary glands, sore and painful; indurations of great hardness and associated with a very dry skin and sharply piercing pains of tabes (wasting due to illness). Use potencies as indicated in metallic lead.

Cerrusite or natural lead carbonate addresses more the structure of the skeleton and all symptoms of demineralization, for example, in osteoporosis and bone metastasis. Use the sixth to the twentieth potency. Natural plumbium silicicum, barysilite or lead silicate is used to stimulate the "I" organization in various deformities of the skeleton, illnesses of the skin and nervous system, as for example in osteoporosis, arteriosclerosis, eczema, or tendency to allergies. Use eighth to the thirtieth potency for this remedy.

Chapter Four

❧

Plants

1. ACHILLEA MILLEFOLIUM Linn.

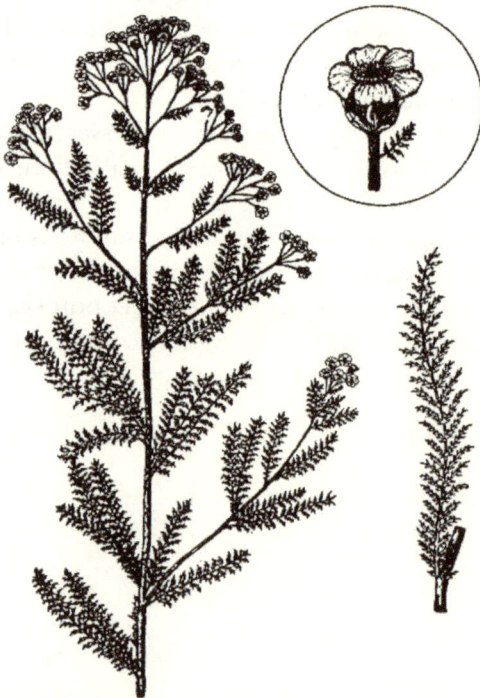

Local Names: *Milfoil, Noble Yarrow, Bloodworth, Carpenter's Weed, Sanguinary, Thousand Leaf, Yarroway*

Properties and Action:

Yarrow has a property that shortens the blood clotting process. It also increases the secretion of gastric juices in healthy individuals.

Conditions Most Used For:

Yarrow is an invaluable remedy for various types of hemorrhages, for example, hemoptysis (spitting of blood).

Other Conditions:

a. Nerve Sense System

Head - Vertigo when one is moving slowly. Sensation as if one had forgotten something. The head seems full of blood. Piercing thrust of pain in the head. **Nose** - Nose bleeding. Piercing pain from the eyes to the root of the nose.

b. Metabolic/Limb System

Female - Convulsion and epilepsy resulting from suppressed menses. Menses come early; profuse and protracted. Hemorrhage from uterus; bright red fluid. Painful varicose veins during pregnancy. **Abdomen** - Great pain in the pit of the stomach. Incarcerated hernia (rupture—the bulging out of a part of any of the internal organs through a weak area in the muscular wall). **Bowel Movement** - Hemorrhage from bowels. Bleeding hemorrhoids. Blood in the urine.

DOSE - Tincture, to third potency.

PARTS UTILIZED - Pounded whole plant, gathered while in flower, in medium-strong alcohol.

2. ALLIUM CEPA Linn.

Local Names: *Cebollas (Spanish); Red Onion (English)*

Properties and Action:

Onion irritates most obviously the various glands in and around the eyes and nose.

Conditions Most Used For:

Onion is best for acute nasal congestion with acrid discharge, laryngeal symptoms, and laryngitis, with violent pain upon coughing. It may also be used for tread-like neuralgic pains in the face, and traumatic chronic neuritis or burning sensation in the nose, mouth, throat, bladder, and skin. This remedy is specially adapted to phlegmatic patients.

Other Conditions:

a. Nerve Sense System

Head - Catarrhal headaches, mostly in the forehead. Headache ceases during menses but returns when menstrual flow disappears. **Eyes** - Red with much burning and tears. Sensitive to light. Eyes are suffused and profusely watery; improvement in the open air. Burning sensation in the eyelids. **Ears** - Ear aches, shooting pains in the eustachian tube. **Nose** - Hay fever. Sneezing, especially when entering a warm room. Copious, watery, and extremely acrid discharge. Feeling of a lump at the root of the nose. Polypus. Singer's cold, becoming worse in a warm room and towards the evening, while becoming better in the open air.

b. Middle/Rhythmic System

Respiratory - Hoarseness of the voice. Tickling feeling in the larynx, or sensation as if the larynx is split or torn. Constricted feeling in the region of the epiglottis (the lid which covers the windpipe). Pain may extend to the ear. Oppressed breathing from pressure in the middle of the chest. Hacking cough while breathing in cold air.

a. Metabolic/Limb System

Stomach - Canine-like hunger. Pain in the pyloric (right below the stomach) region. There is thirst and/or nausea. **Abdomen** - Rumbling of offensive intestinal gases. Belching. Pain in the left hypogastrium (lowest abdominal region). Colic while sitting or moving about. **Rectum** - Diarrhea with very offensive gases. Stitches (sharp pains) or glowing heat in the rectum; itching and skin cracks in the anus. **Urinary** - Sensation of weakness in the bladder and urethra. Increased secretion of urine with acute nasal congestion. Urine is red with much pressure and burning in the urethra. Acute cystitis (inflammation of the bladder). **Extremities** - Lame joints. Arms feel sore and tired. Ulcers form on the heel. Pain in the fingers about the nails. Neuralgia. **Sleep** - Yawning with headache and drowsiness. Gaping while in deep sleep. Waking up at 2 a.m.

DOSE - Third potency.

PARTS UTILIZED - Fresh bulbs in strong alcohol.

3. ALLIUM SATIVUM Linn.

Local Name: *Garlic*

Properties and Action:

Garlic acts directly on the intestinal mucous membrane increasing peristalsis. It has vaso-dilatory (blood vessel dilation) properties.

Conditions Most Used For:

Garlic is best for the following ailments: colitis (inflammation of the large intestine), with pathological flora; hypertension (high blood pressure); indigestion and catarrhal conditions with heartburn from high meat intake; asthma with rough, hoarse voice, and dry cough; hemoptysis (spitting of blood); pulmonary tuberculosis; and hemorrhoids and anal prolapse.

Other Conditions:

a. Nerve Sense System

Head - Heavy, pulsation in the temples, catarrhal deafness. **Mouth** - Saliva tastes sweet after meals and at night. Tongue is pale with red papillae (nipple-like protuberances). **Throat** - Hoarse voice with itching of the larynx and a dry cough. Sensation as if a strand of hair is on the tongue or throat.

b. Middle/Rhythmic System

Respiratory - Constant rattling of mucus in the bronchi. Coughing in the morning is characterized by copious expectoration of a viscid, tenacious mucus of putrid odor. Coughing after meals, seems to come from the stomach. Patient is sensitive to cold air. Bronchi are dilated with fetid expectoration and darting pain in the chest.

c. Metabolic/Limb System

Stomach - Voracious appetite. Burning belching. Least change in the diet causes trouble. **Bowel Movement** - Constipation with constant dull pain in the bowels. **Female** - Pain and swelling of the breast. Eruptions in the vagina, the breast, and the vulva during menses.

DOSE - Third to sixth potency.

PARTS UTILIZED - Fresh bulbs in medium-strong alcohol.

4. ALSTONIA SCHOLARIS Linn.; R.Br.

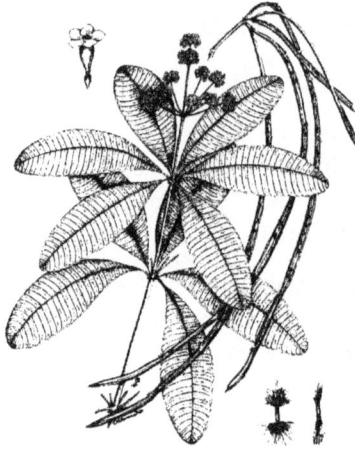

Local Names: *Milky Pine, White Cheese Wood*

Properties and Action:

Milky pine contains a number of alkaloids, one of which is ditamine that gives it its anti-malarial action. It acts mainly on the metabolic system and strengthens it.

Conditions Most Used For:

Milky pine is good in malarial diseases, with diarrhea, dysentery, anemia, and feeble digestion. It is a good tonic (promotes muscular tightness) after an exhausting fever.

Other Conditions:

Metabolic/Limb System

Bowel Movement - Cramp diarrhea. Violent purging, but cramp bowel movement. Dysentery with heat and irritation in the lower bowels. Painless watery feces. Diarrhea caused by bad water and malaria, or immediately after eating. Stool comes with blood. **Extremities** - Rheumatism (apply the tincture externally).

DOSE - Tincture to third potency.

PARTS UTILIZED - Pounded bark in medium-strong alcohol.

5. APIUM GRAVEOLENS Linn.

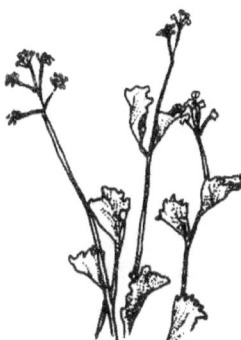

Local Names: *Apyo (Spanish); Chinese Celery (English)*

Properties and Action:

Chinese celery contains a soporific (sleep-causing) active principle.

Conditions Most Used For:

The plant is best for stubborn retention of urine, throbbing headaches, and heartburns. It is also used for swollen throat, face, and hands, and rheumatic pain of the neck and the sacrum (part of the vertebral column).

Other Conditions:

a. Nerve Sense System

Head - Depressed, energetic, restless, nervous, or uneasy; cannot sleep from thinking. Headache, becoming better while eating. Eyeballs feel sunken or itchy. Itching and smarting in the inner canthus of the left eye. **Skin** - Itching blotches; burning, creeping sensation. Profuse discharge from granulating ulcers or wounds. Skin rashes with sudden shaking or trembling. **Sleep** - Unrefreshed feeling after sleep. Sleeplessness. Waking up from 1 to 3 a.m. Not feeling fatigued from the loss of sleep.

b. Middle/Rhythmic System

Respiratory - Tickling dry cough. Intense constriction over the breastbone, with drawing feeling through to the back on lying down. Throat is swollen, breathing is hard. **Abdomen** - Sore; sharp sticking pain with an urge to defecate. Diarrhea; sharp pain in the left lowest region of the small intestines going over to the right. Feeling of nausea increases with pain.

Female - Sharp sticking pains in both the ovarian regions, left ovary feels better when bending over, by lying on the left side, or with legs flexed. Nipples are tender. Growing pains. Dysmenorrhea with sharp, short pains, becoming better when flexing the legs.

DOSE - First to thirtieth potency.

PARTS UTILIZED - Fresh whole plant in strong alcohol.

6. ARECA CATECHU Linn.

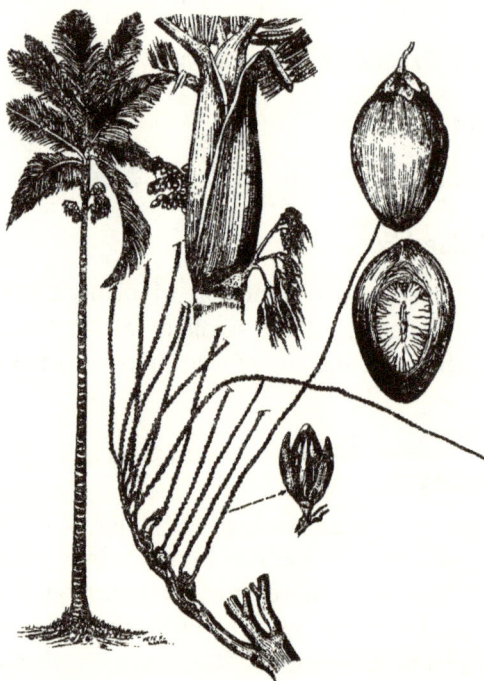

Local Names: *Areca Nut, Betel Nut*

Properties and Action:

Betel nut's alkaloid, *areolin hydrobrom*, contracts the pupil, acting promptly and energetically but short in duration. It also increases the amplitude of pulsation of the heart and promotes the contraction of the intestines.

Conditions Most Used For:

Betel nut is good for glaucoma (pressure of the fluid in the eye increases), or for flushing out worms in the intestines, especially tape worms.

PARTS UTILIZED - Flowers and fresh kernels crushed in medium-strong alcohol. For eye drops, boil the crushed kernel in water in moderate heat for about 10 minutes. Let it cool, and the liquid portion is used as the eye drop or taken internally for worms.

7. ARTEMISIA VULGARIS Linn.

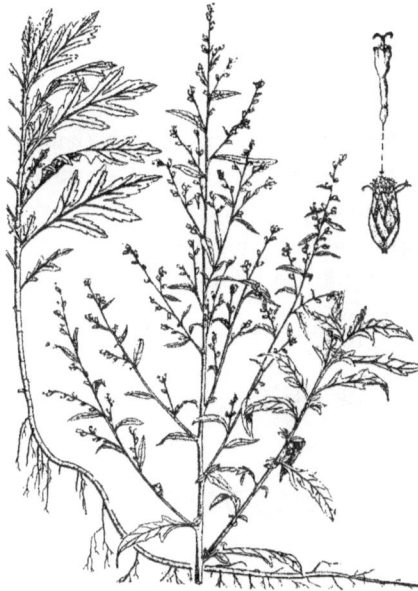

Local Names: *Cintura de San Jose, Santa Maria (Spanish); Motherwort, Wormwood, Moxa, Maidenwort, Felon Herb, Mugwort, St. John's Plant (English)*

Properties and Action:

St. John's Plant has stomachic (gastric stimulant) and tonic (muscular tightness) properties. It is thus a remedy for epilepsy and convulsive diseases of childhood, and for girls undergoing puberty and experiencing difficult menstruation periods.

Conditions Most Used For:

This remedy is given during the convulsive attacks of epilepsy called petit mal (relatively mild attacks). It is also best for other forms of convulsions, such as those that come after a fright and other violent emotions, or after masturbation.

a. Nerve Sense System

Head - Head is drawn back by spasmodic twitching. Mouth is drawn to the left. Congestion of the brain. **Eyes** - Colored lights produce dizziness and vertigo. Pain and blurring of vision, becoming better by rubbing; becoming worse when using eyes. Asthenopia (a strained condition of the eyes, often with headache and dizziness). **Fever** - Profuse sweat that smells like garlic. Several convulsions that come close together.

b. Metabolic/Limb System

Abdomen - Complaints from worms. Gas pains. **Female** - Various menstrual problems such as pre-menstrual syndrome, profuse menses, violent uterine contractions, dysmenorrhea, spasms during menses. **Sleep** - Somnambulism (sleep walking): Getting up at night and walking or working, but remembering nothing in the morning.

DOSE - First to third potency.

PARTS UTILIZED - Fresh whole plant in medium-strong alcohol.

8. ASPARAGUS OFFICINALIS Linn.

Local Name: *Asparagus*

Properties and Action:

Asparagus has a marked and immediate action on the urinary system. It can cause weakness and cardiac depression with a tendency to accumulate fluids in the body.

Conditions Most Used For:

This remedy is best for rheumatism, especially pains on the left shoulder and around the heart. It is also good for most urinary problems.

Other Conditions:

a. Nerve Sense System

Head - Confused. Coryza (acute nasal congestion), with profuse, thin fluid. Aching forehead and root of the nose. Migrainous morning headache with blind spot. **Throat** - Feels rough, with hawking; copious, tenacious mucus.

b. Middle/Rhythmic System

Heart - Palpitation, with a heavy chest. Intermittent pulse, weak pain about the left shoulder and heart that is usually associated with bladder disturbances. **Lungs** - Great difficulty in breathing. Hydrothorax (fluids in the pleural cavity of the lungs).

c. Metabolic/Limb System

Urinary - Frequent urination, with fine stitches in the opening of urethra. Urine is of a peculiar odor. Cystitis (inflammation of the bladder) with pus, mucus, and spasms. Lithiasis (formation of stones in the body). **Extremities** - Rheumatic pains in the back, especially near the shoulder and limbs. Pain at the acromion process (highest and outermost extension of the shoulder) of the left scapula under the clavicle and down the arm, with feeble pulse.

DOSE - Sixth potency.

PARTS UTILIZED - Whole plant with many shoots in strong alcohol.

9. BETA VULGARIS Linn.

Local Name: *Garden Beet*

Properties and Actions:

Beet influences chronic catarrhal states (inflammation of membranes with mucus discharge) and tuberculosis. The salt, betainum hydrocloricum, obtained from the beet seems to be best adapted to tuberculosis patients. Children respond very quickly to the action of the remedy.

DOSE - Second potency or tituration.

PARTS UTILIZED - Air dry the whole plant and grind it into powder.

Titurate in lactose powder or starch. You can also try the crushed whole plant in strong alcohol.

10. CAPSICUM ANUUM Linn.

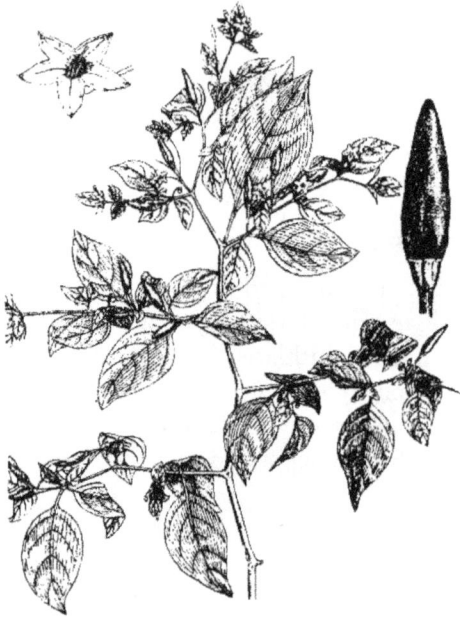

Local Names: *Chile, Chile Picante (Spanish); Red Pepper, Spanish Pepper, Chili, Cayenne Pepper (English)*

Properties and Action:

Cayenne pepper is a general stimulant for persons with lax fiber and weak or diminished vital heat. Such persons are usually fat and indolent, opposed to physical exertion or deviation from their routine. They get homesick easily and have a general uncleanliness of the body. This plant affects the mucus membranes, producing the sensation of constriction.

Conditions Most Used For:

Cayenne pepper is good for older people who have exhausted their vitality, especially by mental work or poor living conditions. They have a bleary-eyed appearance and slow reactions. They fear the slightest draught and have a tendency to develop infections in every inflammatory process. This plant is also preferred in the feeble digestion of alcoholics, in myalgia (pains and jerking of muscles), and in the inflammation of petrous bone. It may also be given in ulcerative glossitis (inflammation of the tongue), pharyngitis, tonsillitis, mastoiditis (inflammation of the bone behind the ear), malaria with great chilliness, chronic urethritis (inflammation of the urethra), and any form of rheumatic pains.

Other Conditions:

a. Nerve Sense System

Head - Bursting headache, becoming worse while coughing. Hot face and red cheeks although it is cold. **Ears** - Burning and stinging pain in and behind the ears. Inflammation of the mastoid. Tenderness over the petrous bone that is extremely sore to the touch. Hearing problems and a mastoid disease before the inflammation. **Mouth** - Herpes labialis. (Apply the mother tincture directly.) Stomatitis (white mouth ulcers). Bad breath. Burning in the tip of the tongue. **Throat** - Hot feeling in the back part of the mouth. Subacute pain of the eustachian tube (tube that connects the pharynx with the middle ear). Pain and dryness in the throat extending to the ears. Sore throat of smokers and drinkers. Burning constriction of the throat, becoming worse between acts of swallowing. Inflamed uvula and palate.

b. Middle/Rhythmic System

Emotional State - Excessive peevishness (hard to please). Homesickness, with sleeplessness and disposition to suicide. The mood is irritable and changeable, alternating between laughing and crying. There is great restlessness, excessive busyness, and anxiety. Wanting to be let alone. **Respiratory** - Constriction of the chest; difficulty in breathing. Hoarseness of the voice. Dry, hacking cough, expelling offensive breaths from the lungs. Feeling as if the chest and the head would fly to pieces. Explosive cough. Threatening gangrene of the lungs. Pain in the distant parts of the body upon coughing—bladder, legs, ears, etc. **Heart** - Pain at the apex of the heart or in the rib region, becoming worse when touched.

c. Metabolic/Limb System

Stomach - Atonic dyspepsia (indigestion). Vomiting; sinking feeling at the pit of the stomach. Much flatulence, especially in debilitated subjects. Intense craving for stimulants. **Bowel Movement** - Feces with bloody mucus, with burning and spasm of the anus; stinging and drawing pain in the back during and/or after defecation. Bleeding piles with soreness of the anus. Thirsty after defecation, with shivering. **Urinary** - Painful urination, frequent, but almost ineffectual urging. Urine comes first in drops, then in spurts; neck of the bladder spasmodically contracted. Burning in the opening of the urethra. **Male** - Coldness of the scrotum (pouch containing testicle), with impotence, loss of sensitivity in the testicles; atrophied testicles. Gonorrhea, with excessive burning, pain in the prostate. **Female** - Uterine hemorrhages while nearing menopause, with nausea. Sticking sensation in the left ovarian region. **Extremities** - Sciatica, becoming worse while bending backwards. Neuralgias; stabbing or tearing pain particularly in the arm and the sciatic nerve. Pain from the hips to the feet, becoming worse while coughing. Intensive pain in the knee. Rheumatic pains with creaking, groaning, cracking, clamping pains and stiffness of the various joints. **Fever** - While feverish, there is great thirst before the chill. Shivering after drinking. Coldness, with ill-humor. Chills begin in the back; becoming better when something hot is placed at the back.

DOSE - Third to sixth potency.

PARTS UTILIZED - Ripe capsules with seeds in medium-strong alcohol.

11. CARICA PAPAYA Linn.

Local Names: *Pawpaw Tree, Papaya*

Properties and Action:

Papaya is used generally for metabolic disorders. It has papain, which is a substance that can aid in the digestion of proteins. Carpain, an alkaloid found in the leaves, can cause a slight drop in blood pressure.

Conditions Most Used For:

Papaya is good for dyspepsia, conjunctivitis, enlarged liver and spleen, and various urinary problems. It may also induce abortion.

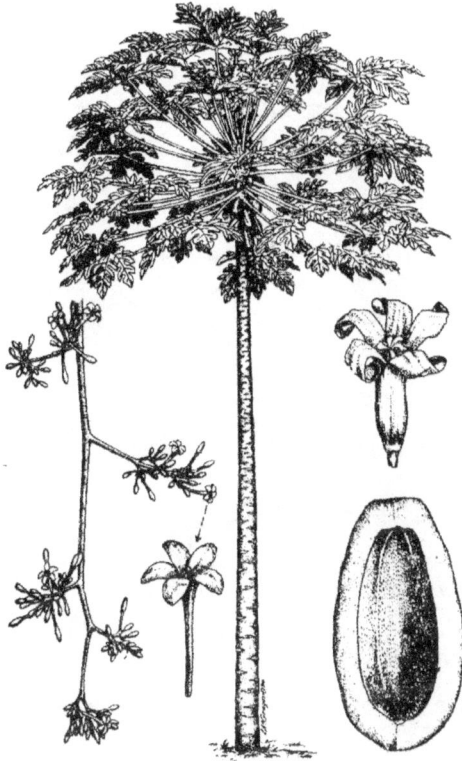

Other Conditions:

Metabolic/Limb System

Abdomen - There is an enlargement of the liver and spleen with fever. Dyspepsia (indigestion), weak digestion with undigested food in the stool in small quantities. White-coated tongue with intolerance to milk. **Female** - Papaya aids menstrual discharge; helps urine contraction and induces abortion when locally applied to the mouth of the uterus.

DOSE - Tincture to third potency.

PARTS UTILIZED - Leaves, flowers, and young fruit in medium-strong alcohol.

12. CENTELLA ASIATICA Linn.

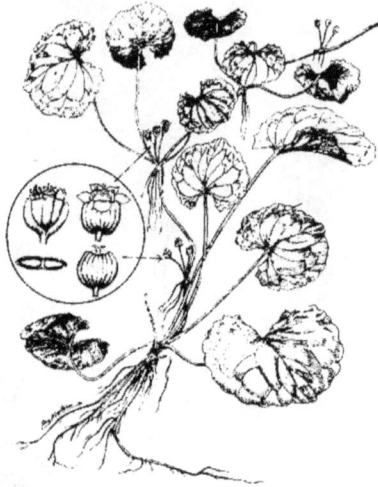

Local Names: *Indian Pennywort, Indian Hydrocotyle*

Properties and Action:

This plant works on the interstitial (spaces between tissues) and connective tissues of the body.

Conditions Most Used For:

Indian hydrocotyle is good for curative disorders that exhibit interstitial inflammation, hypertrophy (enlargement of a tissue or organ), and hardening of the connective tissues and cellular proliferation in any part of the body. The overall picture of this plant's applications includes skin symptoms such as reddening, with itching of the face, neck, chest, back, arms and thighs, with a sensation of heat, stinging, itching, and burning in various places. The skin may also have small pimples and blisters, with desquamation (shedding of skin) or sloughing (dead tissues separating from living ones), and increased infection of existing ulcers. Malformation of the nails may be noticed, as well as neuralgia of the face.

This plant may be of great use in ulcers of the womb, pains in cervical cancer, kidney symptoms and urinary problems. Lupus, psoriasis, leprosy, scleroderma, and hyperkeratosis (multiple warts) are other diseases for which this plant will also be of great help.

Other Conditions:

a. Nerve Sense System

Face - Pain in the left cheekbones and about the orbits. **Skin** - Dry eruptions. Great thickening of the epidermis and exfoliation of scales. Psoriasis gyrate on the trunk, the extremities, and the palms and soles. On the chest are found pimples and circular spots, with scaly edges. Intolerable itching of the soles. Profuse sweat. Syphilitic affection. Acne. Elephantiasis.

b. Metabolic/Limb System

Urinary - Heaviness and pressure in the renal area. Bladder spasms with creeping sensation in the urethra and increased excretion of urine. Inflammation of the neck of the bladder. **Female** - Itching, stinging, heat in the vagina. Profuse leucorrhea (whitish discharge). Violent congestive pains in the uterus. Granular ulceration of the womb. Premature arrival of the menses. Dull pain in the ovarian region. Cervical redness.

DOSE - First to sixth potency.

PARTS UTILIZED - Fresh leaves in medium-strong alcohol.

13. CHENOPODIUM AMBROSIOIDES Linn.; Var. anthelminticum

Local Names: *Quenopodio (Spanish); Jerusalem Oak (English)*

Properties and Action:

The seeds of this plant contain a volatile oil called chenopodium oil. This oil excites and then paralyzes the bodies of various intestinal parasites, especially ascaris. Jerusalem oak can also cause a violent irritation of the gastrointestinal tract and may paralyze the internal muscles and cause constipation.

Conditions Most Used For:

Jerusalem oak is given to those with symptoms of apoplexy (a condition resulting from a decrease in blood flow to the brain, also called stroke). It is also used in cases of hemiplegia (paralysis of one side of the body), aphasia (inability to form words), and affections of the auditory nerves.

Other Conditions:

a. Nerve Sense System

Ears - Inactivity of the auditory nerves. Hearing is better only for high-pitched sounds. There is a comparative deafness to the sound of the human voice, but with great sensitiveness to other sounds, such as the passing of vehicles. Buzzing in the ears. Vertigo due to the impairment of hearing. **Throat** - Tonsils are enlarged.

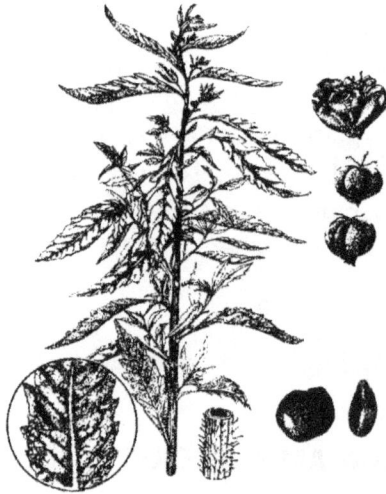

b. Middle/Rhythmic System

Respiratory - Loud, raspy, labored breathing. Pain in the scapula is very marked. **Back** - Intense pain between the angle of the right shoulder blade near the spine, and through the chest.

c. Metabolic/Limb System

Urinary - Urine is copious, yellow, and foamy with acrid sensation in the urethra. Yellowish sediment in the urine. **Bowel Movement** - Constipation.

DOSE - Third potency. The oil of chenopodium is given for hookworm: 10 drops of the oil every 2 hours; given 3 times only.

PARTS UTILIZED - Young fruits with leaves in medium-strong alcohol.

14. CITRUS AURANTIUM Linn.

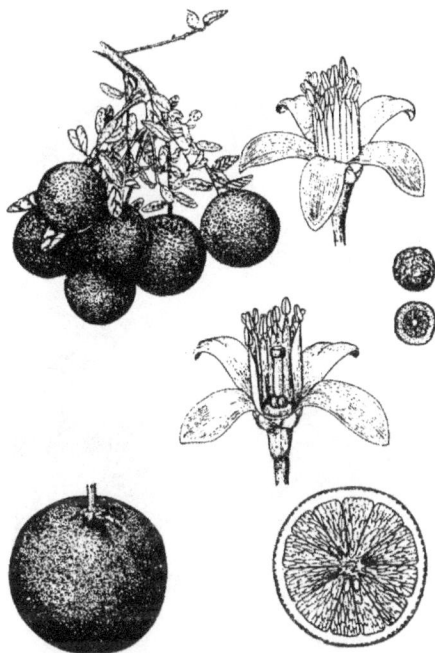

Local Names: *Seville Orange, Sour Orange*

Properties and Action:

Sour orange, especially the boiled dried peel, excites the intestine and increases the flow of bile from the gall bladder and the liver.

Conditions Most Used For:

Sour orange can address headache with nausea, vomiting, and vertigo. It can be used in right-sided facial neuralgias, and in thoracic oppression (the feeling of heaviness on the chest). There is itching, redness, and swelling of the hands. Sleep may be disturbed with frequent and irresistible yawning.

DOSE - Tincture.

PARTS UTILIZED - Crushed whole fruit given raw, or the dried peel ground to a coarse powder in medium-strong alcohol.

15. COFFEA ARABICA Linn.

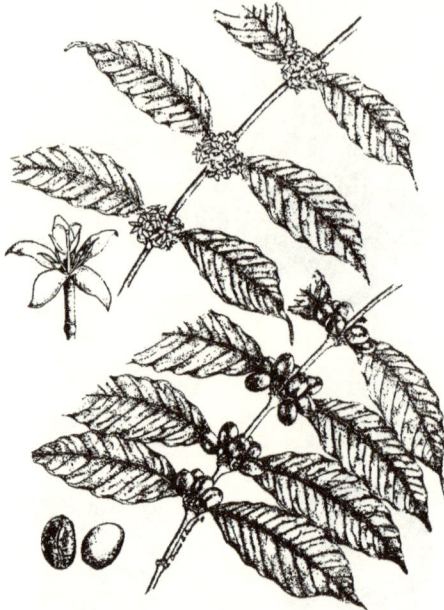

Local Name: *Coffee*

Properties and Action:

Coffee contains caffeine. It is a direct heart stimulant and a diuretic. It raises the blood pressure and increases the pulse rate. It can likewise stimulate the functional activity of all other organs, especially the nervous and vascular systems. In the aged, drinking coffee may increase production of uric acid, causing irritation of the kidneys, and inducing pain in the muscles and joints.

Conditions Most Used For:

Coffee is best for persons who are extremely sensitive to external expression and in the process develop great nervous agitation and restlessness. Neuralgia is also present in various parts of the body with intolerance to the pain, driving one to despair. There is unusual activity of the mind and body. Coffee as remedy can address the bad effects of sudden emotions, such as surprises, joy, etc. It is specially suited to tall, lean, stooping persons with dark complexions, and with choleric and sanguine temperament. The skin may also be hypersensitive. Coffee is also good for dysmenorrhea and paralysis of the bladder.

Other Conditions:

a. Nerve Sense System

Head - Tight or stabbing pain, becoming worse from noise, smell, narcotics, and in the open air. **Face** - Feels hot and dry, with red cheeks. **Mouth** - Toothache; temporarily relieved by holding ice water in the mouth. Eating and drinking hastily with delicate taste. **Sleep** - Wakeful; constant movement on account of mental activity, flow of ideas, with nervous excitability. A person sleeps until 3 a.m., after which he only dozes. Wakes with a start, sleep is disturbed by dreams or itching of the anus.

b. Middle/Rhythmic System

Emotional State - Gay, irritable, excited; senses are alert. Impressionable, especially to outside stimulus. Full of ideas and quick to act. Tossing about in anguish. **Respiratory** - Short, dry cough during measles in nervous and delicate children. **Heart** - Violent irregular palpitation, especially after excessive joy or surprise. Rapid high tension pulse and suppressed urinary functions.

c. Metabolic/Limb System

Stomach - Excessive hunger with intolerance of tight clothing. **Female** - Menses come too early and last long. Dysmenorrhea with large clots of black blood. Hypersensitive vulva and vagina with itching. **Extremities** - Crural (leg or thigh) neuralgia, becoming worse while in motion or in the afternoon and evening; becoming better when pressure is applied.

DOSE - Third to two hundred potency.

PARTS UTILIZED - Dried unroasted beans in coarse powder in strong alcohol. Roasted beans in coarse powder in strong alcohol.

16. CURCUBITA CITRULLUS Linn.

Local Name: *Watermelon*

Properties and Actions:

The seeds are rich in oil and protein. They send an increased supply of blood to the bladder wall and stimulate the epithelium lining. The effect is the soothing of the urinary system.

Conditions Most Used For:

Watermelon seeds are best for painful urination with a sense of constriction and backache.

PARTS UTILIZED - Whole or powdered dry seeds without seed coat, eaten direct.

17. DATURA ARBOREA Linn.

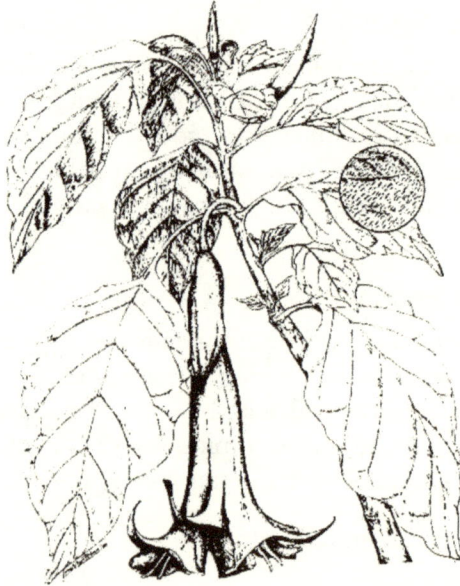

Local Names: *Borrachero, Floripondio (Spanish); Angel's Trumpet (English)*

Properties and Actions:

This is a hallucinogenic plant.

Conditions Most Used For:

Angel's Trumpet may be used in high potencies only for brain diseases, clairvoyance, clairaudience, and vertigo. Persons who hallucinate, hear voices, and are unable to hold themselves firmly in everyday life can be helped by this remedy.

DOSE - Tenth to thirtieth potency.

PARTS UTILIZED - Fresh flowers, leaves, and seeds in pods in medium-strong alcohol.

18. DATURA METEL Linn.

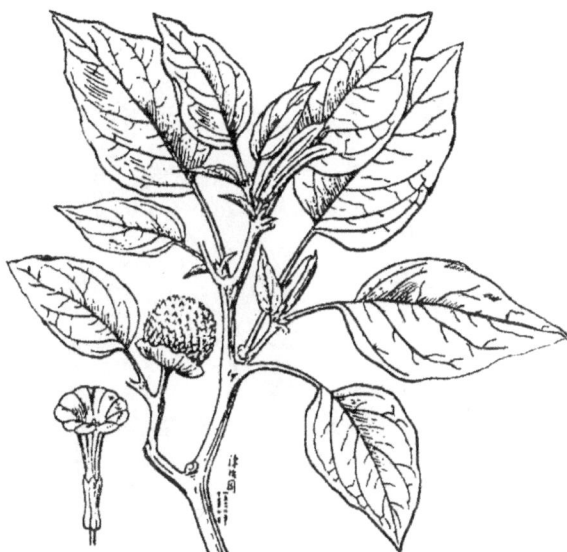

Local Name: *Thorn Apple*

Properties and Action:

This plant causes a soporose condition (unnaturally deep sleep) and later creates delirium and spasms of the body. There is perverted vision and the inability to judge distance. The pupils are extremely dilated. Pulse and body temperature may undergo extreme exaltation and depression.

Conditions Most Used For:

Thorn apple is best for persons with epilepsy, in delirium, or in convulsion. This can also be given to the manic-depressive.

DOSE - Twelfth to thirtieth potency.

PARTS UTILIZED - Fresh leaves, flowers, and unripe seeds in medium-strong alcohol.

19. EUCALYPTUS TERETICORNIS Sm.

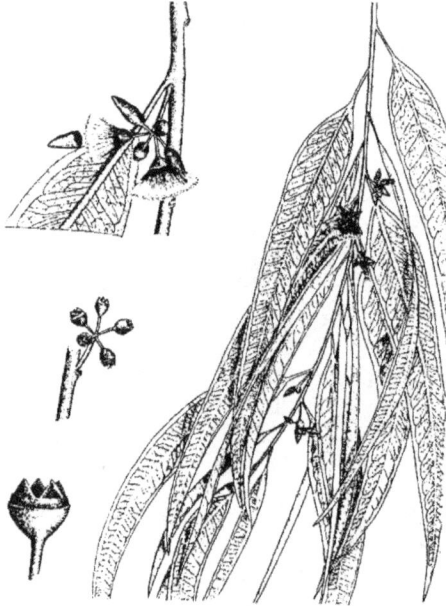

Local Names: *Gray Gum Tree, Blue Gum Tree*

Properties and Actions:

This plant acts as a powerful antiseptic preventing infection and decay and inhibiting the action of microorganisms. It is a stimulating expectorant and an efficient diaphoretic (to increase perspiration). It acts on the mucus surfaces of the air passages, genito-urinary organs, and gastrointestinal tract.

Conditions Most Used For:

Eucalyptus may be given for the following ailments: atonic dyspepsia, gastric and intestinal catarrh, malaria with the accompanying intestinal disturbance, intestinal influenza, fevers especially during a relapse, tracheitis, laryngitis, bronchitis, typhoid fevers, and symptoms of exhaustion and toxemia.

Other Conditions:

a. Nerve Sense System

Head - Exhilaration (highly stimulated). Dull congestive headache. **Nose** - Acute nasal congestion with thin, watery mucus; nose does not stop running; chronic catarrhal, purulent (with pus) and fetid discharge. Sinusitis. **Throat** - White spots in the mouth and throat. Excessive secretion of saliva. Constant sensation of phlegm in the throat. Sore throat. Enlarged, ulcerated tonsils. **Skin** - Herpetic eruptions on the skin with swollen lymph nodes.

b. Middle/Rhythmic System

Respiratory - Asthma, with difficulty in breathing and palpitation. Moist asthma and expectoration of white, thick mucus. Bronchitis in the aged. Irritated cough. Bronchial dilation and emphysema (hardening of the lungs). **Heart** - accelerated but not a strong pulse during high temperature.

c. Metabolic/Limb System

Stomach - Slow digestion with much fetid gas and pulsation in the epigastric arteries. The spleen is hard and contracted. Pain in the epigastrum and upper abdomen is ameliorated by food. Malignant disease of the stomach with vomiting of blood and sour fluid. **Abdomen** - Bowel movement: acute diarrhea preceded by sharp pains. Dysentery, with rectal heat; hemorrhage. Typhoid diarrhea. Intestinal influenza. **Urinary** - Acute nephritis (inflammation of the kidneys) with a complicating influenza. Hematuria (blood in the urine). Urine contains pus and is deficient in urea. Bladder feels loss of expulsive force. Burning and spasms in the bladder; diuresis (frequent urination); urethral cyst. Gonorrhea. **Female** - Leucorrhea (vaginal discharge) acrid, fetid. Ulcer around opening of the urethra. **Extremities** - Rheumatic pains with a pricking sensation in the muscles and joints, tiredness and stiffness of the limbs becoming worse at night.

DOSE - Tincture in one to 20 drops, and lower potencies. Also oil of eucalyptus, in five-drops doses.

PARTS UTILIZED - Freshly gathered leaves, bark, flower, and fruit in medium-strong alcohol.

20. EUGENIA CUMINI Linn.; Druce.

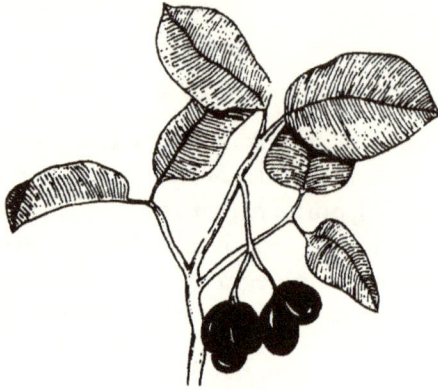

Local Names: *Black Plum, Java Plum*

Properties and Action:

Black plum seeds have the immediate effect of decreasing the sugar in the blood.

Conditions Most Used For:

This is a most useful remedy in the treatment of diabetes mellitus. There is great thirst, weakness, and loss of weight. Prickly heat and small red pimples itching violently in upper part of the body may be present.

DOSE - Tincture to third potency or trituration.

PARTS UTILIZED - Grind the seeds into a fine powder and triturate with lactose or starch. Fresh seeds may be crushed in strong alcohol.

21. FRAGARIA VESCA Linn.

Local Name: *Strawberry*

Properties and Action:

Strawberry acts on the digestive and mesenteric (supporting membranes of some internal organs) glands. It prevents formation of calculi (stones), removes tartar from teeth and prevents attacks of gout. The fruit has refrigerant (removes thirst and reduces fever) properties.

Conditions Most Used For:

Strawberry is good for chilblains (painful swelling of the hands and toes due to cold) which become worse during hot weather. When eaten raw, the strawberry fruit will enhance the whole metabolic system.

Other Conditions:

a. Nerve Sense System

Mouth - Tongue is swollen. **Skin** - Urticaria (a skin condition characterized by itching, burning, stinging, and formation of smooth red patches). Small hemorrhagic spots and streptococci infection of the skin. Swelling of the whole body.

DOSE - Tincture to sixth potency.

PARTS UTILIZED - Fruits (preferably wild) in strong alcohol.

22. HELIANTHUS ANNUUS Linn.

Local Name: *Sunflower*

Properties and Action:

The seeds have a diuretic and expectorant property. They contain 45 to 48 percent fixed oil that is good for cooking. The leaves, flowers, and seeds also contain a glucoside which has a quinine-like action.

Conditions Most Used For:

Sunflower is best for recurrent intermittent fever, acute nasal congestion, and nasal hemorrhage with thick scabs in the nose. Rheumatic pain in left knee. It may also be used for any affliction of the spleen and stomach with nausea and vomiting. It may be applied externally to smoothen the skin or address skin problems.

DOSE - Use tincture to the third potency.

PARTS UTILIZED - Mature flower heads in strong alcohol.

23. INDIGOFERA TINCTORIA Linn.

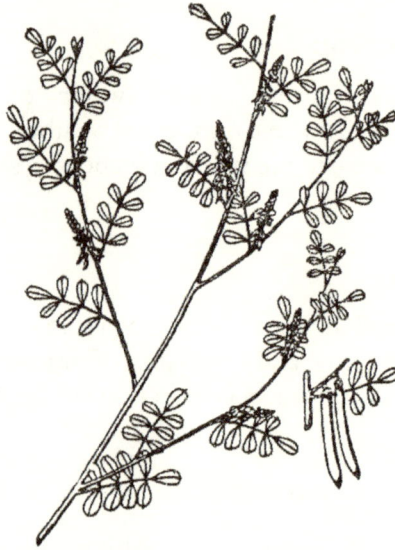

Local Name: *Indigo*

Properties and Action:

Indigo has a marked action on the nervous system. It is an antiseptic (inhibits the growth of or destroys germs) and an astringent (causes contractions and stops discharges).

Conditions Most Used For:

Indigo is of undoubted benefit in the treatment of epilepsy. It is also given in cases of neurasthenia and hysteria. Pure powdered indigo placed on the wound cures snake and spider poisons.

Other Conditions:

a. Nerve Sense System

General nerve conditions - Hysterical symptoms start where pain predominates. There is excessive nervous irritation. Epilepsy accompanied by flashes of heat from the abdomen to the head. Epileptic fits begin with dizziness. Aura begins from a painful spot between the shoulders. **Head** - A feeling of vertigo with nausea. Sensation of a band around the forehead.

Undulating sensation through whole head. Sensation as if the brain were frozen. Head feels frozen. Gloomy feeling; cries at night. Hair feels pulled from the vertex. Convulsions. **Nose** - Excessive sneezing and bleeding from the nose. **Ears** - Pressure and roaring sensation.

b. Metabolic/Limb System

Stomach - Has a metallic taste; belching or bloating. Anorexia (loss of appetite). Flushes of heat rising from the stomach to the head. **Rectum** - Palling feeling of the rectum. One is aroused at night with a horrible itching of the anus. Reflex spasms due to worms. **Urinary** - Constant desire to urinate. Urine is turbid. Catarrh of the bladder. **Extremities** - Sciatica. Pain from the middle of the thigh to the knee. Boring pain in the knee joint becoming better when walking. Pain in the limbs becoming worse after every meal.

DOSE - Third to thirtieth potency.

PART UTILIZED - Fresh leaves in strong alcohol or pure powdered indigo in medium-strong alcohol.

24. JATROPHA CURCAS Linn.

Local Names: *Physic Nut Tree, Big-purge Nut, Purging Nut Tree*

Properties and Action:

This plant addresses more specifically the metabolic-limb system. The seed contains a toxic principle, toxalbumin curcin, and 22 percent oil. It is a drastic purgative.

Conditions Most Used For:

This remedy is most valuable in cholera, diarrhea, and other abdominal symptoms. It will be helpful in cases where measles is suppressed, that is, the rashes are unable to come out.

Other Conditions:

Metabolic/Limb System

Stomach - Hiccoughs, followed by copious vomiting. Nausea with vomiting brought about by drinking, with acrid feeling from the throat.

Great thirst. Heat and burning in the stomach, with crampy, constrictive pain in the epigastrum. **Abdomen** - Distended, with gurgling noises. Pain in the region of the liver and under the right scapula to the shoulder. **Urinary** - Violent urge to urinate. **Bowel Movement** - Diarrhea with sudden, forceful, profuse discharge. Movement is accompanied by cramps, nausea, and vomiting. **Extremities** - Muscle cramps, especially in the calves, legs, and feet. The whole body is cold with pain in the ankles, feet, and toes. Heels are sensitive.

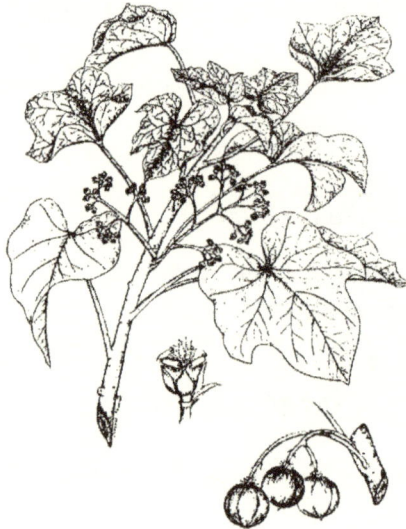

DOSE - Third to thirtieth potency.

PARTS UTILIZED - Fresh roots, bark, leaves and plenty of nuts in medium-strong alcohol.

25. JUNCUS EFFUSUS Linn.

Local Names: *Matting Rush, Common Soft Rush*

Properties and Actions:

This plant is antilithic (preventing the formation of calculi or stones in the body) and is used for urinary problems.

Conditions Most Used For:

Common rush is a diuretic and is used for urinary diseases such as dysuria (painful urination) and ischuria (the retention of urine). In arthritis and lithiasis (the formation of stones in the body), this plant will help dissolve and eliminate uric acid accumulation and prevent gall or kidney stones.

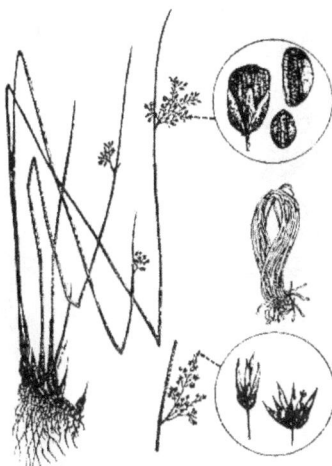

DOSE - Tincture and first potency. A decoction of the whole plant may be drunk as tea.

PARTS UTILIZED - Whole plant in medium-strong alcohol.

26. LYCOPODIUM CLAVATUM Linn.

Local Names: *Licopodio (Spanish); Stag's Horn, Foxtail, Wolf's Claw, Club Moss, Lycopod (English)*

Properties and Action:

The spores must be crushed to release its medicinal properties. It is a specific liver remedy by bringing significant relief and cure in cases of liver damage, liver dysfunction, and even serious degenerative symptoms. Club moss also acts on the urinary and digestive systems.

Conditions Most Used For:

The club moss patient is thin in the upper part of the body, but the abdomen and legs are swollen. There is accumulation of body fluids in the abdomen (ascites) and ulcers on the lower legs, exuding serous fluids. There is weakness and exhaustion with a tendency to depression. The patient has greyish-yellow complexion or yellow patches on the skin. In children, the head is well formed but sickly, with weak muscle development. This is predominantly a right-sided remedy such as right-sided tonsillitis, hernia in the groin, or varicose veins on the right leg. In liver problems, this plant can address jaundice, and hepatic enlargement with greenish, bitter vomiting.

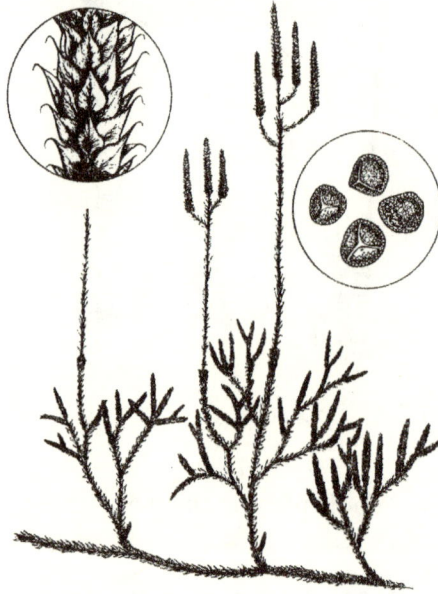

Other Conditions:

a. Nerve Sense System

Fever - Chill between 3 - 4 p.m., followed by sweating. One feels as if lying on ice. One chill is followed by another. **Head** - Patient shakes his head, face and/or mouth without apparent cause. There is a pressing headache at the crown of the head; becoming worse from 4 to 8 p.m., and from lying down or stooping. Vertigo is experienced in the morning on rising. Pain in the temples, as if screws are being turned toward each other. Tearing pain at the back of the head, becoming better with fresh air. Hair is falling out. There is premature baldness and gray hair. Deep furrows on the forehead. **Eyes** - Styes (infection of the gland in the eyelid) near the internal canthus. Ulceration and redness of the eyelids. There is day blindness, but night blindness is more pronounced. Sees only one half of an object. Eyes half open during sleep. Headaches over eyes in severe colds. **Ear** - Thick, yellow, offensive discharge. Eczema about and behind ears. Deafness with or without ringing in the ear. Humming and roaring with difficulty of hearing; every noise causes peculiar echo in the ear. **Nose** - Sense of smell is very acute. Scanty mucus discharge. Ulcerated nostrils. Fluent coryza (acute nasal congestion). **Face** - Grayish-yellow color of the face, with bluish circle around the eyes. Dropping of the lower jaw during a typhoid fever. **Mouth** - Teeth are excessively painful to touch. Toothache, with swelling of the cheeks; relieved by application of warmth. Dryness of the mouth and tongue, without thirst. Tongue is dry, black, cracked, swollen. Mouth waters. Blisters on the tongue. Bad odor from the mouth. Itching, scaly herpes in the comer of the mouth. **Throat** - Inflamed throat, with stitches upon swallowing; becoming better with warm drinks. Ulcers of the tonsils, beginning on the right side. During diphtheria, deposits spread from right to left, becoming worse with cold drinks. Ulceration of the vocal bands. Tubercular laryngitis, especially when ulceration commences. **Skin** - Ulcers and abscesses beneath the skin. Hives, violent itching, fissured eruptions, or acne, becoming worse with warm applications. Chronic eczema associated with urinary, gastric, and hepatic disorders which bleeds easily. Varicose veins. Skin is dry and shrunken, especially on the palms. Psoriasis.

b. Middle/Rhythmic System

Emotional State - Melancholy, apprehensive; afraid to be alone. Extremely sensitive. Little things tend to annoy. Averse to new things. Loss of self-confidence. Constant fear of breaking down under stress. Failing mind power. Weak memory, confused thoughts. Sadness in the morning upon waking. **Respiratory** - Bronchitis with accumulation of mucus, rales (rattling sound), and difficulty in breathing. Pneumonia with difficult expectoration. Tickling cough with constrictive and burning pain in the chest. Cough becoming worse on going downhill. Cough deep and hollow. Expectorated mucus is gray, thick, bloody, purulent, and salty. **Heart** - Aneurism (weakened wall of arteries). Palpitation at night. Patient cannot lie on the left side.

c. Metabolic/Limb System

Stomach - Dyspepsia (digestive disorder) due to starch in the food. Excessive hunger. Desire for sweet things. Food tends to taste sour. Great weakness of digestion. Insatiable appetite, with much bloating. After eating, pressure in the stomach with a bitter taste in the mouth. Eating little creates fullness. Waking up at night feeling hungry. Hiccoughs. Incomplete burning eructations (gas expulsion) which rise only to pharynx; there, it bums for hours. Sinking sensation, worse at night. **Abdomen** - Constant feeling of fermentation going on in the abdomen, like yeast working. Hernia, at the right side. Liver is sensitive. Brown spots on the abdomen. Hepatitis. Pain shooting across lower abdomen from the right to the left. Sour belching. **Bowel Movement** - Diarrhea. Inactive intestinal canal. Ineffectual urging. Feces: hard, difficult, small, incomplete. Hemorrhoids; very painful to touch, aching. **Urinary** - Pain in the back before urinating but ceases after. Urine is slow in coming, must strain oneself. Polyuria (excessive urination) during the night. Urine with heavy red sediment. Child cries before urinating. **Male** - Impotence. No erectile power. Premature emission. Enlarged prostate. Condylomata (wart-like growth in the anus or genitals). **Female** - Menses are too late; last too long and are profuse. Vagina is dry. Coition (sexual intercourse) is painful. Pain in the right ovary. Varicose veins of the genitals. Leucorrhea (vaginal discharge) acrid, with burning sensation in the vagina. Discharge of blood from the genital during bowel movement. **Back** - Burning between the scapula like hot coals. **Extremities** - Numbness and/or drawing and tearing in the limbs, more pronounced at rest or at night. Limbs twitch and jerk. One foot hot while the other cold. Chronic gout, with chalky deposit in the joints. Profuse sweat of the feet. Pain in the heel on treading, as on a pebble. Painful calluses on the soles with the toes and fingers contracted. Sciatica, worse on the right side. Cramps in the calves and toes at night while in bed. Heaviness of the arms. Tearing pain in the shoulder and elbow joints. **Sleep** - Startled, or making involuntary movements while asleep. Dreams of accident. Drowsy during the day.

DOSE - Both the lower and higher potencies are credited with excellent results. For purposes of aiding excretion or detoxification, the second or third potency, a few drops 3 times a day is already effective. In individuals who do not respond well to the low potencies, the 6th to 200th potency and higher, in not too frequent doses, may be given.

PARTS UTILIZED - Crushed fresh leaves with plenty of spores in medium-strong alcohol. Dried version titurated in lactose is better.

27. MANGIFERA INDICA Linn.

Local Name: *Mango*

Properties and Action:

Mango tends to promote better circulation and relaxes the mucus membranes of the alimentary canal.

Conditions Most Used For:

Mango is one of the best general remedies for passive hemorrhages in the uterus, kidneys, stomach, lungs, and intestines. It is also used in rhinitis, pharyngitis, and other acute throat troubles, especially with suffocating sensation. Mango can also address varicose veins, drowsiness, and poor circulation where the muscles are too relaxed.

Other Conditions

a. Nerve Sense System

Skin - Itching of the palms of the hands. Skin looks as if sunburnt, swollen. White spots on the skin with intense itching. Lobes of the ears and lips are swollen.

b. Metabolic/Limb System

Abdomen - Catarrhal and serous discharges with chronic intestinal irritation.

DOSE - Use the tincture or boil the leaves and drink as tea.

PARTS UTILIZED - Mature leaves, bark and resin in medium-strong alcohol.

28. MENTHA x Cordifolia

Local Names: *Peppermint, Marsh Mint, Mint*

Properties and Actions:

Mint stimulates the cold perceiving nerves so that just after taking it, a current of air at ordinary temperature feels cold. It has a marked action on the respiratory organs and the skin.

Conditions Most Used For:

This plant is useful in colds with gas in the stomach and intestines.

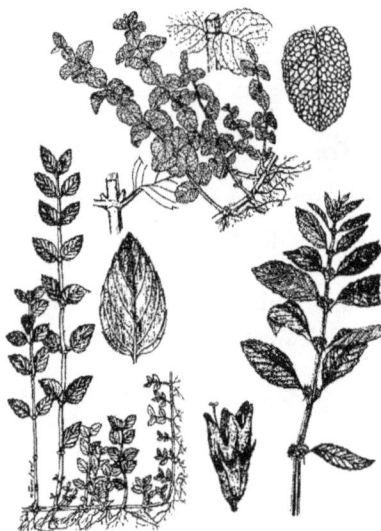

Other Conditions:

a. Nerve Sense System

Skin - Every scratch become a sore. Itching of the arm and hand when writing. Pruritus vaginae (intense itching of the skin on and around the vagina). Herpes zoster (acute, infectious, inflammatory skin disease).

b. Middle/Rhythmic System

Respiratory - Voice is husky. Tip of the nose is sore to touch. Throat is dry and sore. Dry cough becomes worse from air coming into the larynx, or from tobacco smoke, fog, or while talking. Trachea is painful to touch.

c. Metabolic/Limb System

Abdomen - Bloated abdomen and sleep is disturbed. Infantile colic. Bilious colic with great accumulation of gas.

DOSE - Tincture, 1 to 20 drops, to thirtieth potency. Mint may be applied locally in pruritus vaginae.

PARTS UTILIZED - Crushed fresh whole plant in medium-strong alcohol.

29. MOMORDICA CHARANTIA Linn.

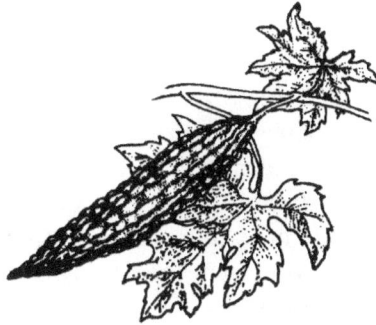

Local Names: *Balsam Apple, Balsam Pear, African Cucumber, Bitter Gourd*

Properties and Action:

The leaves and fruits of the bitter gourd contain a bitter alkaloid (momordicin) and a glucoside responsible for its chief action on the metabolic system.

Conditions Most Used For:

Bitter gourd addresses gripping, colic, pain in the back and stomach with painful and excessive menses. There is accumulation of flatus (gas in the stomach and intestines) and dropsy (accumulation of body fluids).

Other Conditions:

a. Nerve Sense System

Head - Dizziness, but the contents of head feel light. There may be mist before the eyes.

b. Metabolic/Limb System

Abdomen - Rumbling, gripping, colicky pains that start from the back and spread over the abdomen. **Female** - Painful menstruations followed by gushes of blood. Pain at a small point of the back coming towards the front of the pelvis.

DOSE - Tincture to sixth potency.

PARTS UTILIZED - Crushed roots, stem, leaves, flowers, and young fruit in medium-strong alcohol. The wild variety is more effective.

30. NICOTIANA TABACUM Linn.

Local Name: *Tobacco*

Properties and Action:

Tobacco induces nausea, dizziness, death-like pallor, vomiting, icy coldness, and sweat accompanied by intermittent pulse. It has a marked antiseptic quality that is an antidote to cholera germs. This plant may further cause the complete exhaustion of the entire muscular system by inducing vigorous peristaltic activity. This situation may then lead to diarrhea and produce hypertension and arteriosclerosis.

Conditions Most Used For:

Tobacco is used in gastralgia (pains in the stomach), enteralgia (gas pains in the intestines), sea-sickness, and cholera infantum. It has been proven to be the most effective homeopathic drug for angina pectoris (severe attacks of pain over the heart) that is accompanied by coronaritis (inflammation of the arteries supplying the heart muscles), and hypertension. It may also be given in various forms of neuralgias.

Other Conditions:

a. Nerve Sense System

Head - Vertigo upon opening of the eyes; headaches, with deathly nausea coming in periodically. Sudden pain, as if one's head is struck by a hammer. Nervous deafness. Secretion from the eyes, nose, and mouth is increased. **Eyes** - Dim sight, one sees as if through a veil; cross-eyed. Amaurosis (blindness); muscae olitantes (spots before the eyes). Rapid blindness without lesion, followed by venus hyperemia (increased blood flow) and atrophy of the optic nerve. **Face** - Pale, blue, pinched, sunken, and covered with cold sweat. **Throat** - Nasopharyngitis and tracheitis with hemming, morning cough, and sometimes vomiting. Hoarseness of the voice of public speakers.

b. Middle/Rhythmic System

Emotional State - There is a sensation of excessive wretchedness, very despondent, forgetful, and discontented. There is fear of death. **Heart** - Palpitation of heartbeat when lying on the left side. Intermittent, feeble, or imperceptible pulse. Angina pectoris, pain in the precordial (area overlying the heart) region. Pain radiates from the center of the sternum.

Tachycardia (rapid beating of the heart coming on in sudden attacks). Bradycardia (slow heart rate). Acute dilation of the heart caused by shock or violent physical exertion. **Respiratory** - Difficult, violent constriction of the chest. Precordial oppression, with palpitation and pain between the shoulders. Dyspnea (difficult breathing), with tingling sensation down the left arm when lying on the left side. Cough followed by hiccough. Cough dry, teasing, must take in a mouthful of cold water to relieved.

c. Metabolic/Limb System

Stomach - Incessant nausea, becoming worse with the smell of tobacco smoke; vomiting at the least motion. If during pregnancy, there is much spitting. Sea-sickness; terrible faint, sinking feeling at the pit of the stomach. Gastralgia; pain from the cardiac region and extending to the left arm. **Abdomen** - feels cold but wants the abdomen uncovered. Painful distention. Incarcerated hernia. **Bowel Movement** - Constipated with the rectum paralyzed, or prolapsed (out of place). Diarrhea, with nausea and vomiting, exhaustion, and cold sweat; stool looks like sour milk, thick, curdled and watery. Rectal tenesmus (spasms). Cholera with icy coldness of the body. **Urinary** - Renal colic; violent pain along the ureter, at the left side. **Extremities** - Legs and hands are icy cold; limbs tremble. Paralysis follows apoplexy (stroke). Gait shuffling, unsteady. Feebleness of the arms. **Sleep** - Insomnia with dilated heart, with cold, clammy skin and anxiety. **Fever** - Chills, with cold sweat.

DOSE - Third to thirtieth potency.

PARTS UTILIZED - Unfermented dried leaves in medium-strong alcohol.

31. PIPER NIGRUM Linn.

Local Names: *Pepper, Peppercorn*

Properties and Action:

Pepper contains an acrid resin and an oleoresin that give the pungent taste and aromatic odor. Taken internally, it is a stomachic (gastric stimulant), carminative (aid to digestion) and induces the secretion of bile. It is a rubefacient (causing redness, e.g., skin) and a counter-irritant.

Conditions Most Used For:

Pepper is best for the sensation of burning and pressure anywhere in the body.

Other Conditions:

a. Nerve Sense System

Head - Heavy headache, as if the temples were pressed in; pressure in the nasal and facial bones. Eyes and face inflamed, burning and red. Eyeballs aching. Nose itches, sneezes or bleeds. Lips are dry and cracked. **Throat** - Sore, feels raw, burns. Burning pain in the tonsils.

b. Middle/Rhythmic System

Emotional State - Sad, apprehensive, unable to concentrate; startles at any noise. **Respiratory** - Difficulty in breathing, cough with pain in the chest in spots. **Heart** - Palpitation, cardiac pain, with slow intermittent pulse. **Female** - Great flow of milk in lactating mothers.

c. Metabolic/Limb System

Stomach/Abdomen - Flatulence with gastric discomfort. Feeling of fullness. Tympanites (abdominal distention due to gas). Colic and cramps. Great thirst. **Urinary** - Burning in the bladder and urethra. Difficult urination. Bladder feels full, swollen; frequent urging but without success. **Male** - Priapism (continued erection of the penis without sexual desire).

DOSE - First to the sixth potencies.

PARTS UTILIZED - Dried unripe berries in strong alcohol.

32. PLANTAGO MAJOR Linn.

Local Names: *Llantin (Spanish); Plantain, Ribwort, Wild Saso, Cart Tract Plant, Way Bread, Broad Leaf Plantain (English)*

Properties and Action:

The plant contains potassium salt, citric acid, a glucoside, and enzymes invertin and emulsin. This makes broad leaf plantain astringent (causes contraction and stops discharges) and an emollient (relaxing and soothing agent).

Conditions Most Used For:

This plant has considerable clinical reputation in the treatment of earache, toothache, and enuresis (inability to control urination). It may also be used when there is a sharp pain in the eyes, pain from a decaying tooth, or an inflammation of the middle ear.

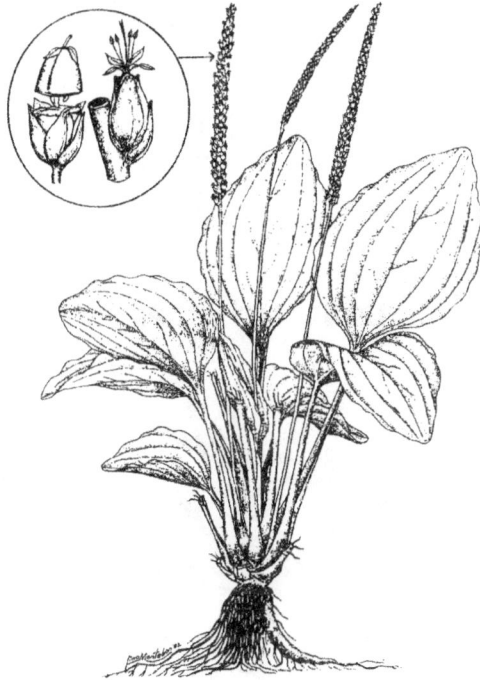

Other Conditions:

a. Nerve Sense System

Head - Periodical prosopalgia (facial pains), becoming worse at 7 a.m. to 2 p.m., accompanied with flow of tears. Photophobia (aversion to light) with pains that radiate to the temples and lower face. Eyeballs are very tender to touch. Pain plays between teeth and ears. **Ears** - Hearing is acute, with pain experienced with every sound. Neuralgic earache; pain goes from one ear to the other through the head. Otalgia (earache), with toothache. **Nose** - Sudden, yellowish, watery discharge. **Mouth** - Teeth ache and are sensitive and sore to touch. Swelling of the cheeks. Salivation; teeth feel too long, becoming worse in cold air and upon contact. Toothache, becoming better while eating. Profuse flow of saliva. Toothache with reflex neuralgia of the eyelids. Pyorrhea alveolaris (infection of the gums). **Skin** - Urticaria, itching and burning; papule (small red raised area on the skin).

b. Metabolic/Limb System

Bowel Movement - Urge to defecate; going often but unproductive. Piles (hemorrhoids) so bad, one can hardly stand. Diarrhea, with brown watery stool. **Urinary** - Profuse flow of urine; bed-wetting. **Sleep** - Insomnia produced by heavy smoking, accompanied by depression and aversion to the smell of smoke.

DOSE - Tincture and lower potencies. This plant may be applied locally as in the case of toothaches, earaches, and wounds.

PARTS UTILIZED - Fresh leaves in medium-strong alcohol.

33. POLYGONUM HYDROPIPER Linn.

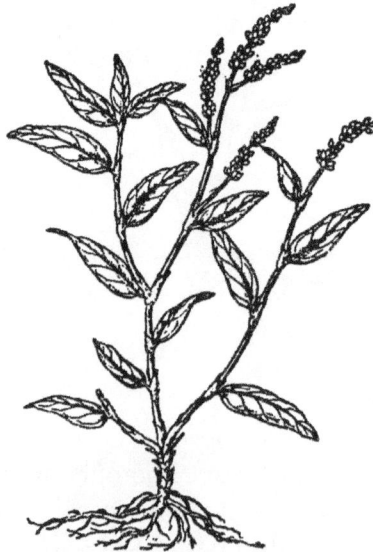

Local Names: *Hydropiper, Smartweed (English)*

Properties and Action:

Smartweed has a hemostatic (to stop hemorrhages) property and is also a sedative.

Conditions Most Used For:

Smartweed is best in cases of metrorrhagia (vaginal bleeding unrelated to the monthly period), and amenorrhea (stoppage of normal menstrual periods) in young girls.

Other Conditions:

a. Metabolic/Limb System

Stomach - Burning in the stomach followed by feeling of coldness in its pit. **Abdomen** - Gripping pain, with great rumbling, nausea, and liquid feces. Flatulent colic. Hemorrhoids and rectal pockets. **Extremities** - Varicose veins. Superficial ulcers and sores on the lower extremities. **Urinary** - Painful constriction at the neck of the bladder. **Female** - Aching pains in the hips and loins. Sensation as if the hips were being drawn together. Sensation of weight and tension within the pelvis. Shooting pains through the breast.

DOSE - Tincture.

PARTS UTILIZED - Pounded fresh whole plant in medium-strong alcohol.

34. PUNICA GRANATUM Linn.

Local Name: *Pomegranate*

Properties and Action:

The pomegranate bark and rind contains a number of alkaloids, glucosides, and tannins that act as a vermifuge (to expel tapeworms), and as an astringent (causes contraction and stops discharges).

Conditions Most Used For:

Pomegranate is useful in salivation, with nausea, and vertigo. It is also used in the spasm of the glottis (the space between the vocal cords).

Other Conditions:

a. Nerve Sense System

Head - Feels empty. Sunken eyes; pupils dilated; weak sight. Vertigo is very persistent. **Skin** - Itching in the palms of the hands. Sensation as if pimples would break out. Yellowish complexion.

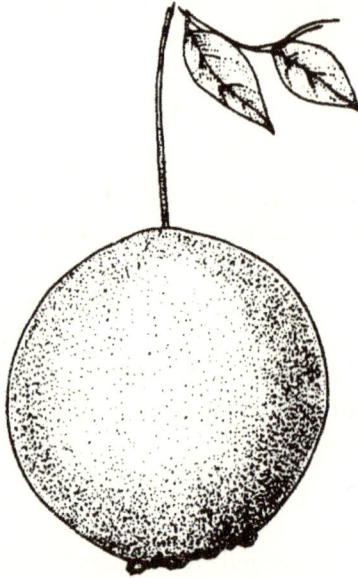

b. Middle/Rhythmic System

Chest - Oppressed, with sighing; even clothing seems oppressive. Pain between shoulders as if heavy load is being carried.

c. Metabolic/Limb System

Stomach - There is a feeling of constant hunger. Poor digestion. Loses flesh. Vomiting at night. **Abdomen** - Pain in the stomach and abdomen; becoming worse about the umbilicus. Swelling resembling umbilical hernia. **Female** - Dragging in the vaginal region, as if hernia would protrude. **Bowel Movement** - Ineffectual urging. Itching at the anus. **Extremities** - Pain in all the finger joints. Tearing in the knee joint. Convulsive movements of the arms or legs.

DOSE - First to third potency.

PARTS UTILIZED - Fresh bark and rind of fruit crushed in medium-strong alcohol. Dried powdered form is titurated in lactose.

35. RAPHANUS SATIVUS Linn.

Local Name: *Radish*

Properties and Action:

Radish produces pain and stitches in liver and spleen. It increases the production of bile and the secretion of saliva. These symptoms will not appear if salt is used with the radish.

Conditions Most Used For:

Radish is used when there is great accumulation and confinement of flatulence (abdominal gas). It is also given in cases of seborrhea (excessive oiliness of the skin caused by glandular upsets); in pemphigus (one of the most severe and rare types of oral ulceration); in hysteria; and in nymphomania (excessive sexual desire in the female).

Other Conditions:

a. Nerve Sense System

Head - Headache, brain feels tender and sore. Edema (swelling) of the lower eyelids. Mucus in the posterior nares. **Throat** - Hot ball feeling from the throat and the uterus, stopping there. Heat and burning in the throat.

b. Middle/Rhythmic System

Emotional State - Sadness, with an aversion to children, especially girls. **Chest** - Pain in the chest which extends to the back and to the throat. Heavy lump and coldness in the center of the chest.

c. Metabolic/Limb System

Stomach - Putrid belching. Burning in the epigastrum, followed by hot belching. **Abdomen** - Retching and vomiting, loss of appetite. Distended, plenty of gas, hard. No gas is emitted, upward or downward. Griping pain about the navel. Vomiting of fecal matter. **Bowel Movement** - Stool is liquid, frothy, profuse, brown, with colic, and pad-like swelling of the intestines. **Female** - Nervous irritation of the genitals. Menses are very profuse and long-lasting. Nymphomania, with aversion to her own sex and to children. Insomnia due to strong sexual urge. **Urinary** - Urine is turbid, with yeast-like sediment. Urine is more copious, thick like milk.

DOSE - Third to thirtieth potency.

PARTS UTILIZED - Fresh roots in medium-strong alcohol.

36. RICINUS COMMUNIS Linn. BOFAREIRA

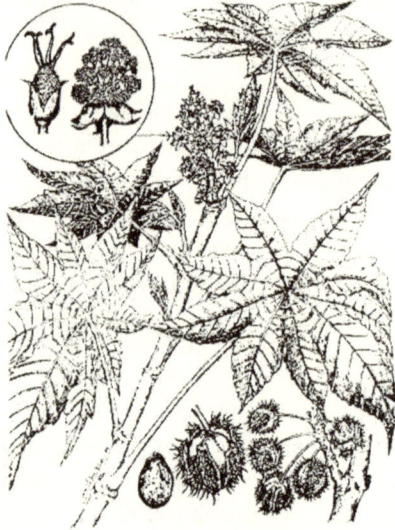

Local Name: *Castor Oil Plant*

Properties and Action:

Castor oil plant has marked action on the gastrointestinal tract. It also increases the quantity of milk in nursing women.

Conditions Most Used For:

This plant may be used in case of vomiting and the purging of bowels from the intestines.

Other Conditions:

a. Nerve Sense System

Head - Experiences of vertigo, occipital pain, congestive symptoms, and buzzing in the ears. The face is pale with twitching of the mouth. **Mouth** - Dry. Paresis (acid taste).

b. Metabolic/Limb System

Stomach - Anorexia (loss of appetite) with great thirst, burning in the stomach. Nausea, profuse vomiting, pit of the stomach is sensitive. **Abdomen** - Rumbling with the contraction of the rectal muscles; colic, incessant diarrhea with purging. **Bowel Movement** - Rice water stools with cramps and chilliness. Bowels are loose, incessant, painless, but with painful cramps in the muscles of the extremities. Anus inflamed. Stools green, slimy, and bloody. **Fever** - Emaciation (to become abnormally lean), somnolence (induced drowsiness).

DOSE - Third potency. Five drops are given every four hours to increase the flow of milk. Crushed leaves may be applied locally on the breast.

PARTS UTILIZED - Crushed seeds in strong alcohol.

37. RUMEX CRISPUS Linn.

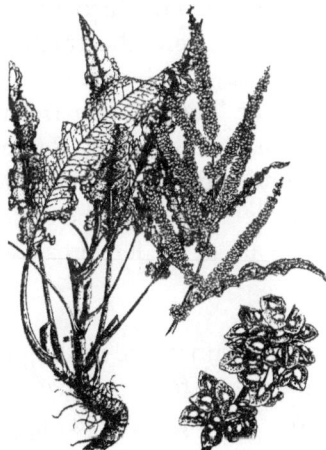

Local Names: *Yellow Duck, Curly Duck*

Properties and Action:

Curly duck induces pains which are numerous and varied, but neither fixed nor constant anywhere in the body. It diminishes the mucous secretion, and at the same time increases the sensibility of the membranes of the larynx and trachea. Its action upon the skin is marked by intense itching. The lymphatic vessels are also enlarged and their secretion perverted.

Conditions Most Used For:

Curly duck is best for coughs that are caused by an incessant tickling in the throat. This tickling runs down to the bronchial tubes. The cough is immediately induced by the mere touching of the throat-pit. Cough becomes worse from encountering the least cold air. All coughing ceases by covering up the body and head with bed clothes.

Other Conditions:

a. Nerve Sense System

Mouth - Tongue is coated and sore at the edges. Sensation of a lump in the throat. **Skin** - Itching of the skin is intense, especially on the lower extremities; becoming worse from exposure to cold air especially when undressing. Urticaria; contagious prurigo (a chronic inflammatory skin disease).

b. Middle/Rhythmic System

Respiratory - Nose is dry. Tickling in the throat-pit causes cough. Copious mucous discharge from the nose and the trachea. Dry, teasing cough, preventing sleep. Cough is aggravated by pressure, talking, and especially by inspiring cool air and at night. Thin, watery, frothy expectoration by the mouthful; later becoming stringy and tough. Rawness of the larynx and the trachea. Valuable in advanced phthisis (tuberculosis). Soreness behind the sternum, especially on the left side or in the region of the left shoulder. Raw pain under the clavicle. Pain in the left breast after meals.

c. Metabolic/Limb System

Stomach - Sensation of a hard substance in the pit of the stomach with hiccough, pyrosis (burning in the stomach), nausea. Eating meat causes eructation (belching), pruritus (itching). Jaundice appears after the excessive use of alcohol. Chronic gastritis; aching pain in the pit of the stomach and shooting pain in the chest; extending towards the throat-pit, becoming worse from any motion or talking. **Bowel Movement** - Feces is brown and watery. Diarrhea occurs early in the morning with cough. Itching of the anus, with the sensation as if a stick is in the rectum. Piles (hemorrhoids).

DOSE - Third to sixth potency.

PARTS UTILIZED - Crushed fresh roots in medium-strong alcohol.

38. SACCHARUM OFFICINARUM Linn.

Local Name: *Sugar Cane*

Properties and Action:

Sugar cane is an antiseptic (inhibits the growth of germs). It combats infection and putrefaction. It dissolves fibrin (a protein produced by the blood to stimulate clotting) and stimulates the secretion of other chemicals in the tissue. Thus, this plant may be used to rinse wounds to induce healing. Sugar cane is also an oxytocic (makes the uterus contract). It can be most helpful if sugar is given to mothers who are undergoing difficult childbirth (as long as there is no mechanical obstruction) due to uterine inertia.

Conditions Most Used For:

The sugar is considered a sustainer and developer of the muscles of the heart. Hence it is very useful in a variety of cardiovascular troubles. The sugar acts as a nutrient and a tonic (muscular tightener) in most wasting (weakening) disorders, such as anemia and neurasthenia, by giving weight and energy. *Tuba* is given to fat, bloated, large-limbed children, who are cross, peevish, whining, capricious, and want dainty things but refuse substantial food. There is edema (swelling) of the feet. Headache is experienced every seven days. The sight is dimmed and the cornea are opaque.

DOSE - Thirtieth potency and higher. The juice may be applied locally in case of gangrene. In epilepsy, blood with reduced sugar content irritates the nervous system, which leads to convulsions. One ounce of lump sugar in the morning then could help prevent epileptic convulsions. In the case of difficult labor in childbirth, dissolve 25 grams of sugar in water, and give several times every half hour.

PARTS UTILIZED - Fresh sugar cane juice in strong alcohol.

39. SMILAX CHINA Linn. and SMILAX LEUCOPHYLLA Blume.

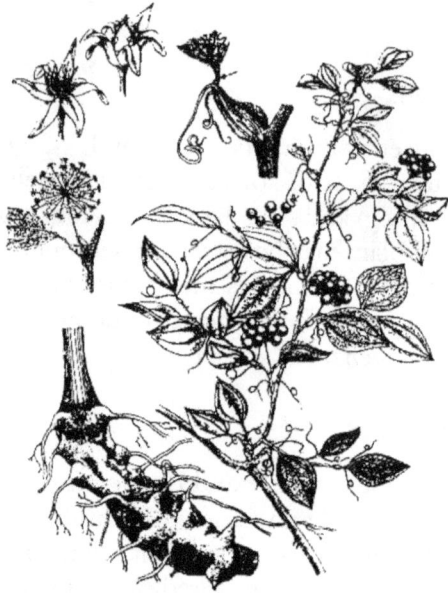

Local Names: *Chinese Root, Chinese Sarsaparilla, Sarsaparilla*

Properties and Action:

Sarsaparilla is a depurative (purifies), diaphoretic (increases perspiration), and demulcent (soothes irritated or inflamed mucous membranes).

Conditions Most Used For:

Sarsaparilla is used in renal colic, marasmus (extreme malnutrition), and periosteal (a membrane of fibrous connective tissues covering all bones) pains due to venereal disease. It is good for skin eruptions following the advent of hot weather or as a result of vaccinations, boils, and eczema. Sarsaparilla also addresses urinary problems.

Other Conditions:

a. Nerve Sense System

Head - Pains in the head cause depression. Shooting pain from above the right temporal region. Pains from the occiput to the eyes. Words reverberate in the ear to the root of the nose. Influenza. Scalp is very sensitive. Eruptions on the face and the upper lip. Moist eruption on the scalp. **Mouth** - Tongue is white; aphthea (white spots) is present; saliva is profuse with metallic taste but no sensation of thirst. The breath is fetid. **Skin** - Emaciated (abnormally lean), shriveled, lies in folds, dry, and flabby. Herpetic eruptions or ulcers. Rash from exposure to open air; dry, itching, comes on in spring; becomes crusty. Rhagades (skin cracks) on the hands and feet. Skin is hard, indurated. Summer skin diseases.

b. Middle/Rhythmic System

Emotional State - Despondent, sensitive, easily offended, ill-humored and taciturn (uncommunicative).

c. Metabolic/Limb System

Abdomen - Rumbling and fermenting sensation. Colic and backache at the same time. Much flatus; cholera infantum. **Urinary** - Urine is scanty, slimy, flaky, sandy, bloody. Renal colic. Severe pain at the conclusion of urination. Urine dribbles while sitting. Bladder is distended and tender. Spasms of the bladder; urine passes in thin feeble stream. Child screams before and while passing urine. Sand on the diaper. **Male** - Bloody seminal emissions. Intolerable odor of the genitals. Herpetic eruptions on the genitals. Itching on the scrotum (pouch of the testicles) and the area between the genitals and the anus. Syphilis, squamous eruption and bone pains. **Female** - Nipples are small, withered and retracted. Before menstruation, there is itching and humid eruption on the forehead. Moist eruption in the right groin before the menses. Menses are late and scanty. **Extremities** - Pain from the right knee downward. Paralytic, tearing pains. Rheumatism with pains in the bones, becoming worse at night. Trembling of the hands and feet. Burning on the sides of the fingers and toes. Onychia (ulceration around the ends of the fingers and toes), cutting sensation under the nails. Blisters on the hands.

DOSE - First to sixth potency.

PARTS UTILIZED - Coarsely powdered dried roots in medium-strong alcohol.

40. SOLANUM LYCOPERSICUM Linn.

Local Name: *Tomato*

Properties and Action:

The plant contains solanin, fixed oils, and other compounds that promote gastric secretion, purify the blood, and stimulate a torpid (sluggish) liver.

Conditions Most Used For:

Tomato is used for rheumatism and influenza where there are severe aching pains all over body. The head always shows signs of acute congestion. It is good for hay fever that is aggravated by breathing in the least dust. Frequent urination and profuse watery diarrhea also call for the use of this remedy.

Other Conditions:

a. Nerve Sense System

Head - Bursting pain, beginning in the occiput and spreading all over. The whole head and the scalp feel sore and bruised even after pain has ceased. **Eyes** - Dull, heavy; pupils are contracted; eyeballs feel contracted; aching in and around the eyes. Eyes are suffused (spread and diffused). **Nose** - Profuse, watery coryza; nasal discharge drops down the throat. Itching in the anterior chamber becoming worse when breathing in any dust, becoming better when indoors.

b. Metabolic/Rhythmic System

Heart - Decrease in pulse rate with anxiety and apprehensiveness. **Respiratory** - Voice is husky. Hoarseness of voice with a constant desire to clear the throat. Expulsive cough that is deep and harsh. Dry, hacking cough coming on at night and keeping one awake. Pain and heaviness in the chest, extending to the head.

c. Metabolic/Limb System

Urinary - Constant dribbling of urine in the open air. One must rise at night to urinate. **Extremities** - Aching pain throughout the back. Dull pain in the lumbar region. Pain deep in the middle of the right arm. Rheumatic pain in the right elbow and wrist, and hands of both sides. Tingling along right ulnar nerve (nerve of the arm). Intense aching in the lower limbs. Right leg and thigh neuralgia.

DOSE - Third to thirtieth potency.

PARTS UTILIZED - Whole fresh plant in medium-strong alcohol.

41. SOLANUM NIGRUM Linn.

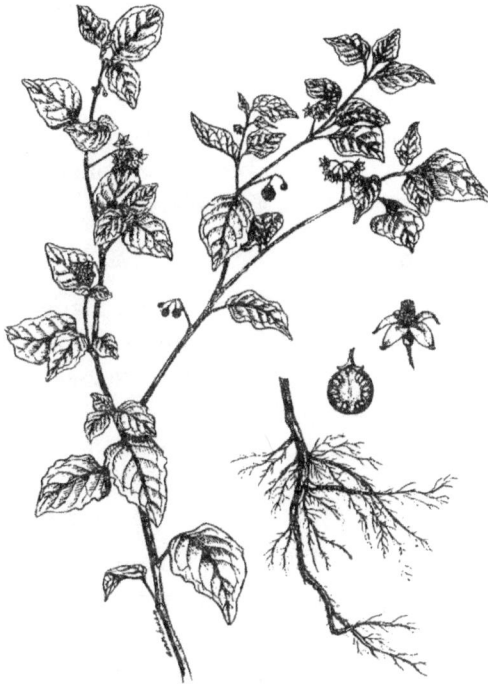

Local Names: *Black Nightshade, Common Nightshade, Deadly Nightshade*

Properties and Action:

This plant has a marked action on the head and eyes, bringing about restlessness of a violent, convulsive nature, and disorientation.

Conditions Most Used For:

This plant is best for meningitis (inflammation of the lining of the brain and spinal cord), encephalomalacia (softening of the brain due to deficient blood supply) and any form of brain irritation.

Other Conditions:

a. Nerve Sense System

Head - Furious delirium. Vertigo with terrible headache and the complete cessation of the mental faculties. Night terrors. **Nose** - Acute coryza; profuse, watery discharge from the right nostril while the left nostril is clogged up. Nasal congestion is accompanied by chilly sensations, alternating with heat. **Eyes** - Pain over both eyes. Alternating dilation and contraction of the pupils; weak sight with floating spots.

b Middle/Rhythmic System

Respiratory - Pain in the left chest that is sore to touch. Constrictive feeling in the chest, with difficulty in breathing; cough with tickling in the throat. Expectorated mucus is thick and yellow.

c. Metabolic/Limb System

Fever - There is alternation of coldness and heat. Scarlet fever; eruption in spots, large and vivid. **Abdomen** - Chronic intestinal toxemia (poisoning). In ergotism (a condition resulting from the excessive eating of grains infested with the ergot fungus), with tetanic (tetanus) spasm and stiffness of the whole body.

DOSE - Second to thirtieth potency.

PARTS UTILIZED - Crushed fresh whole plants in medium-strong alcohol.

42. SYMPHYTUM SP.

Local Name: *Comfrey*

Properties and Action:

The root of the comfrey plant contains essential oil and alkaloids, allantoin, choline, the glycoside consolidin, tannins, and resins. They stimulate the growth of epithelium (cellular tissues) of ulcerated surfaces (like wounds and lesions) and promote callus formation.

Conditions Most Used For:

Comfrey is given for fractures of all kinds, especially the long bones of the legs, particularly when the sites of the fracture are very painful. It also addresses the pain that persists after the fracture has healed, or the sensitivity of stumps after an amputation.

Other Conditions:

a. Nerve Sense System

Head - Pain in the occiput, top and forehead; changing places. Pain comes down the bone of the nose. Inflammation of the inferior maxillary bone, hard, red, swelling. **Eyes** - Pain in the eye after a blow of a blunt object. Traumatic injuries of the eye. Ulceration of the eyeball with spasmodic closing of the eyelids.

b. Metabolic/Limb System

Abdomen - Ulcers of the stomach and the duodenum (first 8 inches of the small intestines). **Extremities** - Neuralgia of the knees and ankles. Injury to the tendons and ligaments. Sensitivity of the bones at the site of a fracture. Psoas (two muscles of the loin that connects the spinal column and the thighbone) abscess following tubercular disease of the spine.

DOSE - Tincture up to sixth potency. Externally as a dressing for sores, ulcers, and wounds.

PARTS UTILIZED - Crushed fresh whole plant with plenty of roots gathered before flowering, in medium-strong alcohol.

43. TARAXACUM OFFICINALE Weber V.

Local Names: *Irish Daisy, Blowball, Milk Gowan, Dandelion*

Properties and Action:

The plant contains a bitter alkaloid (taraxacin) and other compounds that act together as a general stimulant to the kidneys and liver.

Conditions Most Used For:

Dandelion is used foremost as a liver remedy: gastric headaches, bilious attacks, with characteristically mapped tongue and jaundice skin.

Other Conditions:

a. Nerve Sense System

Head - Sensation of great heat on the top of the head. Sterno-mastoid muscle (behind the ear) very painful to touch. **Mouth** - Mapped tongue. Tongue covered with a white film; feels raw; comes off in patches, leaving red, sensitive spots. Salivations of the mouth. **Skin** - Profuse sweat at night.

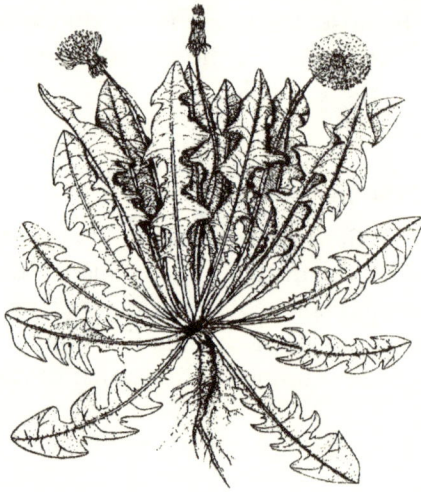

b. Metabolic/Limb System

Stomach - There is loss of appetite, bitter taste and eructations (belching). **Abdomen** - Liver is enlarged and indurated (hardened). Sharp stitches in the left side. **Bowel Movement** - Sensation of bubbles bursting in the bowels. Tympanites (abdominal distention due to gas) with difficult evacuation of gases. Flatulence. **Urinary** - Cancer of the bladder. **Extremities** - Very restless limbs. Neuralgia of the knee; becoming better with pressure. Limbs are painful to touch. Fever. Chilliness after eating, becoming worse by drinking; finger tips are cold. Bitter taste. Heat in the face, in the toes, without thirst. Sweating on falling asleep.

DOSE - Tincture, to third potency. In cancer, about 7 milliliters of the fluid extract (by decoction) should be given four times each day.

PARTS UTILIZED - Whole plant gathered when coming into flower in medium-strong alcohol.

44. THEA SINENSIS Linn.

Local Name: *Tea*

Properties and Actions:

Tea has caffeine and theobromine and very small quantities of other alkaloids that act as nerve stimulants. It produces headaches and is an antidote to tobacco.

Conditions Most Used For:

Tea is used for nervous sleeplessness, heart troubles, palpitation, and dyspepsia (indigestion) of old tea drinkers.

Other Conditions:

a. Nerve Sense System

Head - Cold, damp feeling at the back of the head. Sick headache radiating from one point. Temporary mental exaltation. Hallucination of hearing.

b. Middle/Rhythmic System

Heart - Anxious oppression. Precordial (area overlying the heart) distress. Palpitation; unable to lie on the left side. Fluttering. Pulse is rapid, irregular and intermittent. **Emotional State** - Ill-humored. Restless.

c. Metabolic/Limb System

Stomach - Sinking sensation of the epigastrum (upper middle portion of the abdomen). Faint, going away feeling in the stomach. One craves acidic food and drinks. There is the sudden production of gases in large quantities. **Abdomen** - Liability to hernia. **Female** - Soreness and tenderness in the ovaries. **Sleep** - Sleepy in the daytime but sleepless at night, with vascular excitement and restlessness, and dry skin. Horrible dreams cause no horror.

DOSE - Third to thirtieth potency.

PARTS UTILIZED - Dried crushed leaves in medium-strong alcohol, or fresh whole plant in strong alcohol.

45. VERBENA OFFICINALIS Linn.

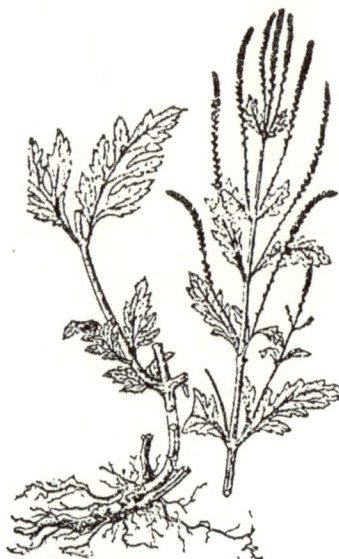

Local Name: *Blue Verbain*

Properties and Action:

This plant is an astringent (causes contraction and stops discharges) and a tonic (induces muscular tightness). It promotes the absorption of blood and alleviates pain in bruises. It also affects the skin and nervous system.

Conditions Most Used For:

Verbain is used in nervous depression, general body weakness, and when there is irritation and spasms in any part of the body. It is one of the remedies for passive congestion and intermittent fever. It is also helpful in epilepsy, insomnia, and mental exhaustion. In epilepsy, it brightens up the patient's mental power. It is applied directly to the skin in cases of vesicular erysipelas (infection of the skin with streptococci).

DOSE - Single dose of the tincture. In epilepsy, however, it must be continued for a long time. Verbain made into a tea is a good diuretic drink to eliminate toxins.

PARTS UTILIZED - Crushed fresh whole plant in medium-strong alcohol.

46. ZEA MAYS Linn.

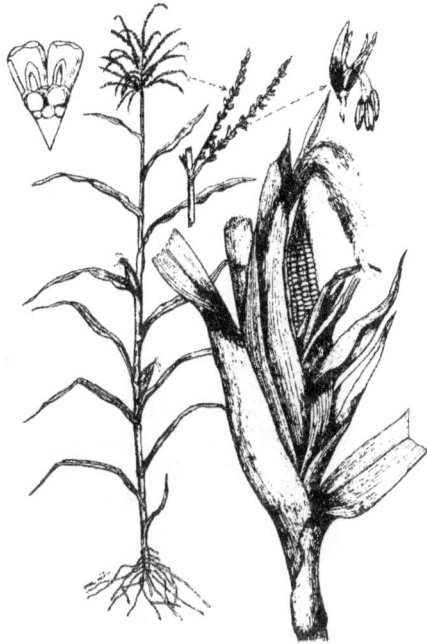

Local Names: *Maiz (Spanish); Maize, Indian Corn (English)*

Properties and Action:

Corn silk has a marked action on the urinary system. Though only a weak diuretic, it promotes the excretion of chlorides.

Conditions Most Used For:

Corn silk is best given to those who are suffering from chronic nephritis, hypertension, diabetes, and organic heart disease with much edema of lower extremities and scanty urination.

Other Conditions:

a. Metabolic/Limb System

Urinary - Suppression and unnecessary retention of urine. Dysuria (painful urination). Renal lithiasis (stone formation); nephritic colic (spasms); blood and red sand in the urine. Tenesmus (spasm of the bladder) after urinating.

Vesical (bladder) catarrh. Cystitis (inflammation of the bladder). Enlarged prostate. Uric and phosphatic (containing phosphoric acid). Gonorrhea.

DOSE - Tincture in ten- to fifty-drop doses.

PARTS UTILIZED - Corn silk in medium-strong alcohol.

47. ZINGIBER OFFICINALE Bose.

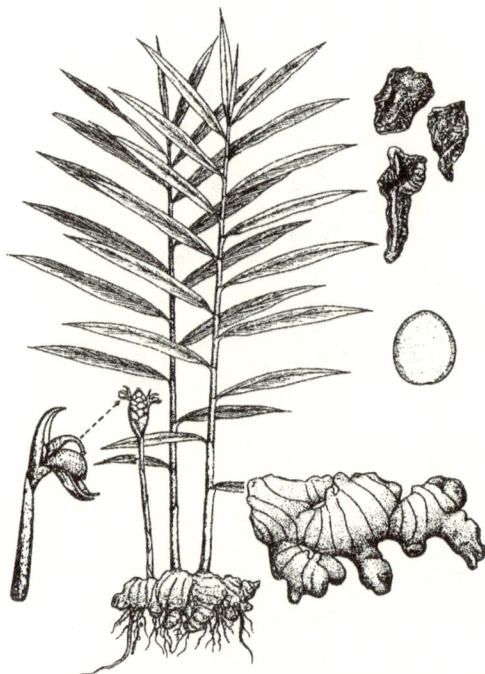

Local Names: *Gengibre (Spanish); Ginger (English)*

Properties and Actions:

Ginger contains a variety of oils, zingiberene being one of them. These oils give ginger a stomachic (gastric stimulant) and an antirheumatic (if given externally) quality.

Conditions Most Used For:

Ginger is best for the states of debility in the digestive tract, sexual system, respiratory troubles, and the complete cessation of the function of the kidneys.

Other Conditions:

a. Nerve Sense System

Head - Hemicrania (one-sided headache); sudden glimmering before the eyes. Head feels confused and empty. Pain over the eyebrows. **Nose** - Feels obstructed and dry. Intolerable itching with red pimples.

b. Middle/Rhythmic System

Respiratory - Hoarseness of voice. Sharp pain below the larynx; breathing is difficult. Asthma but without anxiety, becoming worse towards the morning. Scratching sensation in the throat; stitches in the chest. Cough is dry, hacking, and copious.

c. Metabolic/Limb System

Stomach - Taste of food remains for a long time, especially that of bread and toast. Stomach feels heavy, like containing a stone. Stomach disorders resulting from eating melons and from drinking impure water. Stomach acidity. Heaviness in the stomach upon awakening with gases and rumbling, great thirst and emptiness. Pain from the pit to under the sternum, becoming worse by eating. **Bowel Movement** - Colic, diarrhea, with extremely loose bowel movements. Diarrhea from drinking bad water, with much flatulence, cutting pain in the abdomen. Hot, sore, painful anus during pregnancy. Chronic intestinal catarrh. Anus is red and inflamed. Hemorrhoid is hot, painful, and sore. **Urinary** - Frequent desire to urinate. Stinging, burning in the orifice (opening). Yellow discharge from the urethra. Urine is thick, turbid, of strong odor and suppressed. Complete suppression of urinary functions after a typhoid fever. After urinating, urine continues to ooze in drops. **Male** - Itching of prepuce (foreskin of the penis). Enhanced sexual desire. Painful erections or emissions. **Extremities** - Very weak feeling in all the joints. The back is lame. Cramps in the sole and palms of the hands and feet.

DOSE - First to sixth potency.

PARTS UTILIZED - Powdered root in strong alcohol, or fresh root in strong alcohol.

Chapter Five

🌿

Animals

1. APIS MELLIFERA

Local Name: *Honey Bee*

Properties and Action:

The sting of the honey bee causes the edema of skins and mucous membranes. Once processed as a potentized remedy, it acts on the outer parts of the skin, and coatings of inner organs and serous membranes (lining tissues of the body that are moistened by a fluid resembling the serum of the blood).

Conditions Most Used For:

The remedy is given to any swelling or puffing up of various parts of the body, such as in edema (accumulation of fluids), stinging pains, soreness, intolerance of heat, and others. The above conditions tend to become worse at the slightest touch, and towards the afternoon.

Other Conditions:

a. Nerve Sense System

Head - Irritation of the meninges (the tissue that nourishes the brain). Serous meningitis. The whole brain feels very tired. Vertigo with sneezing, becoming worse on lying down or closing the eyes. Heat, throbbing pains, becoming better on applying pressure, but worse while in motion. Sudden piercing pains. Pain around the orbits of the eyes. Serous exudation (discharge), edema, and sharp pains. Suppurative (infection), inflammation of the eyes. Keratitis (inflammation of the cornea of the eye). Styes (inflammation of the glands in the eyelids). **Ears** - External ear is red, inflamed, and sore with stinging pains. **Nose** - Coldness of the tip of the nose. Nose is red, swollen, inflamed, with sharp pains. **Face** - Swollen, red, with piercing pain. Waxy, pale, edematous (watery). Erysipelas (skin infection) with stinging burning edema. **Mouth** - Tongue is fiery red, swollen, sore, and raw, with blisters. Scalding (injured by burning) in the mouth and throat. Tongue feels scalded, red hot, trembling. Gums and lips are swollen, especially the upper portion. Membrane of the mouth and throat is glossy, as if varnished. Red, shining, and puffy, like erysipelas (infection of the skin with streptoccoct). Cancer of the tongue. **Throat** - Constricted, stinging pains. Uvula swollen, sac-like. Throat is swollen, inside and out; tonsils are swollen, puffy, fiery red, beginning on the right side. Ulcers on the tonsils. Sensation of a fish bone in the throat.

b. Middle/Rhythmic System

Emotional State - Apathy, indifference, and unconsciousness. Awkwardness; tendency to drop things readily. Stupor (state of decreased feeling), with sudden sharp cries. Stupor alternating with erotic mania. Sensation of dying. Listless; cannot think clearly or concentrate the mind to study. Jealous, fidgety, hard to please. Tearful. There is fright, rage, vexation, or grief. **Respiratory** - Hoarseness; dyspnea (breathing is hurried and difficult). Edema of the larynx. One feels as if he cannot draw another breath. Suffocation; short, dry cough. Hydrothorax (watery fluids in the pleural cavity of the lungs).

c. Metabolic/Limb System

Stomach - Sore feeling. Thirstless. Vomiting of food. Craving for milk. **Abdomen** - Sore, bruised upon pressure and when sneezing. Extremely tender. Dropsy of the abdomen. Peritonitis (inflammation of the lining tissue of the abdominal cavity). Swelling in the right groin. **Bowel Movement** - Involuntary discharge on every motion; anus seems open. Bloody but painless. Hemorrhoids, with stinging pain. Diarrhea: watery, yellow; like cholera infantum type. Cannot urinate without defecation. Feces dark, fetid, becoming worse after eating. Constipation; feels as if something would break upon straining. **Urinary** - Burning and sore when urinating. Suppressed, frequent and involuntary with stinging pain; scanty, highly colored. Incontinence (inability to control urination). Glomerolunephritis (inflammation of the kidneys). **Female** - Edema of the labia with soreness and stinging pains. Ovaritis; worse in the right ovary. Menses are suppressed with cerebral and head symptoms especially in young girls. Dysmenorrhea, with severe ovarian pains. Ovarian tumors. Metorrhagia (vaginal bleeding unrelated to the monthly period) profuse, with a heavy abdomen, faintness, stinging pain. Bearing down, as if menses were to appear. Metritis (inflammation of the uterus with stinging pains). Great tenderness over the abdomen and uterine region. **Extremities** - Edematous. Synovitis (inflammation of the lining of a joint). Felon (infection of the far end and inner surface of a finger) is beginning. Knee is swollen, shiny, sensitive, sore, with stinging pain. Feet are swollen and stiff. Feet feel too large; rheumatic pain in the back and limbs. Hands and tips of the fingers are numb. **Skin** - Swelling after insect bites; sore, sensitive. Erysipelas with sensitiveness, swelling, and a rosy hue. Carbuncles, with burning, stinging pain. Hives (skin rashes) with intolerable itching. Sudden puffing up of the whole body. **Sleep** - Very drowsy. Dreams are full of care and toil. Screams and sudden starting characterize sleep. **Fever** - Afternoon chill with thirst becoming worse on motion and with heat. External heat, with suffocating feeling. Sweat is slight with sleepiness. Perspiration breaks out and dries up frequently. Sleep after a recurrence of fever.

DOSE - Tincture to thirtieth potency. During swelling of tissues, use the lower potencies. Sometimes the action of the remedy is slow. It may take several days for its effect to be noticed.

PARTS UTILIZED - Live honey bees in medium-strong alcohol.

2. BLATTA ORIENTALIS

Local Name: *Cockroach*

Properties and Action:

The chemicals extracted from the tincture of cockroach have a specific action on the vagus nerve (the tenth cranial nerve) providing parasympathetic innervation (nerve supply) to the larynx, lungs, heart, esophagus, and most of the abdominal organs.

Conditions Most Used For:

The extract of this animal is a remedy for bronchial asthma, cough with difficulty in breathing, bronchitis, and tuberculosis which are aggravated in bad, rainy weather. This remedy dissolves the mucus and reduces the number of attacks. It acts best in stout and obese patients.

DOSE - The lower potencies are preferred during an attack. In chronic cases, the higher potencies are used. One should stop taking this remedy when an improvement of the condition is already achieved.

PARTS UTILIZED - Whole cockroaches in strong alcohol.

3. FORMICA RUFA

Local Name: *Large Black Wood Ants*

Properties and Action:

The chemicals found in the tincture of wood ants have a marked deterrent influence on the formation of polypi and uric acid deposits.

Conditions Most Used For:

This is a good arthritic medicine, even in gout and rheumatism of the arteries where the right side shows more symptoms than the left. *Formica rufa* is also used in tuberculosis, neuralgias, hematuria (passing of blood in the urine), albuminuria (albumin in the urine) chronic nephritis (inflammation of the kidneys) and carcinoma (a particular type of cancer).

Other Conditions:

a. Nerve Sense System

Head - Vertigo. Brain feels too heavy and large. Sensation as if a bubble will burst in the forehead. Headache with cracking sound in the left ear. Coryza (acute nasal congestion). Rheumatic iritis (inflammation of the iris). Nasal polypi. **Ears** - Ringing and buzzing. Parts around the ear feel swollen. Polypi. **Skin** - Red, itching and burning. Nettle rash. Nodes around the joints. Profuse sweating without relief.

b. Middle/Rhythmic System

Respiratory - Hoarseness of the voice with dry, sore throat. Cough is worse at night, with an aching forehead and chest pains. Pleuritic (membrane that covers the lungs) pains in the lungs.

c. Metabolic/Limb System

Stomach - Constant pressure at the cardiac end of the stomach and a burning pain there. Nausea, with headache and vomiting of yellowish bitter mucus. Pain tends to shift from the stomach to the vertex (crown of the head). Gas from the stomach stagnates. **Bowel Movement** - In the morning, the passage of small quantities of gas is difficult; afterwards diarrhea-like urging in the rectum persist. Pain in the bowels before movement, with shuddering chilliness. Constriction in the anus. Drawing pain around the navel before defecation. **Urine** - Bloody, albuminous, with much urging and quantities of urates (a salt of uric acid). **Extremities** - Rheumatic pains; stiff and contracted joints. Muscles feel strained and torn from their attachment. Weakness of the lower extremities. Paraplegia (loss of motion and sensation in the legs and lower part of the body). Pain in the hips.

DOSE - Sixth to thirtieth potency.

PARTS UTILIZED - Live ants in medium-strong alcohol.

4. LAC DEFLORATUM

Local Name: *Skimmed Milk*

Properties and Action:

Skimmed milk is a remedy for illnesses with faulty nutrition.

Conditions Most Used For:

Skimmed milk is best given to those suffering from toxoplasmosis (an illness caused by a protozoa), which is often accompanied by hard stool and anal fissures.

Other Conditions:

a. Nerve Sense System

Head - Headache in the morning upon rising, moving from the forehead to the occiput with accompanying visual disturbance, nausea, and vomiting, becoming worse during menstruation, while becoming better by applying pressure or by bandaging head tightly. Headaches with a profuse flow of urine during pains. Car- or sea-sickness.

b. Metabolic/Limb System

Bowel Movement - Constipation. Stools are hard, large, requiring great straining. Movement is painful, lacerating the anus.

DOSE - Sixth to thirtieth potency.

PARTS UTILIZED - Take fresh unpasteurized skimmed milk and potentize in weak alcohol.

5. MEDUSSA

Local Name*: Jellyfish*

Properties and Action:

Upon direct contact with the tentacles of this variety of jellyfish, one experiences stinging pain and the skin reacts by developing small sacs filled with fluids.

Conditions Most Used For:

Jellyfish is used in any case of edema (unnecessary retention of fluids) and skin problems, for example, when the whole face is puffed. The skin shows numbness, burning, pricking heat, and vesicular eruptions (small sac filled with fluids), especially on the face, arms, shoulders, and breasts. The extract of this animal is also good for nettle rashes.

DOSE - Tincture to sixth potency.

PARTS UTILIZED - Whole jellyfish in strong alcohol.

Bibliography

Books

Aeppli, Willi. *The Care and Development of the Human Senses.* Forest Row, UK: Steiner Waldorf School Fellowship; 1998.

Arms, Suzanne. *Immaculate Deception: A New Look at Women and Childbirth.* New York: Bantam Books; 1977.

Augros, Robert and Stanciu, George. *The New Story of Science: Mind and the Universe.* New York: Bantam Books; 1984.

Bauman E et al. *The Holistic Health Book.* Compiled by the Berkeley Holistic Health Center. Berkeley: AND/OR Press; 1978.

Beinfield, Harriet and Korngold, Efrem. *Between Heaven and Earth: A Guide to Chinese Medicine.* New York: Ballantine Books; 1991.

Berger, Stuart M. *What Your Doctor Didn't Learn in Medical School.* New York: Avon Books; 1989.

Bianchi, Ivo. *Principles of Homotoxicology.* Baden Baden: Aurelia-Verlag; 1988.

Bing, Elizabeth. *Six Practical Lessons for an Easier Childbirth.* New York: Bantam Books; 1977.

Boericke, William. *Pocket Manual of Homeopathic Materia Medica.* Philadelphia: Boericke and Runyon and Tafel, Inc.; 1927.

Brazelton, Berry T. *Raising Children Toxic Free.* New York: Avon Books; 1995.

Bresantz, Hagen and Klingborg, Arne. *The Goetheanum: Rudolf Steiner's Architectural Impulse.* London: Rudolf Steiner Press; 1979.

Callen, Michael. *Surviving Aids.* New York: Harper Colllins; 1991.

Carpenter, Malcolm B. *Core Text of Neuroanatomy.* 4th ed. Baltimore: Williams & Wilkins; 1991.

Carter, James P. *Racketeering in Medicine: The Suppression of Alternatives.* Norfolk, VA: Hampton Roads Publishing Co. Inc.; 1992.

Castaneda, Carlos. *The Teachings of Dun Juan: A Yaqui Way of Knowledge.* New York: Pocket Books; 1971.

Caufield, Catherine. *Multiple Exposures.* London: Seeker and Warburg; 1989.

Childs, Gilbert. *Steiner Education in Theory and Practice.* Edinburgh: Floris Books; 1991.

Chopra, Deepak. *Quantum Healing: Exploring the Frontiers of Mind/Body Medicine.* New York: Bantam Books; 1989.

_____. *Ageless Body, Timeless Mind.* New York: Harmony Books; 1993.

Clarke, John Henry. *A Dictionary of Practical Materia Medica.* Vols. 1-3. London: The Homeopathic Publishing Co.; 1925.

Co, Leonardo L. *Common Medicinal Plants of the Cordillera.* Baguio City, Philippines: Community Health Education, Services and Training in the Cordillera Region (CHESTCORE); 1989.

Collier, Joe. *The Health Conspiracy.* London: Century Hutchinson Ltd.; 1989.

Cordero, A. A. *Proven Drugless Remedies for Acute Diseases.* 1414 Roxas Blvd, Ermita, Manila: Science of Nature Healing Center.

Coultier, Harris L. *Homoepathic Influences in 19th Century Allopathic Therapeutics: A Historical and Philosophical Study.* St. Louis, MO: Formur, Inc. Publishers; 1973.

Cowan, Thomas et al. *The Fourfold Path to Healing: Working with the Laws of Nutrition, Therapeutics, Movement and Meditation in the Art of Healing.* Washington, DC: New Trends Publishing, Inc.; 2004.

Crook, William. *The Yeast Connection.* New York: Vintage Books; 1986.

Davisson, Charles T. *Is Clinical Medicine a Science? Applications of Some Ideas of Owen Barfield in Clinical Medicine* [thesis]. Yale University School of Medicine; 1978.

Davy, John. *Work Arising from the Life of Rudolf Steiner.* Rudolf Steiner Press; 1975.

Diamond, Harvey and Diamond, Marilyn. *Fit For Life.* New York: Warner Books Inc.; 1987.

Dossey, Larry. *Healing Words.* San Francisco: Harper San Francisco; 1993.

Dudley, Nigel. *Good Health on a Polluted Planet.* London: Thorsons; 1991.

Duesberg, Peter. *Is AIDS Virus a Science Fiction?* Berkeley: University of California; 1990.

Dunselman, Ron. *In Place of Self: How Drugs Work.* UK: Hawthorn Press; 1995.

Edwards, David A. *Theory and Practice of Biological Medicine.* Reno, NV: International Biological Research Institute; 1995.

Emoto, Masaru. *The True Power of Water.* New York: Atria Books; 2005.

Fawcett, Ann and Smith, Cynthia. *Cancer Free: 30 Who Triumph Over Cancer Naturally.*

Compiled by East-West Foundation Japan Publication Inc.; New York.

Ferencz, Benjamin B. *Planethood: The Key to Your Survival and Prosperity.* Vision Books; 1988.

Fischer, Jeffrey A. *Breakthroughs in Health and Longevity by the Year 2000 and Beyond.* New York: Pocket Books; 1992.

Garb, Solomon. *Undesirable Drug Interaction.* New York: Springer; 1975.

Gloeckler, Langhammer, and Wiechert. *Education–Health for Life.* Dornach, Switzerland: Goetheanum [Medical and Pedagogical Sections]; 2006.

Gloeckler, Michaela and Goebel, Wolfgang. *A Guide to Child Health.* Edinburgh: Floris Books; 2003.

Gold, Cybele and Gold, E. J. *Joyous Childbirth: Manual for Conscious Natural Childbirth.* New York: Signet Book; 1977.

Goleman, Daniel. Emotional Intelligence. New York: Bantam Books; 1996.

Graedon, Joe. *The People's Pharmacy.* New York: Avon Books; 1976.

Griffin, Mark. *AIDS: The Apprenticeship.* 20, route du Vallon, CH 1224 Chene- Bougeries, Switzerland.

Hansmann, Henning. *Education for Special Needs.* Edinburgh: Floris Books; 1992.

Hauschka, Rudolf. *Nutrition.* Spock, Marjorie and Richards, Mary, trans. London: Rudolf Steiner Press; 1983.

Heidemann, Christel. *Meridien Therapie: Die Wiederherstel-lung der Ordnung lebendiger Prozesse.* 3. unveranderte Auflage; 1988.

Heller, Tom, Bailey, Lorna, and Pattison, Stephen, eds. *Preventing Cancers.* Open University Press; 1992.

Hodgkinson, Neville. *Will to Be Well: The Real Alternative Medicine.* London: Hutchinson Publishing Group; 1984.

Honorof, Ida and McBean, E. *Vaccination The Silent Killer: A Clear and Present Danger.* Honor Publications, Sherman Oaks, CA; 1977.

Husemann, Friedrich and Wolff, Otto. *The Anthroposophical Approach to Medicine.* Vol 1. Spring Valley, NY: The Anthroposophic Press; 1982.

_____. *The Anthroposophical Approach to Medicine.* Vol 2. Hudson, NY: The Anthroposophic Press; 1987.

_____. *The Anthroposophical Approach to Medicine.* Vol 3. Hudson, NY: The

Anthroposophic Press; 1989.

Illich, Ivan. Limits to medicine. In *Medical Nemesis: The Expropriation of Health*. Penguin Books; 1977.

Jarvis D. C. *Folk Medicine*. New York: Faucett Publication, Inc.; 1967.

Kaptchuk, Ted and Croucher, Michael. *The Healing Arts*. British Broadcasting Corp.; 1986.

Kavanaugh, Philip. *Magnificent Addiction: Discovering Addiction as Gateway to Healing*. Lower Lake, CA: Asian Publishing; 1992.

Kenmmore, Peter E. *Integrated Pest Management: A Model for Asia*. FAO Rice IPC Programme; FAO, P.O. Box 1864, Manila, Philippines; 1991.

Kidel, Mark and Rowe-Leete, Susan, eds. *The Meaning of Illness*. London: Routledge; 1988.

Kimbrell, Andrew. *The Human Body Shop: The Engineering and Marketing of Life*. Penang, Malaysia: Third World Network; 1993.

King, Francis X. *Rudolf Steiner and Holistic Medicine*. Maine: Nicolas-Hays, Inc.; 1986.

Koepf, Herbert et al. *Bio-Dynamic Agriculture*. Spring Valley, NY: The Anthroposophic Press; 1976.

Kolisko, Lily. *Physiologischer und Physikalischer Nachweis der Wirksamkeit Kleinster Entitaten*. Stuttgart, Adelheidweg 4: Herausgegeben durch die Arbeitsgemeinschaft anthroposophischer Arzte; 1921.

_____. *Spirit in Matter*. Bournemouth: Kolisko Archive Publication.

Kuhlewind, Georg. *From Normal to Healthy: Paths to the Liberation of Consciousness*. Great Barrington, MA: Lindisfarne Press; 1988.

Lamaze, Fernand. *Painless Childbirth: The Lamaze Method*. New York: Pocket Books; 1972.

Lappe, Frances Moore. *Diet for a Small Planet*. New York: Ballantine Books; 1971.

Large, Martin. *Who is Bringing Them Up? Television and Child Development: How to Break the T.V. Habit*. UK: Hawthorn Press; 1980.

LeVert, Suzanne. *Melatonin: The Anti-Aging Hormone*. New York: Avon Books; 1995.

Lievegoed, Bernard. *Phases: Crisis and Development in the Individual*. London: Rudolf Steiner Press; 1979.

_____. *Man on the Threshold: The Challenge of Inner Development*. UK: Hawthorn Press; 1985.

Lucas, Richard. *Nature's Medicine: The Folklore, Romance, and Value of Herbal Remedies*. New

York: Parker Publishing Company, Inc.; 1966.

Mander, Jerry. *Four Arguments for the Elimination of Television.* New York: Quill; 1977.

Mann, Felix. *Acupuncture: The Ancient Chinese Art of Healing.* 2nd ed. London: William Heinemann Medical Books Ltd.; 1971.

Martin, Eric. *Hazards of Medications: A Manual on Drug Interaction, Incompatibilities, Contraindications and Adverse Effects.* Philadelphia: J. B. Lippincott; 1995.

Matsen, Jonn. *The Mysterious Causes of Illnesses.* Canfield, Ohio: Fischer Publishing Corp.; 1987.

McKeown, T. *The Role of Medicine: Dream, Mirage or Nemesis?* Princeton, NJ: Princeton University Press; 1979.

McTaggart, Lynne. *What Doctors Don't Tell You.* New York: Avon Books; 1998.

Meek, Jennifer. *Sick Earth Symdrome and How to Survive it.* London: Optima Book; 1992.

Mees, L. *Blessed by Illness.* New York: Anthroposophic Press; 1990.

Mendelsohn, Robert S. *Confessions of a Medical Heretic.* New York: Warner Books Inc.; 1980.

_____. *Male Practice: How Doctors Manipulate Women.* Chicago: Contemporary Books, Inc.; 1982.

_____. *How to Raise A Healthy Child In Spite of Your Doctor.* Chicago: Contemporary Books, Inc.; 1984.

Murphy, Jamie. *What Every Parents Should Know About Immunization.* Boston: Earth Healing Products; 1994.

Nicholls, Philipp A. *Homeopathy and the Medical Profession.* London: Croom Helm Ltd.; 1988.

Olsen, Kristin Gottschalk. *The Encyclopedia of Alternative Health Care.* New York: Pocket Books; 1990.

Otto, James H. et al. *Modern Health.* New York: Holt, Rinehart and Winston Publisher; 1985.

Pearce, Joseph Chilton. *Magical Child: Rediscovering Nature's Plan for Our Children.* New York: Bantam Books; 1977.

_____. *The Biology of Transcendence: A Blueprint of the Human Spirit.* Vermont: Park Street Press; 2002.

Perlas, Nicanor III. *Overcoming Illusions About Biotechnology.* Penang, Malaysia: Third World

Network; 1994.

_____. *Shaping Globalization: Civil Society, Cultural Power and Threefolding*. CADI, unit 718 CityLand MegaPlaza, Ortigas, Pasig City, Philippines; 2000.

Pokert, Manfred. *The Essentials of Chinese Diagnostics*. Zurich: Chinese Medicine Publications Ltd.; 1983.

P.S.I. & Associates, Inc. *Home Medical Dictionary*. Miami: Ottemheimer Publisher, Inc.; 1992.

Quisumbing, Eduardo. *Medicinal Plants of the Philippines*. Quezon City: Katha Publishing Co., Inc.; 1978.

Reckeweg, Hans-Heinrich. *Homotoxicology: Illness and Healing through Anti-Homotoxic Therapy*. Albuquerque: Menaco Publishing Co. Inc.; 1980.

_____. Materia medica. In: *Homoeopathia Antihomotoxica*. Vol 1. Baden-Baden: Aurelia-Verlug.

Renzenbrink, Udo. *Diet and Cancer: An Anthroposophical Contribution to Cancer Prevention*. London: Rudolf Steiner Press; 1988.

Rhodes, Philip. *An Outline History of Medicine*. London: Butterworths; 1985.

Richter, G. *Art and Human Consciousness*. Spring Valley, NY: Anthroposophic Press; 1985.

Rowland, David. *Vascular Cleansing: A New Hope for Heart Disease*. Uxbridge: Canadian Nutrition Institution Inc.; 1986.

Ruesch, Hans. *Naked Empress or The Great Medical Fraud*. Klosters, Switzerland: Civis Publication.

Sadler, T. W. *Langman's Medical Embryology*. 7th ed. Baltimore: Williams & Wilkins; 1995.

Sagan, Carl. *The Dragons of Eden*. New York: Ballantine Books; 1977.

Salter, Joan. *The Incarnating Child*. Gloucestershire: Hawthorn Press; 1987.

Sardello, Robert. *Freeing the Soul From Fear*. New York: Riverhead Books; 2001.

_____. *The Power of Soul: Living the Twelve Virtues*. Charlottesville, VA: Hampton Roads Publishing Company; 2002.

_____. *Love and the Soul: Creating a Future for Earth*. Berkeley, CA: Goldenstone Press, Heaven & Earth Publishing, and North Atlantic Books; 2008.

Schad, Wolfgang. *Man and Mammals: Towards a Biology of Form*. Scherer, Carrol, trans. New York: Waldorf Press; 1977.

Scheffer, Mechthild. *Bach Flower Therapy: Theory and Practice.* Thorsons Publisher, Inc.; 1993.

Scheibner, Viera. Vaccination: *100 Years of Orthodox Research Shows that Vaccines Represent a Medical Assault on the Immune System.* Victoria: Australian Print Group; 1993.

Schindler, Maria. *Goethe's Theory of Colour.* Sussex: New Knowledge Books; 1964.

Schmidt, Gerhard. *The Dynamic of Nutrition.* Wyoming, Rhode Island: Bio-dynamic Literature; 1980.

_____. *The Essentials of Nutrition.* Wyoming, Rhode Island: Bio-dynamic Literature; 1987.

Schrag, Peter and Divoky Diane. *The Myth of the Hyperactive Child and Other Means of Child Control.* New York: Pantheon Books; 1975.

Schwenk, Theodore. *Sensitive Chaos: The Creation of Flowing Forms in Water and Air.* London: Rudolf Steiner Press; 1965.

_____. *The Basis of Potentization Research.* Spring Valley, NY: Mercury Press; 1988.

Scully, Diana. *Men Who Control Women's Health: The Miseducation of Obstetrician-Gynecologists.* Boston: Houghton Mifflin Company; 1980.

Siegel, Bernie. *Love, Medicine and Miracles: Lessons Learned About Self-Healing from A Surgeon's Experience with Exceptional Patients.* New York: Harper and Row, Publishers; 1990.

Sigman, Aric. *Remotely Controlled.* London: Vermillion; 2005.

Sorokin, P. A. *Social and Cultural Dynamics.* 4 vols. New York: Bedminster Press; 1963.

Sousa, Marion. *Childbirth At Home.* New York: Bantam Books; 1976.

Steiner, Rudolf. *Knowledge of Higher Worlds and Its Attainment.* Spring Valley, NY: Anthroposophic Press; 1947.

_____. *The Course of My Life.* Bell's Pond, Hudson, NY: The Anthroposohic Press; 1951.

_____. *The Arts and Their Mission.* New York: Anthroposophic Press; 1964.

_____. *A Lecture on Eurythmy.* London: Rudolf Steiner Press; 1967.

_____. *A Theory of Knowledge Implicit in Goethe's World Conception.* Spring Valley, NY: Anthroposophic Press; 1968.

_____. *Theosophy: An Introduction to the Supersensible Knowledge of the World and the Destination of Man.* New York: Anthroposophical Press; 1971.

_____. *Occult Science: An Outline.* New York: Anthroposophic Press; 1972.

_____. *Spiritual Science and Medicine*. London: Rudolf Steiner Press; 1975.

_____. *Agriculture*. London: Bio-Dynamic Agriculture Association; 1977.

_____. *Cosmic Memory: Prehistory of Earth and Man*. San Francisco: Harper and Row Publisher; 1981.

_____. *The Philosophy of Spiritual Activity*. New York: Anthroposophic Press; 1986.

Steiner, Rudolph and Wegman, Ita. *Fundamentals of Therapy*. London: Rudolf Steiner Press; 1925.

Stiefvater, Eric. *What Is Acupuncture? How Does It Work?* Sussex, England: Health Science Press, Rustlington; 1971.

Szasz, Thomas. *Pharmacracy: Medicine and Politics in America*. New York: Syracuse University Press; 2003.

Treichler, Rudolf. *Soulways*. UK: Hawthorn Press; 1989.

Twentyman, Ralph. *The Science and Art of Healing*. Edinburgh: Foris Books; 1989.

Ulett, George A. *Principles and Practice of Physiologic Acupuncture*. St. Louis, MO: Warren H. Green, Inc.; 1982.

Ullman, Dana. *Homeopathy: Medicine for the 21st Century*. Berkeley: North Atlantic Books; 1988.

Vithoulkas, George. *Homeopathy: Medicine of the New Man*. New York: Avon Books; 1971.

Vogel, Heinz Hartmut. *The Skin: The Development Morphology, Physiology, and Pathology of the Skin with Indications for the Treatment of Skin Diseases*. D7325 Eckwaelden/Bad Boll, West Germany: WALA Literature; 19–.

Wachsmuth, Guenther. *The Etheric Formative Forces in Cosmos, Earth and Man: A Path of Investigation into the World of the Living*. London: Anthroposohical Publishing; 1932.

Waldron, K. W. Johnson I. T., and Fenwick G. R., eds. *Food and Cancer Prevention: Chemical and Biological Aspects*. Cambridge, UK: The Royal Society of Chemistry; 1993.

Weiner, Michael and Goss, Kathleen. *The Complete Book of Homeopathy*. New York: Bantam Books; 1982.

Winn, Marie. *The Plug-In Drug*. Penguin Books; 1977.

Wolf, Adolf Hungry. *The Good Medicine Book: The Wisdom of the Old Ones—Their Legends, Crafts and Sacred Ways*. New York: Warner Communications Company; 1973.

The American Homeopathic Pharmacopea. 10th ed. Philadelphia: Boericke and Tafel; 1926.

The Essentials of Chinese Acupuncture. Beijing: Foreign Languages Press; 1979.

Journals

Adler J et al. Clone hype. *Newsweek* Nov 8, 1993:42-44.

_____. AIDS minus HIV. *Lancet* 1992(Aug);340:280.

AIDS may not develop for 20 years in HIV sufferers. *Philippine Star* July 31, 1994:19.

Altrow AB. Rethinking cancer. *Lancet* 1994(Feb);343:494-495.

Amato. Molecular divorce gives strange vibes. *Science News* 1986(Nov):277-278.

Argentine Episiotomy Trial Collaborative Group. Routine versus selective episiotomy: a randomised controlled trial. *Lancet* 1993(Dec);342:1517-1518.

Arshad SH et al. Effect of allergen avoidance on development of allergic disorders in infancy. *Lancet* 1992(June);339:1493-1497.

Austoker J. Cancer prevention in primary health care: diet and cancer. *British Medical Journal* 1994(June);308:1610-1614.

_____. Cancer prevention in primary care: screening for ovarian, prostatic, and testicular cancers. *British Medical Journal* 1994(July);309:315-320.

Bailar JC III, Smith EL. Progress against cancer? *New England Journal of Medicine* 1986(May);314:1226-1232.

Barker JP et al. Fetal nutrition and cardiovascular disease in adult life. *Lancet* 1993(April);341:938-941.

Barret JFR et al. Absorption of non-haem iron from food during normal pregnancy. *British Medical Journal* 1994(July);309:79-82.

Begley S. Beyond vitamins. *Newsweek* April 25, 1994:42-47.

_____. The end of antibiotics? Medicine: A 'nightmare' in the making. *Newsweek* March 7, 1994:44.

Benjamin CM et al. Joint and limb symptoms in children after immunization with measles, mumps and rubella vaccines. *British Medical Journal* 1992(April);304:1075-1078.

Birchall JD, Chappel JS. Aluminum, chemical physiology and Alzheimer's disease. *Lancet* 1988(October):1008-1010.

Black WE et al. Advances in diagnostic imaging and overestimation of disease prevalence and the benefits of therapy. *New England Journal of Medicine* 1993(April);328:1237-1243.

Bray GP. Liver failure induced by paracetamol. *British Medical Journal* 1993(Jan);306:157-158.

Brennan TA et al. Incidence of adverse events and negligence in hospitalized patients. *New England Journal of Medicine* 1991(Feb);324:370-376.

Breast Cancer Prevention Collaborative Group. Breast cancer: environmental factors. *Lancet* 1992(Oct);340:904.

Bucher HC, Schimidt JG. Does routine ultrasound scanning improve outcome in pregnancy? Meta-analysis of various outcome measures. *British Medical Journal* 1993(July);307:13-17.

Buckman R, Lewith G. What does homeopathy do and how? *British Medical Journal* 1994(July);309:103-106.

Buenaviste J et al. Human basophil degranulation triggered by very diluted anti-serum against IgE. *Nature* 1988(June);333:816-818.

Bunin GP et al. Relation between maternal diet and subsequent primitive neuroectodermal brain tumours in young children. *New England Journal of Medicine* 1993(Aug);329:536-541.

Carpenter L. Cancer in laboratory workers. *Lancet* 1991(Oct);338:1080-1081.

100,000 Chinese dying from wrong medicine: UPI release. *Philippine Star* May 23, 1995.

Christie C et al. The 1993 epidemic of pertusis in Cincinnati: resurgence of disease in a highly immunized population of children. *New England Journal of Medicine* 1994;331:16-21.

Coghlan A. Biotechnology faces trial by jury. *New Scientist* 1994(Nov):5.

Collier JG, Herxheimer A. Roussel convicted of misleading promotion. *Lancet* 1987(Jan):113-114.

Collier JG. Rules of conduct and the pharmaceutical industry. *Lancet* 1984(Jan):453.

Collier JG. New L. Illegibility of drug advertisements. *Lancet* 1984(Jan):341-342.

Collier JG, Pilkington TRE. Human insulin: a misleading advertisement. *British Medical Journal* 1984;xx:289-291.

Combe C, Aparicio M. Body building, high protein diet, and progressive renal failure in chronic glomerulonephritis. *Lancet* 1993(Feb);341:380.

Cowley G. Are supplements still worth taking? *Newsweek* November 25, 1994:45.

_____. Red meat and prostate cancer. *Newsweek* October 25, 1993:48B.

_____. What high tech can't accomplish. *Newsweek* October 4, 1993:42

Czeizel A et al. Smoking during pregnancy and congenital limb deficiency. *British Medical Journal* 1994(Feb);308:1473-1476.

Daems WF. The process as a factor in quality. *Man and Remedy: WELEDA Newsletter for Physicians* May 1986.

Davenas E et al. Effect on mouse peritoneal macrophages of orally administered very high dilutions of silica. *European Journal of Pharmacology* 135(4t,7):313-319.

Dickson D. Critics still lay blame for AIDS on lifestyle, not HIV. *Nature* 194(June);369:434.

Dietary fibre: importance of function as well as amount. *Lancet* 1992(Nov);340:1133-1134.

Dorfman P, Lasserre MN, Tetau M. Preparation for birth by homeopathy: experimentation by double blind versus placebo. *Cahiers de Biotherapie* 1987(April);94:77-81.

Dossley L. Science and healing. *Resurgence* 161:21-25.

DOST warns on 'misinformation' in current biotechnology debate. *Business World* September 9, 1994.

Duesberg PH, Schwartz JR. Latent virus and mutated oncogenes: no evidence of pathogenicity. *Progress in Nucleic Acid Research and Molecular Biology* 1992;43:135-205.

Early warnings, early worries. *Economist* June 18, 1996:89-91.

East Anglian Multicenter Controlled Trial. Treatment of active Crohn's disease by exclusion diet. *Lancet* 1993(Nov);342:1131-1134.

Easterbrook PJ et al. Publication bias in clinical research. *Lancet* 1991(April);337:867-872.

Esmail A, Everington S. Racial discrimination against doctors from ethnic minorities. *British Medical Journal* 1993(March);306:691-692.

Eysenck HJ. Psychosocial factors, cancer, and ischaemic heart disease. *British Medical Journal* 1992(Aug);305:457-459.

Fat diet raises risk of lung cancer among non-smokers, study says. *Philippine Star* December 2, 1993.

FDA eyes painkiller warnings for heavy drinkers. *Philippine Star* July 8, 1993.

Farquharson J et al. Infant cerebral cortex: phospolipids fatty acid composition and diet. *Lancet* 1992; 340:810-813.

Ferley JP et al. A controlled evaluation of a homeopathic preparation in the treatment of influenza-like symptoms. *British Journal of Clinical Pharmacology* 1989;27:329-335.

Fischer P, Ward A. Complementary medicine in Europe. *British Medical Journal* 1994(July);309:107-110.

de Francisco A et al. Acute toxicity of vitamin A given with vaccines in infancy. *Lancet* 1993(Aug);342:526-527.

Frequent prenatal ultrasound: time to think again. *Lancet* 1993(Oct);342:878-879.

Fugh-Bernan A, Epstein S. Tamoxifen: disease prevention or disease substitution? *Lancet* 1992(Nov)340:1143-1145.

Gantley M et al. Sudden infant death syndrome: links with infant care practices. *British Medical Journal* 1993(Jan);306:16-20.

Garenne M et al. Child mortality after high titre measle vaccine: prospect study in Senegal. *Lancet* 1991(Nov);338:903-907.

Garrow J. Starvation in hospitals. *British Medical Journal* 1994(April);308:934.

Gelman D et al. How will the clone feel? *Newsweek* November 8, 1993:46-47.

Gene test. *New Scientist* November 12, 1994:40-44

Gerber M. The psycho-motor development of African children in the first year, and the influence of maternal behavior. *Journal of Social Psychology* 1958;47:185-195.

_____. The state of development of newborn African children. *Lancet* 1957(June):1216-1219.

Gibson RG, Gibson SLM, MacNeil AD et al. Homeopathy therapy in rheumatoid arthritis: evaluation by double blind controlled trial, *British Journal of Clinical Pharmacology* 1980;9:453-459.

Gibson RG et al. Salicylates and homeopathy in rheumatoid arthritis: preliminary observation. *British Journal of Clinical Pharmacology* 1978;6:391-395.

Goodwin JS et al. The effect of marital status on stage treatment, and survival of cancer patients. *Journal of the American Medical Association* 1987(Dec);258:3125-3130.

Graham NMH et al. Adverse effects of aspirin, acetaminopehn, and ibuprofen on immune function, viral shedding, and clinical status in rhinovirus-infected volunteers. *Journal of Infectious Diseases* 1990;162:1277-1282.

Guillermo IIM et al. Vitamin A supplementation and child survival. *Lancet* 1992(Aug);340:267-671.

Gustafson TL et al. Measle outbreak in a full, immunized secondary-school population.

New England Journal of Medicine 1987;316:771-774.

Guttentag OE. Homeopathy in the light of modern pharmacology. *Clinical Pharmacology and Therapeutics* xxxx(7);966:426.

Hall A. Lessons from measle vaccination in developing countries. *British Medical Journal* 1993(Nov);307:1294-1295.

Halliwell B. Free radicals and vascular disease: how much do we know? *British Medical Journal* 1993(Oct);307:885-886.

Hampton JR, Julian DG. Role of pharmaceutical industry in major clinical trials. *Lancet* 1987;2:1258-1259.

Haney DQ. Fungal infection emerge as major health threat. *Philippine Star* November 28, 1993.

Hassan W, Oldham R. Reiter's syndrome and reactive arthritis in health care workers after vaccination. *British Medical Journal* 1994(July);309:94.

Hedegaard M et al. Psychological distress in pregnancy and pre-term delivery. *British Medical Journal* 1993(July);307:234-239.

Hedlund JU et al. Risk of pneumonia in patients previously treated in hospital for pneumonia. *Lancet* 1992(Aug);340:396-397.

Herroben L et al. Central nervous system demyelination after immunization with recombinant hepatitis B vaccine. *Lancet* 1991(Nov);338:1174-1175.

Hersh BS et al. A measle outbreak at a college with prematriculation immunization requirement. *American Journal of Public Health* 1991;81:360-364.

Hideo O et al. Long-term effects of a cholesterol free diet on serum cholesterol levels of Zen monks. *New England Journal of Medicine* 1992(Feb)326:416.

High protein diet may promote kidney cancer. *Philippine Star* August 4, 1994:21.

Hishida O et al. Clinically diagnosed AIDS cases without evident association with HIV type 1 and 2 infections in Ghana. *Lancet* 1992(Oct);340:971-972.

Hubbard R, Wald E. The eugenics of normalcy: the politics of gene research. *The Ecologist* 1993(Sep-Oct);23:185-191.

Hunter D. Breast cancer: nutritional factors. *Lancet* 1992(Oct);340:905.

Idjradinita P et al. Adverse effects of iron supplementation in weight gain on iron-replete young children. *Lancet* 1994(May);343:1252-1254.

Jacobs J et al. Treatment of acute childhood diarrhea with homeopathic medicine: a randomized clinical trial in Nicaragua. *Pediatrics* 1994;93:719-725.

Jacobus CH et al. Hypervitaminosis 0 associated with drinking milk. *New England Journal of Medicine* 1992(April);326:1173-1177.

Jensen B, Pakkenberg B. Do alcoholics drink their neurons away? *Lancet* 1993(Nov);342:1201-1204.

Kenmore PE. Integrated pest management: a model for Asia. *FAG Rice IPC Programme* 1991; FAO, P.O. Box 1864, Manila, Philippines.

Kilburn KH. Epidemics then and now: chemicals replace microbes and degeneration oust infections. *Archives of Environmental Medicine* 1994(Jan-Feb);49(1):3-5.

Kimmond S et al. Umbilical cord clamping and pre term infants: a randomized trial. *British Medical Journal* 1993(Jan);306:1722-1725.

Kjeldsen-Kragh J et al. Controlled trial of fasting and one-year vegetarian diet in rheumatoid arthritis. *Lancet* 1991(Oct);338:899-902.

Kleijnen J, Knipschild P, ter Riet G. Clinical trials of homeopathy. *British Medical Journal* 1991(Feb);302:316-323.

Kluger MJ, Ringler DH. Fever and survival. *Science* 1975(April);188:166-168.

_____. Fever: effect of drug-induced anti-pyresis on survival. *Science* 1976(July);193:237-239.

Kyle W. Simian retroviruses, poliovaccine and origin of AIDS. *Lancet* 1992(March);339:600-601.

Lauren J. et al. Acquired immunodeficiency syndrome without evidence of infection with HIV type 1 and 2. *Lancet* 1992(Aug);340:273-274.

Lauritsen K et al. Withholding unfavorable results in drug company sponsored clinical trials. *Lancet* 1987;1:1091.

Leape LL et al. The nature of adverse events in hospitalized patients. *New England Journal of Medicine* 1991(Feb);324:377-384.

Lee HP et al. Dietary effects of breast cancer risk in Singapore. *Lancet* 1991(May);337:1197-2000.

Lewith G, Brown PK, Tyrell DAJ. Controlled study of the effects of homeopathic dilution of infuenza vaccine on antibody titres in man. *Complementary Medicine Research* 1989;3:22-24.

Life, industrialized. *New York Times* February 22, 1988.

Lissau I, Sorensen TLA. Parental neglect during childhood and increased risk of obesity in young adulthood. *Lancet* 1994(Feb);343:324-326.

Lucas A, Cole TJ. Breast milk and neonatal necrotising enterocolitis. *Lancet* 1990(Dec);336:1519-1523.

Lucas A et al. Breast milk and subsequent intelligence quotient in children born pre-term. *Lancet* 1992(Feb);339:261-264.

Maddox J. Is molecular biology yet a science? *Nature* 1992(Jan);355:201.

Mauricio L. Four Kidney Institute doctors facing murder charges. *Philippine Star* August 25, 1994:1, 3.

McKinley S, McKinley J. The questionable contribution of medical measures to the decline of mortality in the United States in the twentieth century. *Milbank Memorial Fund Quarterly* 1997(Summer):405-430.

McWhirter JP, Pennington CR. Incidence and recognition of malnutrition in hospitals. *British Medical Journal* 1994(April);308:945-948.

Miller E et al. Risk of asceptic meningitis after measles, mumps and rubella vaccines in UK children. *Lancet* 1993(April);341:979-981.

Mittra L. Breast screening: the case for physical examination without mammography. *Lancet* 1994(Feb);343:342-344.

Mortimer PP. The fallibility of HIV western blot. *Lancet* 1991(Feb);337:286-287.

Murphy BK. The politics of AIDS. *Third World Resurgence* 47:33-40.

Mayaux MJ, Guihard-Moscato ML, Schwarz D et al. Controlled clinical trial of homeopathy in post operative ileus. *Lancet* 1988(xx):528-529.

Nash MJ. Stopping cancer in its tracks. *Time Magazine* April 25, 1994:38-44.

Neri LC. Aluminum, Alzheimer's disease and drinking water. *Lancet* 1991(Aug);337:390.

Neunham JP et al. Effects of frequent ultrasound during pregnancy: a random controlled trial. *Lancet* 1993(Oct);42:887-890.

Nosocomial infection with respiratory syncytial virus. *Lancet* 1992(Oct);340:1071-1073.

Obomsawin R. Traditional life styles and freedom from the dark seas of disease. *Community Development Journal* 1983(18);2:xx.

Olsson R et al. Centrolobular liver cell Necrosis: myocardial infarction and hyperamylasaemia after high dose of corticosteriods. *British Medical Journal* xxxx;308:454.

Otani H et al. Long-term effects of a cholesterol-free diet on serum cholesterol levels of Zen monks. *New England Journal of Medicine* 1992(Feb);326:446.

Otten MW Jr et al. Epidemic poliomyelitis in the gambia following the control of poliomyelitis as an edemic disease. *American Journal of Epidemiology* 1992;135:381-392.

Pablos-Mendez et al. Infectious prions or cytotoxic metabolites? *Lancet* 1993(Jan);341:159-161.

Pediatrician warns of Habitual soft drinks consumption. *Philippine Star* November 9, 1993.

Perlas N. When what could go wrong, did go wrong. *Third World Resurgence* 1993;38:8.

_____. The second scientific revolution and the Center for Alternative Development Initiatives. 110 Scout Rallos St., Quezon City, Philippines.

Perneger TV et al. Risk of kidney failure associated with the use of acetaminophen, aspirin, and nonsteriodal antiinflammatory drugs. *New England Journal of Medicine* 1994(Dec);331:1675-1679.

Philips D et al. Psychology and survival. *Lancet* 1993(Nov);342:1142-1145.

Philips D, King EW. Death takes a holiday: mortality surrounding major social occasions. *Lancet* 1988(xxx);xx:728-732.

Pillay D et al. Parvovirus B19 outbreak in a children's ward. *Lancet* 1992(Jan);339:107-109.

Pittet D et al. Nosocomial blood stream infection in critically ill patients: excess length of stay, extra cost and attributable mortality. *Journal of the American Medical Association* 1994(May);271:1598-1601.

Pisacane A et al. Breast feeding and multiple sclerosis. *British Medical Journal* 1994(Feb);308:1411-1412.

Polish LB et al. Nosocomial transmission of hepatitis B virus associated with the use of a spring-loaded finger-stick device. *New England Journal of Medicine* 1992(March);326:721-725.

Ponninghaus JM et al. Efficacy of BCG against leprosy and tuberculosis in Northern Malawi. *Lancet* 1992(March);339:636-639.

Purdey M. Degenerative nervous diseases and chemical pollution. *The Ecologist* 1994;24(3):100-105.

Reiley D. Young doctors' views on alternative medicine *British Medical Journal* 1983(July);287:337-339.

Reiley D et al. Is evidence for homeopathy reproducible? *Lancet* 1994(Dec);344:1601-1606.

Reiley D et al. Is homeopathy a placebo response? Controlled trial of homeopathy potency, with pollen in hayfever as model. *Lancet* 1986(Oct):881-886.

Reiley D et al. Is homeopathy a placebo response? A controlled trial of homeopathic immunotherapy (HIT) in atropic asthma. *Complementary Therapies in Medicine* 1993;1(suppl):24-25.

Riebel L. A homeopathic model of psychotherapy. *Journal of Humanistic Psychology* 1984(Winter);24:9-48.

Rivellese A et al. Long term metabolic efficacy of two dietary methods of treating hyperlipidaemia. *British Medical Journal* 1994(Jan);308:227-231.

Root-Bernstein RS. Do we know the cause of AIDS? *Perspectives in Biology and Medicine* 1990(Summer);33(4):480-500.

Sainte L, Haynes JD, Gerswin G. Inhibition of whole blood dilutions on basophil degranulation. *International Journal of Immunotherapy* 1986(2):247-250.

Saracci R et al. Cancer mortality in workers exposed to cholophenoxy-herbicides and chlorophenols. *Lancet* 1991(Oct);338:1027-1032.

Schardt D. Phytochemicals: plants against cancer. *Philippine Star* August 20, 1994:27, 29.

Schjelderup W. The principle of holography: a key to holistic medicine. *American Journal of Acupuncture* 1982(April-June):167-171.

Schmidt J. Epidemiology of mass breast cancer screening: a plea for valid measure of benefit. *Journal of Clinical Epidemiology* 1990;43(3):215-225.

Shann F. Antipyretics in severe sepsis. *Lancet* 1995(Feb);343:338.

Scientists clarify biotech misinformation. *Daily Inquirer* September 11, 1994.

Simmons NA et al. Case against antibiotic prophylaxis for dental treatment of patients with joint prothesis. *Lancet* 1992(Feb);339:301.

Simms D, Silveria WR. Post traumatic stress disorders in children after television programmes. *British Medical Journal* 1994(Feb);8:389-390.

Singh RB et al. Randomized controlled trial of cardioprotective diet in patients with recent acute myocardial infarction: results of one-year follow-up. *British Medical Journal* 1992(April);304:1015-1019.

Therapies by cancer patients receiving conventional treatment. *British Medical Journal* 1994(July);309:86-89.

UK National Case Control Study Group. Breast feeding and risk of breast cancer in young Women. *British Medical Journal* 1993(July);307:17-20.

Watts GF et al. Effects on coronary artery disease of lipid lowering diet plus cholestyramine: The St. Thomas Artherosclerosis Regression Study (STARS). *Lancet* 1992(March);339:563-569.

Weatherball DJ. The inhumanity of medicine. *British Medical Journal* 1994(Dec);309:1671-1672.

WHO Programme for the Control of Acute Respiratory Infections: the management of fever in young children with acute respiratory infections in developing countries. Geneva: World Health Organization WHO/ARI 1993(30).

Willett WC et al. Intake of trans fatty acids and risk of coronary heart disease among women. *Lancet* 1993(March);341:581-585.

Windle W. Brain damage by asphyxia at birth. *Scientific America.* October 1969.

Witt MD et al. Conflict of interest: dilemmas in biomedical research. *Journal of the American Medical Association* 1994(Feb);271:547-551.

Van der Meer JTM et al. Efficacy of antibiotic prophylaxis for prevention of native-valve endocarditis. *Lancet* 1992(Jan);339:136-137.

Yao AC et al. Effect of gravity on placental transfusion. *Lancet* 1969(xxx):505-508.

_____. Distribution of blood between infants and placenta after birth. *Lancet* 1969(xxx):871-873.

Yankner BA. B Amyloid and the pathogenesis of Alzheimer disease. *New England Journal of Medicine* 1991;325:1849-1857.

About the Author

As a university student, Joaquin G. Tan (more commonly called "Jake") had an inner yearning to engage in a socially relevant profession. This was fully awakened when he got involved in student activism in the early 1970s. The most famous slogan used then was "serve the people," pertaining to the underprivileged ones. Fortunately, his exposure to the Liberation Theology of Latin America and the writings of Paulo Freire provided a different perspective and motivation of service that saved him from toeing the line of the predominantly Marxist university student environment. The following thoughts, however, continued to persist: What is the best way to express this yearning? What is the best approach or intervention, so that the change introduced can have a life of its own and eventually transform society peacefully?

After graduation from university with a degree in Marine Fisheries, he was disappointed to realize that knowledge learned from school was not appropriate to serve the basic needs of most poor communities (but rather for big capital-oriented industries). In 1977, together with a number of friends who were formerly activists, coming mostly from the University of the Philippines Student Catholic Action (or UPSCA), they founded one of the first private non-government organizations (NGOs) that worked directly with poor communities using the methods of community organizing and appropriate technology (inspired by Saul Alinsky and E.F. Schumacher respectively). This was achieved in spite of martial law.

Alongside this, he became a vegetarian after getting to know Buddhism and while being a student of the Kaballah in a correspondence course. This experience later gave him the understanding of how to incorporate nutrition as part of preventive medicine, or of the process of healing. Vegetarianism was further reinforced by the ideas of political vegetarian Frances Moore Lappe's "Diet for a Small Planet." The core principles inherent in these worldviews are: change must first come from within, and it should be expressed in the appropriate transformation of one's lifestyle (essential to transforming society and lessen the burden on the finite aspect of the planet).

While in the rural areas of the Philippines, Jake sought out local healers to converse with them about their practice and ask questions like, "What makes people ill and how can they be healed?" From a number of local healers he interviewed, it appeared that people's illnesses come from subtly perceptible entities, such as fear, shame, and an individual's corresponding negative reactions, inabilities, attitudes, and thoughts like helplessness or destitution that eventually find their way as dis-ease into the physical body. Healing, too, has a non-material side to it, like the life forces in plants, or human touch and intentions like love, respect, positivity, tolerance, and understanding. Together with other self-taught modalities, Jake still uses the principles and some modes of treatment (particularly with plants) that he learned from indigenous healers to address ailments of his family and friends. He would rather bring his family members to a local healer than to a regular orthodox doctor, if and when he cannot manage the illness himself.

These experiences and viewpoints fueled a conflict among his colleagues as to the appropriate direction NGO work should aim for. The conflict eventually cut short his involvement with this particular NGO, and in 1985 he started on a search for other worldviews and models of interventions that could authentically begin the process of change.

This search brought him to read, among others, the works of Alice Bailey, the inspiration behind the World Peace Movement and Planetary Synthesis. In search of a comprehensive explanation to the ancient and other mysteries of life, he read through the works of Erich von Daniken and other similar writers, and became a member of the Ancient Astronaut Society. Their worldviews and explanations of the meaning and mysteries of life, however, fell short of his expectations.

In May 1987, while hosting a workshop on permaculture, he encountered anthroposophy, biodynamic agriculture, and Waldorf education through Nicanor Perlas III. From that time on, he made anthroposophy his guiding star. He read the works of Rudolf Steiner at every possible opportunity. Anthroposophy satisfactorily answered many of his questions and pro-vided a consistent and coherent worldview, the meaning and direction of the evolution of life and of the earth, as well as concrete alternatives to the current systems in society.

Mr. Perlas also brought in a new dimension to social change: the problem of materialistic science itself. Social change initiatives can only genuinely transform society if the fundamental assumptions of society (as articulated by materialistic science) are questioned, enlarged, extended, or replaced by the emerging new sciences (especially anthroposophy) which are holistic, encompassing, and coherent (capable of understanding life, human beings, and human societies), rather than just relying on explanations given by materialistically-inspired sciences. The applied sciences of biodynamic agriculture, Waldorf education and anthroposophical medicine are ready examples of the developed, open-ended but dynamic expressions of these transformed aspects of social life. They can therefore be introduced and adapted to any culture.

In February 1989, he joined his wife, Bella—trained in Waldorf education—in Melbourne, Australia. Jake took care of their two children while they were there. It was during this time when he and his family met a woman who was visiting the school one Sunday morning. She worked in the plant laboratory of the WALA Heilmittel GMBH in Eckwaelden, Germany. She narrated her experience of how anthroposophic remedies are being made with the conscious participation of spiritual beings! This conversation made quite an impression on Jake. When the Tans were denied their visas to England for Jake to pursue a course in Rural Development at Emerson College, he contacted this German acquaintance for possible training in the WALA. In 1992, the door opened for him to study in Germany. While spending about six months with the WALA, he learned about the five-week seminar on anthroposophic medicine at Arlesheim, Switzerland. He was allowed to join this event, which was for medical doctors only, even though his only formal training in a medically-related field was a basic course in acupuncture which he took before leaving for Australia.

Being in this seminar was a kind of knowledge (spirit) recalling for him, which was why he was able to quickly grasp the basic principles and therapeutics of anthroposophic medicine. It was a blessing and a big advantage that he studied the basic foundations of anthoposophy and that he had not undergone formal training in orthodox medicine before taking the course. He did not have the usual mental blocks most orthodox doctors experience in understanding how anthroposophic medicine works. Additionally, he was able to fully comprehend and realize how *anthroposophy is the unifying principle/framework* behind all the other schools of thought in medicine (as described in this book).

In 1993, a few months after returning to the Philippines, he organized a seminar entitled "You Can Be Your Own Doctor." This seminar became a hit, especially among local NGOs looking for alternatives to the current system. Almost every month, for a number of years, he either conducted the seminar in coordination with various NGOs in various parts of the country, or organized it himself in metro Manila. The seminar promoted self-reliance, as well as personal and community empowerment—qualities that were still present but in dire need of renewal in most Filipino communities. Moreover, the seminar encapsulated the kind of social intervention that can authentically begin the process of change and inspire current and future generations.

In 1995, he wrote the book, *Healing Ourselves: A Guide to Creative, Responsive, and Self-Reliant Medicine,* to reach more people who are seeking other ways to better understand health and illnesses. He continued to cultivate a small practice where friends and individuals seeking other ways of working with their ailments could come and consult to find relief, and possibly true healing from their predicaments.

In addition, he built a small laboratory to make homeopathic remedies for those who consulted him, and for other aspiring anthroposophical doctors or homeopaths who could not make the preparations themselves.

In 2002, eight years after pioneering the first Steiner school in the Philippines with several other anthroposophists, Jake and Bella began conducting teacher training courses in Waldorf education on early childhood and anthroposophy together with other local resource persons. They have given workshops in two Kolisko conferences that were held in different parts of the world. Since 2005, the couple has been giving lectures and workshops in the Asia-Pacific region—Taiwan, Hong Kong, mainland China, and other countries whose interest is to deepen their understanding of child development, nutrition and health, Steiner education, and anthroposophy.

Now and again, Jake takes part as a faculty member of the International Post-Graduate Medical Training Courses (IPMT) in the Philippines, sponsored by the Medical Section of the Goetheanum.

Though still in the process of accreditation, Jake's work has been identified and acknowledged by the Philippine Institute for Traditional and Alternative Health Care (PITAHC) of the Department of Health— the government body that prepares the implementing guidelines for the procedure of obtaining proper legal recognition of alternative modalities of healing (and their practitioners). Furthermore, he has actively taken part in a series of public hearings on acupuncture and homeopathy for non-medical practitioners. These consulting bodies drew up and approved the national certification of practitioners of the said modalities, the certification of their training programs, training centers and clinics, and their code of ethics.

These endeavors are more aptly termed hitherto as *socially engaged spirituality*, i.e., consciously bringing the ethical and moral principles of social life (among others factors) into the process of change.

www.ingramcontent.com/pod-product-compliance
Lightning Source LLC
Chambersburg PA
CBHW032030090426
42733CB00029B/74